Dermoscopy of the Hair and Nails

This new edition of a bestselling text almost amounts to a completely new book, with over 750 figures of common and uncommon disorders, including new chapters on trichoscopy of hair transplantation, teletrichoscopy, and trichoscopy of the shaved scalp. The chapters also list the key clues that are important to help the practitioner reach the correct diagnosis about problems with hair or nails.

"Numerous high-quality photos are helpful in demonstrating key features" (Doody's Reviews) [of the previous edition]

Dermoscopy of the Hair and Nails

Third Edition

Antonella Tosti, MD
Fredric Brandt Endowed Professor of Dermatology,
Dr. Phillip Frost Department of Dermatology and Cutaneous Surgery,
University of Miami Miller School of Medicine Miami, Florida, USA

Andrea Sechi, MD, PhD
Dermatology, Fondazione IRCCS Ca' Granda, Ospedale Maggiore Policlinico,
Milan, Italy

CRC Press
Taylor & Francis Group
Boca Raton London New York

CRC Press is an imprint of the
Taylor & Francis Group, an **informa** business

Third edition published 2026
by CRC Press
2385 NW Executive Center Drive, Suite 320, Boca Raton FL 33431

and by CRC Press
4 Park Square, Milton Park, Abingdon, Oxon, OX14 4RN

CRC Press is an imprint of Taylor & Francis Group, LLC

ISBN: 9781041020028 (hbk)
ISBN: 9780429351433 (ebk)

DOI: 10.1201/9780429351433

Typeset in Times
by Deanta Global Publishing Services, Chennai, India

Contents

Preface

Dear friends, it took me a few years before finishing the third edition of this book and I can tell this is a completely new book, full of the pictures that I have been taking in these last years from common and uncommon disorders.

I believe that after reading this book you will be confident in diagnosing most hair and nail disorders using your dermatoscope. This book reflects my opinion and my knowledge, and I personally think that listing all the possible dermoscopic findings that you can find in a disease is absolutely not helping in making the correct diagnosis. So what you will find in this book are the clues that are important for you to reach the correct diagnosis.

Acknowledgments

I have to thank Dr. Colombina Vincenzi who helped me during these years in taking and selecting the best images for the book.

Antonella Tosti

1 Trichoscopy Patterns

Table 1.1 sets out the important follicular and interfollicular patterns in diseases of the hair.

HAIR AND SCALP DERMOSCOPIC PATTERNS

- Follicular
- Interfollicular (epidermal, vascular, and pigment related)
- Hair shaft
- Hair roots through the scalp

FOLLICULAR PATTERNS

- Yellow dots
- Pinpoint white dots
- Red dots
- Blue-gray dots arranged in a target pattern
- Follicular staining
- Keratotic plugs
- Gray white halos
- Peripilar signs
- Empty follicles
- Follicular pustules
- Loss of follicular openings
- Peripilar scales/casts

Yellow Dots (Figures 1.1–1.5)

- Yellow dots are round or polycyclic yellow to yellow-pink dots.
- Yellow dots can be empty or contain miniaturized, vellus, dystrophic, or broken hair shafts.
- Yellow dots correspond to dilated infundibular ostia filled with sebum and keratin debris.
- In alopecia areata, they are numerous and can present different shades of color, ranging from scalp color, especially in children, to bright yellow pinkish-yellow and brown-yellow. They might or might not contain different types of broken hairs and sometimes present a keratotic plug.
- In androgenetic alopecia yellow dots correspond to follicles with advanced miniaturization and preserved sebaceous gland activity. Yellow dots are usually sparse and more numerous in the frontal region. They often contain miniaturized hairs.
- In trichotillomania yellow dots are irregularly distributed and often contain black dots, broken hairs of different length, or fine black hair residues.
- Yellow dots are also seen in alopecia areata incognito, chemotherapy alopecia, pressure alopecia, permanent alopecia after chemotherapy, endocrine alopecia, and congenital hypotrichosis.
- Yellow dots are not or less visible in patients with dark phototypes.
- 3D yellow dots are typical of dissecting cellulitis of the scalp; these resemble soap bubbles.
- Yellow dots can occasionally be seen in scarring alopecias, particularly in frontal fibrosing alopecia.

Pinpoint White Dots (Figures 1.6–1.9)

- Pinpoint white dots are characteristic of the black scalp and are seen both in normal and pathological conditions.
- Pinpoint white dots are regular, small circular structures interspersed between the hair follicles (starry sky distribution).
- Pinpoint white dots correspond to follicular and sweat gland openings.
- Pinpoint white dots corresponding to follicular openings are bigger than pinpoint white dots corresponding to sweat gland openings.
- Pinpoint white dots are increased in number in all types of alopecias.

DOI: 10.1201/9780429351433-1

TABLE 1.1
Important Follicular and Interfollicular Patterns in Diseases of the Hair

	Alopecia areata	Alopecia areata incognito	Androgenetic alopecia	Chemotherapy/ radiotherapy alopecia	Contact dermatitis	Dermatomyositis	Loose anagen hair syndrome	Pemphigus vulgaris	Permanent/Persistent alopecia after chemotherapy	Pressure alopecia	Psoriasis
Follicular Patterns											
Yellow dots	X	x	x	X					X	X	
Loss of pinpoint white dots*											
Red dots											
Blue-gray dots											
Keratotic plugs											
Gray white halos											
Peripilar signs			X								
Empty follicles	x	x	X	X			x		X	x	
Follicular pustules											
Loss of follicular openings											
Peripilar casts/scales								x			x
Interfollicular Pattern											
Scales: interfollicular					X	X		X			X
Vessels: arborizing vessels					x	X					
Vessels: red dot vessels and twisted loops					x			x			X
Vessels: dilated capillaries						X					
Rectangular structures							X				
Hair powder											
Extravasation					X			X			
Loss of honeycomb pattern											
White patches											
Hair shaft pattern											
Hair diameter diversity	x	x	X						x		
Thinned short regrowing hairs	x	X	X						x	x	
Thick short regrowing hairs	X			X			x			x	
Pigtail hairs	X	X	x	x				x	x		
Thick circle hairs	x			x				x			
Hair tufting											
Exclamation mark hairs	X			x						x	
Broken hairs	X			X						x	
Black dots	X			X						X	
Question mark hairs											
Flame hairs	x			x						x	
Comma/ corkscrew/ morse-code/ zig-zag hairs											
Tulip and tulipoid hairs	x			x						x	
Coudability hairs	X			x							
Monilethrix-like hairs	X			x							
Pili torti											
Tubular hair casts								X			X
Anagen hair roots											

X: Trichoscopic finding detected in a huge amount
x: Trichoscopic findings detected in a mild/moderate amount
X/x: Salient features/trichoscopic clues of the disease
*: specific for skin of color

Rosacea	Seborrheic dermatitis	Telogen effluvium	Tinea capitis	Trichotillomania	Acne keloidalis nuchae	Cicatrical central centrifugal alopecia	Discoid lupus erythematosus	Dissecting cellulitis of the scalp	Erosive pustular dermatosis of the scalp	Folliculitis decalvans	Fibrosing alopecia in pattern distribution	Frontal fibrosing alopecia	Lichen planopilaris	Morphea	Traction alopecia
		x		x				X (3D)				x			
							X			x					
							X								
							X						X		
							X	x							
						X									
		X		x				x							x
	x		x		x			x	x	X					x
					X	X	X	X	X	X	X	X	X	X	x
x	x		X		x		x			X	X	X	X		x
	X		X			X	x			X	x		X		
X	X						X	x	x						
								x		X					
x							X		x						
				X											
									X	X					
							X								
						X	X	X	X	X	x	X	X	X	x
						x					X				x
						x		x			X				x
		X	X	X				x							x
				x				x							
					x	x	x	x		x	x	x	x		
					x					X			X		
			X	X	x	x	x	x	x	x	x	x	x	x	x
			X	X	x	x		X		x		x	x	x	x
				X											
				X											
			X												
				X											
					x	x	x	x	x	x	x	x	x	x	x
	X		X							X			X		X
									X				x		

- In non-scarring alopecia, pinpoint white dots are evenly distributed and might contain miniaturized or broken hairs.
- In scarring alopecia, pinpoint white dots are irregularly distributed and associated with white patches indicative of follicular scarring. In discoid lupus erythematosus pinpoint white dots are greatly reduced or absent.

Red Dots (Figures 1.10, 1.11)

- Red dots are a characteristic pattern of discoid lupus erythematosus.
- Red dots correspond to a dilated infundibulum, surrounded by extravasated erythrocytes and dilated vessels.
- Presence of red dots has been associated with the possibility of hair regrowth with treatment.
- Red dots are commonly seen in discoid lupus erythematosus in black scalp; when the scalp is hypopigmented they are not associated with regrowth.
- Red discoloration of follicular openings without peripheral vessels can be seen in the scalp of patients affected by hypopigmentary disorders as albinism or vitiligo.
- Red discoloration of follicular openings can be detected in the glabella of patients with frontal fibrosing alopecia (glabellar red dots).

Blue-Gray Dots Arranged in a Target Pattern (Figure 1.12)

- Blue-gray dots arranged in a target pattern are seen in lichen planopilaris in pigmented scalp.
- They correspond to melanophages in the papillary dermis due to pigmentary incontinence.
- The blue-gray dots are seen at the site of destroyed hair follicles and should be differentiated from interfollicular speckled or mottled blue-gray dots observed in discoid lupus erythematosus.

Follicular Staining (Figures 1.13, 1.14)

- Hair dyes can cause black or brown dots on the scalp.
- These dots are due to the dye residues on the scalp surface and within hair follicles.
- Anthralin, used for alopecia areata treatment, can also cause brown/black dots associated with follicular openings.

Keratotic Plugs (Figures 1.15, 1.16)

- Keratotic plugs are a typical feature of discoid lupus erythematosus and can be seen in both active and chronic lesions.
- Keratotic plugs correspond to hyperkeratosis and plugging of infundibula by keratotic material.
- Isolated keratotic plugs filling enlarged follicular ostia are a feature of dissecting cellulitis of the scalp, especially in the dark skin phototypes.

Gray White Peripilar Halos (Figure 1.17)

- Gray white peripilar halos are a specific feature of central centrifugal cicatricial alopecia.
- They appear as a white-grayish circle of 0.3–0.5 mm in diameter surrounding a single hair or more commonly a group of two–three hairs emerging from the same ostium.
- Gray white peripilar halos are found around pigmented and non-pigmented hairs, either in early or late-stage disease.
- Gray white peripilar halos correspond to lamellar perifollicular fibrosis.
- Gray white peripilar halos should be differentiated from pinpoint white dots, which are interfollicular.

Peripilar Sign (Figure 1.18)

- Peripilar sign is a feature seen in androgenetic alopecia, particularly in early androgenetic alopecia.
- Corresponds to perifollicular inflammation in the upper follicle.
- Peripilar sign in early androgenetic alopecia appears as a slightly depressed brown halo surrounding the follicular opening.
- Peripilar signs in patients with dark skin phototype are more pigmented.

Empty Follicles (Figure 1.19)

- Empty follicles correspond to empty follicular openings on the scalp.
- Empty follicles are a common feature in non-scarring alopecias such as androgenetic alopecia and telogen effluvium.
- Empty follicles can be detected also in the initial reversible stages of scarring alopecias like dissecting cellulitis and traction alopecia.
- They differ from yellow dots due to the lack of sebum retention within the follicular unit ostia.

Follicular Pustules (Figure 1.20)

- Follicular pustules are small, inflamed, pus-filled lesions that develop around hair follicles.
- Follicular pustules can be found both in non-scarring and scarring hair disorders, including seborrheic dermatitis, acneiform eruptions of the scalp, tinea capitis, and folliculitis decalvans.
- Examining the vascular pattern around these pustules can aid in differentiating between the conditions.

Loss of Follicular Openings (Figure 1.21)

- Loss of follicular openings indicates an irreversible cicatricial process. This feature is common to all types of scarring alopecias.

Peripilar Scales/Casts (Figures 1.22, 1.23)

- Peripilar scales can only be appreciated with dry or polarized dermoscopy.
- Peripilar scales (hair casts) are seen in several cicatricial alopecias including: lichen planopilaris and its variants, discoid lupus, and folliculitis decalvans.
- Hair casts can surround a single hair or multiple hair shafts and might be associated with presence or absence of interfollicular scales.
- In lichen planopilaris and its variants the hair casts usually surround a group of two to four hair shafts.
- In folliculitis decalvans, the hair casts typically surround more than 6 and up to 100 hair shafts.
- Hairs surrounding scalp scars can also present peripilar casts.

INTERFOLLICULAR PATTERNS

- Scales/crusts
- Vessels
  - Simple red loops
  - Arborizing vessels
  - Twisted red loops
  - Giant capillaries
- Hair powder
- Rectangular structures
- Honeycomb pigment
- White patches
- Scalp deposits/staining

Scales/Crusts (Figures 1.24, 1.25)

- Interfollicular scales are indicative of parakeratotic disorders such as psoriasis and seborrheic dermatitis, but can also be found in tinea capitis, folliculitis decalvans, and discoid lupus.
- Extensive scaling is characteristic of pemphigus foliaceus and discoid lupus.
- Exudative crusts result from the clotting of serous exudate and have a typical yellowish color.
- These are detected in contact dermatitis, pemphigus, folliculitis decalvans, erosive pustular dermatosis, dissecting cellulitis, and in superinfections, where

pustules and lakes of pus are associated findings.
- In erosive pustular dermatosis and pemphigus vulgaris they often overlie eroded plaques or nodules.

Vessels (Figures 1.26–1.30)

- Better appreciated utilizing an interface solution.
- The skin's blood supply originates from perforating vessels that rise from the muscles and subcutaneous fat to form the lower horizontal plexus at the dermal-subcutaneous interface.
- From this lower plexus, paired arterioles and venules ascend to create direct connections with the subpapillary plexus in the papillary dermis.
- Capillary loops arise from the subpapillary plexus which is situated 1–2 mm below the skin's surface.
- The orientation of these capillary structures, whether horizontal or perpendicular to the skin surface, affects their response to diascopy.
- Simple red loops and arborizing vessels are seen in normal scalp.
- Prominent arborizing vessels are seen in seborrheic dermatitis, contact dermatitis, and rosacea.
- Arborizing vessels blanch with pressure, indicating a horizontal orientation parallel to the skin surface.
- Twisted capillary loops are characteristic for psoriasis and are also seen in folliculitis decalvans.
- Twisted capillary loops generally do not blanch, because of perpendicular orientation to the skin.
- Stretched linear vessels converging to hair follicle opening can be detected in folliculitis decalvans.
- The vessel's size can be roughly established by comparing vessels with hair shaft. If the size of the vessel is larger than the size of the shaft, this indicates enlarged vessels.
- Single "caterpillar-shaped" enlarged vessels are seen in scalp rosacea.
- Giant enlarged vessels are a sign of connective tissue disorders, reflecting changes in the microvasculature of the deeper vascular plexus.
- In lupus erythematosus thick giant branching vessels are seen both in cases of scarring and non-scarring alopecia. Active lesions show thicker vessels compared to inactive lesions.
- In dermatomyositis vessels are enlarged, tortuous, and bushy as those of proximal nail fold.

Hair Powder (Figure 1.31)

- Hair powder corresponds to residue of destroyed hair shafts due to mechanical manipulation.
- It is a typical finding of trichotillomania.
- Hair powder is found in the interfollicular scalp, and it can be wiped out with a cotton gauze, as it has no attachment with the previous damaged hair.

Rectangular Structures (Figure 1.32)

- Rectangular structures are pigmented structures with a rectangular shape found in loose anagen hair syndrome.
- They are probably produced by the residues of the inner root sheath.

Honeycomb Pigment (Figures 1.33, 1.34)

- This is a typical feature of sun-exposed or pigmented scalp
- Homogeneous mosaic of contiguous brown regularly sized lines encircling hypopigmented areas.
- The hyperchromic lines correspond to the rete ridge melanocytes, and the hypochromic areas correspond to the melanocytes residing in the suprapapillary epidermis.
- The honeycomb pattern is typically seen in the normal sun-exposed or pigmented scalp and is preserved in all non-scarring and scarring alopecias

except for discoid lupus erythematosus, where it is disrupted.

White Patches (Figure 1.35)

- White patches are a common feature in scarring alopecias.
- Appear as irregular ivory-white areas devoid of hairs and follicular openings and correspond to dermal fibrosis.

Scalp Deposits/Staining (Figures 1.36–1.39)

- Scalp deposits result from environmental particles like dust, the application of camouflage products, or topical therapies.
- "Dirty dots" refer to small residue of environmental debris and are prevalent in children and the elderly due to their low sebum production.
- Camouflage products are employed to mask areas of reduced hair density and may appear as powder or fibers.
- Scalp deposits may also arise from residues of topical medications.
- Semi-permanent dyes stain the interfollicular scalp, whereas permanent dyes often also penetrate the follicular openings.
- Micropigmentation is a cosmetic tattoo aimed to mimic the shape of hair follicles. Dark gray, black, or red dots are evenly spaced across the interfollicular scalp; they are larger than real hair follicles.

HAIR SHAFT FEATURES SEEN IN HAIR DISEASES

- Hair diameter diversity
- Short regrowing hairs
- Circle hairs
- Hair tufting
- Broken hair
  - Exclamation mark hairs*
  - Broken hairs
  - Cadaverized hairs or "black dots"
  - Question mark hairs
  - Comma hairs
  - Flame hairs
  - Corkscrew hairs
  - Morse hairs
  - Zigzag hairs
  - Trichorrhexis nodosa (proximal and distal)
  - Tulip hairs
  - Trichoptilosis
- Hair shaft abnormalities
  - Coudability hairs
  - Pseudomonilethrix
  - Pili torti
  - Pili annulati
  - Pili trianguli and canaliculi
- Hair shaft disorders associated with hair fragility
  - Monilethrix
  - Trichorrhexis invaginata
- Encircling structures
  - Tubular hair casts
  - Nits
  - Pseudonits
  - Hair shaft deposits
  - Hair casts beyond the scalp
- Hair roots through the scalp

*Tapered hairs: This term includes exclamation mark hairs, coudability hairs, and monilethrix-like hairs.

Hair Diameter Diversity (Figure 1.40)

- Hair diameter diversity (anisotrichosis) is a typical feature of androgenetic alopecia.
- Diagnosis of androgenetic alopecia is indicated by more than 20% diversity with hair shafts of different thickness.
- Corresponds to hair follicle miniaturization.
- Hair diameter diversity is also seen in alopecia areata, where miniaturization occurs in clusters, and in central centrifugal cicatricial alopecia.
- Hair diameter diversity impacts the cumulative hair thickness and density, which correlates with disease severity in androgenetic alopecia.

- Miniaturization in androgenetic alopecia does not affect all the follicles of the follicular unit until end-stage disease.

Short Regrowing Hairs (Figure 1.41)

- Short regrowing hairs are classified according to their thickness as normal (> 0.03 mm) or thin.
- Short regrowing hairs of normal thickness are seen in normal scalp, in regrowing patches of alopecia areata, where they are clustered, and in telogen effluvium, where they are interspersed with long terminal hairs. They are also observed in trichotillomania, tinea capitis, and temporal triangular alopecia.
- Regrowing hairs of normal thickness are indicative of hair regrowth and positive prognosis; on trichoscopy they usually stand vertically (upright) with a thick, pigmented base and a tapered end.
- Thin short regrowing hairs are often light, as the shaft is hypopigmented, and bended or circled. These hairs are a feature of androgenetic alopecia and chronic alopecia areata.
- Presence of more than 10% or more than six thin short regrowing hairs in the frontal scalp at ×20 magnification is a criterion for diagnosing early androgenetic alopecia.

Circle Hairs (Figures 1.42–1.46)

- Circle hairs are classified based on the thickness of the shaft, distinguishing between those with thinned shafts and those with normal thickness.
- Circle hairs with reduced thickness are often referred to as pigtail hairs due to their resemblance to the tail of a pig.
- Pigtail hairs are commonly found in alopecia areata, alopecia areata incognito, and androgenetic alopecia; they are less frequently observed in acute telogen effluvium.
- A high density of pigtail hairs is suggestive of alopecia areata, including alopecia areata incognito.
- Circle hairs of normal thickness can be found isolated in different hair conditions, including scarring alopecias, hair shaft disorders, and scalp scars.
- Circle hairs of normal thickness are divided according to their shape and their attachment to the scalp into embedded, rolled, knotted, long circle hairs, and pili torti circle hairs.
- Embedded circle hairs have either the proximal or the distal extremity underneath the scalp skin, or underlie the skin for their entire length.
- In dissecting cellulitis of the scalp embedded circle hairs might be seen within follicular clefts.
- Rolled hairs are short, convoluted hairs that form a simple or doubled spiral.
- Knotted circle hairs are caused by friction.
- Long circle hairs can occasionally be found in the normal scalp.
- Circle hairs of normal thickness can also be found on the body (see Chapter 14).

Hair Tufting (Figures 1.47–1.50)

- Hair tufting describes the clustering of multiple hairs emerging from a single follicular opening.
- Hair tufts are surrounded by peripilar scales in scarring alopecias (lichen planopilaris, fibrosing alopecia in a pattern distribution, discoid lupus, and folliculitis decalvans), where they represent a clue for diagnosis.
- In folliculitis decalvans hair tufts emerge from a common opening with a shape that resembles a volcano.
- Presence of more than six hairs in the tuft suggests diagnosis of folliculitis decalvans; in lichen planopilaris the number of hairs in the tuft is usually less than four.
- Tufting of vellus hairs is occasionally seen in the hairline of patients affected by male pattern hair loss (MPHL).

Exclamation Mark Hair (Figure 1.51)

- Exclamation mark hair is a fractured hair with a dark, frayed, and thick tip.
- Its proximal portion is thin and hypopigmented.
- Corresponds to a telogen hair with a broken tip.
- Exclamation mark hairs are the hallmark of alopecia areata, and correlate with disease activity.
- Exclamation mark hairs are best detected in the scalp surrounding the patches of alopecia areata.
- A few exclamation mark hairs may be seen in anagen effluvium, including chemotherapy-induced alopecia, early dissecting cellulitis of the scalp, and pressure alopecia.

Broken Hairs (Figures 1.52–1.54)

- Broken hairs are hair shafts fractured at different levels from the scalp's emergence.
- They are a prominent pattern of several non-scarring alopecias, including alopecia areata, anagen effluvium, tinea capitis, trichotillomania, friction alopecia, and active traction alopecia.
- A few broken hairs are commonly seen in scarring alopecia, including folliculitis decalvans, lichen planopilaris, and frontal fibrosing alopecia.

Black Dots (Figures 1.55, 1.56)

- Black dots are fractured hairs, broken before emerging from the scalp.
- Black dots are seen in patients with dark hairs.
- The density of black dots corresponds to the severity of inflammation, with a higher number found in acute conditions and fewer in chronic or less inflamed states.
- Numerous black dots are commonly found in alopecia areata, anagen effluvium, dissecting cellulitis of the scalp, tinea capitis, and trichotillomania.
- Few isolated black dots are seen in scarring alopecias, particularly lichen planopilaris and frontal fibrosing alopecia.

Question Mark Hair (Figure 1.57)

- Question mark hair (hook hair) is a short hair with a coiled thin tip, resembling a question mark.
- Question mark hair is a specific finding of trichotillomania, since it is produced by the mechanical distortion caused by hair-pulling forces.
- Question mark hairs are usually few in number.

Flame Hairs (Figures 1.58, 1.59)

- Flame hairs are wavy, cone-shaped hair residues resembling a flame, and they present a tapered proximal shaft and expanded flame-like distal end.
- Flame hairs are seen in many non-scarring alopecias including alopecia areata, chemotherapy alopecia, radiation alopecia, and trichotillomania.
- Their formation results from acute injury to the hair matrix and keratogenous zone due to severe mechanical pulling in trichotillomania, ongoing trauma to hairs in traction alopecia, acute damage to anagen follicles from chemotherapy, radiotherapy, or alopecia areata.

Comma Hair (Figure 1.60)

- Comma hair is a short, broken hair, which is bent, resembling a comma.
- Comma hair is typical for tinea capitis, resulting from the hair shaft being weakened and curved due to fungal hyphae infiltration.
- Comma hair is seen both in endothrix and ectothrix infections.
- Comma hair is seen in patients of all ethnicities.

Corkscrew Hair (Figure 1.61)

- Corkscrew hair is a spiralized broken hair, which resembles a corkscrew.
- Corkscrew hair is seen in tinea capitis in association with comma hairs.
- Corkscrew hair is seen both in endothrix and ectothrix infections.

Morse-Code Hairs (Figure 1.62)

- Morse-code-like hairs, also known as "bar-code-like hairs," refer to hairs characterized by horizontal white bands across their length that look like Morse code.
- Morse-code hairs are typical of endothrix tinea capitis.
- The white bands make the hairs appear empty, translucent, and weakened and correspond to localized areas of heavy fungal infection within the hair shaft.
- The horizontal bands may lead to hair bending and breakage since they represent the weakest point within the hair shaft.

Zigzag Hairs (Figure 1.63)

- Zigzag hairs are Z-shaped broken hairs.
- Zigzag hairs are seen in tinea capitis.

Trichorrhexis Nodosa (Figures 1.64, 1.65)

- Trichorrhexis nodosa can affect either the proximal or distal shaft.
- Trichorrhexis nodosa is characterized by multiple areas of hair shafts weakness and breakage.
- Proximal trichorrhexis nodosa is associated with friction, and the affected hairs are broken a few millimeters to a centimeter above scalp level. The broom hair is a short, broken hair with a frayed tip that is typical of friction.
- Distal trichorrhexis nodosa is characterized by grayish-white or yellowish nodules along the hair shaft and a broken, frayed tip.

Tulip Hairs (Figure 1.66)

- Tulip hair is characterized by a distal dark rounded tip, resembling the shape of a tulip flower.
- Tulip hairs are seen in trichotillomania, anagen effluvium, including alopecia areata, and in the recipient scalp after hair transplantation.

Trichoptilosis

- Trichoptilosis represents the longitudinal splitting of the distal hair shaft (split ends).
- In long hairs, trichoptilosis is indicative of excessive heat and mechanical stress to the hair shaft.
- Central splitting of the hair shaft is common in African hair.

COUDABILITY HAIR (FIGURE 1.67)

- Coudability hair is a hair of normal length with a narrowing in its proximal portion.
- It is typical of active alopecia areata, where it is usually found at the periphery of enlarging patches, but can also be found in other types of anagen effluvium.

PSEUDOMONILETHRIX HAIRS (FIGURE 1.68)

- Pseudomonilethrix hairs are hair shafts presenting irregular narrowing.
- Breakage can occur at the site of narrowing.
- They are seen in alopecia areata, and less frequently in chemotherapy-induced alopecia.

PILI TORTI (FIGURE 1.69)

- Pili torti are hairs whose shaft is flattened at irregular intervals and twisted along its longitudinal axis.
- Pili torti are seen in several hair shaft disorders, in scarring alopecias, or as a normal finding in the scalp.

- In cicatricial alopecia, pili torti are often broken and are due to the perifollicular fibrosis.
- Inherited pili torti are very rare and associated with genetic disease.

PILI ANNULATI (FIGURE 1.70)

- Pili annulati are an inherited condition usually asymptomatic.
- Pili annulati have regular alternating light and dark bands along the hair shaft.
- The white bands correspond to air-filled cavities within the hair shaft's cortex.

PILI TRIANGULI AND CANALICULI

- Pili trianguli and canaliculi are hair shafts with a longitudinal groove and a triangular cross-section.
- Pili trianguli and canaliculi are typical of uncombable hair syndrome.

MONILETHRIX (FIGURE 1.71)

- Monilethrix hairs exhibit a regular pattern of elliptical nodes/constrictions devoid of medulla, alternating with fusiform expansions with medulla.
- Breakage occurs at the internodal level.
- Vellus hairs can also be involved.

TRICHORRHEXIS INVAGINATA

- Trichorrhexis invaginata, also known as "bamboo hair," is a hair shaft abnormality where the distal portion invaginates into the proximal portion of the hair shaft.
- In trichorrhexis invaginata the breakage at the site of invagination creates the "golf tee" and the "matchstick" pattern. See Chapter 6.
- Trichorrhexis invaginata is pathognomonic of Netherton syndrome.

TUBULAR HAIR CASTS (FIGURE 1.72)

- Tubular hair casts, which may resemble nits, are firm, shiny, movable tubular structures surrounding the hair shaft.
- They consist of hyperkeratotic or parakeratotic cells from the outer root sheath that wrap around the hair shafts.
- Most of the tubular casts are located proximally.
- Tubular hair casts can be found in traction alopecia, psoriasis, seborrheic dermatitis, folliculitis decalvans, pemphigus vulgaris, and lichen planopilaris.
- In traction alopecia their presence at the margins of the alopecic patch indicates that the hairstyle is creating traction.

NITS (FIGURE 1.73)

- Nits are signs of scalp infestation by pediculosis capitis.
- Nits are attached to one side of the hair shaft and are hard to detach.
- Viable nits are brown with a convex distal end and usually found close to the scalp surface.
- Empty nits are translucent with a flat distal end.

PSEUDONITS (FIGURE 1.74)

- White Piedra presents with multiple, oval, whitish masses along the hair shafts caused by *Trichosporon asahii.*
- Black Piedra is caused by a pigmented fungus named Piedraia hortae. It is characterized by brown or black, hard concretions tightly bound to the hair shafts, ranging from round to elongated nodules, which give the impression of a hair shaft studded with black stones.

HAIR SHAFT DEPOSITS (FIGURE 1.75)

- Hair shaft deposits are concretions of hair styling products along the hair shafts, known as "pseudo-casts."
- Residues from dry shampoos, hair sprays, gels, and mousses are the primary contributors to these deposits.
- They present a whitish or yellow coloration and, unlike tubular hair casts, are less movable and may be misinterpreted as nits.

HAIR CASTS BEYOND THE SCALP (FIGURE 1.76)

- Trichomycosis palmellina is a superficial infection caused by *Corynebacterium* spp. The hair shaft of axillary, pubic, scrotal, and intergluteal areas is surrounded by granular waxy and yellowish concretions.
- Multiple myeloma can produce cutaneous spicules plugging follicular ostia and yellowish-white movable hair casts, composed by amorphous eosinophilic material formed by precipitated monoclonal dysproteins.
- Trichodysplasia spinulosa is characterized by bright white, long, keratin-based spicules protruding from the borders of follicular openings.
- Empty or viable nits of Phthirus pubis can be found at the base of pubic hairs in adults or eyelashes in children, presenting as ovaloid whitish/brownish structures on one side of the shaft, with a flat or convex distal end.
- Seborrheic dermatitis often affects the eyelashes and, rarely, the vellus hairs of the face, leading to the formation of greasy, cylindric casts.
- Demodex folliculorum can affect the face and/or the eyelashes producing hyaline encircling structures attached to the base of the shaft.

HAIR ROOTS THROUGH THE SCALP (FIGURE 1.77)

- Hair roots visible through the scalp are observed when the scalp becomes thin or atrophic.
- These can be detected in congenital or acquired disorder, particularly scalp atrophy due to steroids, aplasia cutis congenita, and erosive pustular dermatosis of the scalp.
- Aplasia cutis congenita shows a typical radial arrangement of hair shaft and elongated hair bulbs at the patch margins.
- Erosive pustular dermatosis of the scalp and steroid-induced scalp atrophy both show hair bulbs through a translucent skin due to the epidermal atrophy.

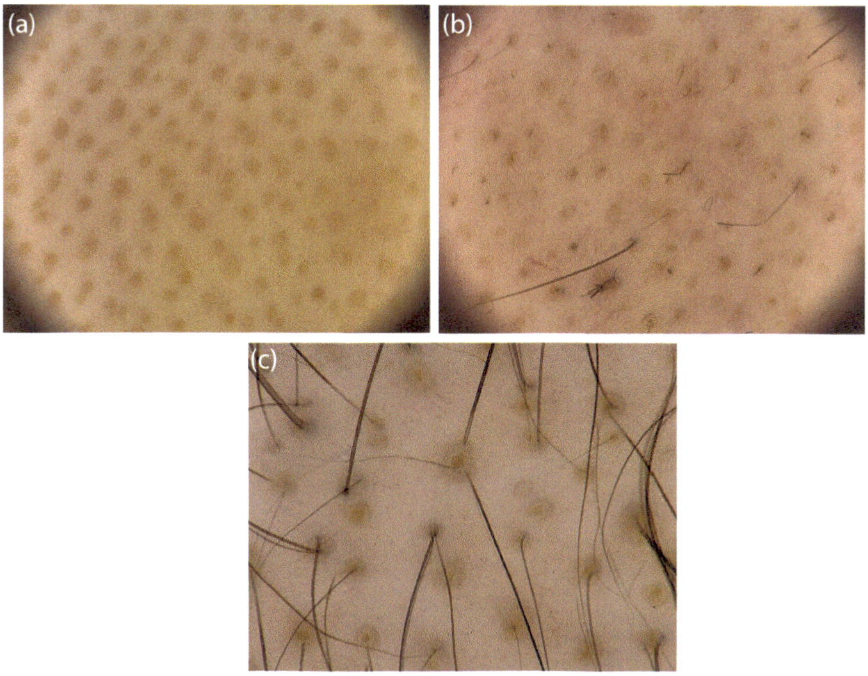

FIGURE 1.1 Yellow dots in alopecia areata. ×20 Diffuse, evenly distributed yellow dots in alopecia areata totalis. Dots have a round or polycyclic shape and different sizes (a); ×20 yellow dots with broken hairs of different lengths in active alopecia areata (b); ×20 yellow dots in alopecia areata incognito (c).

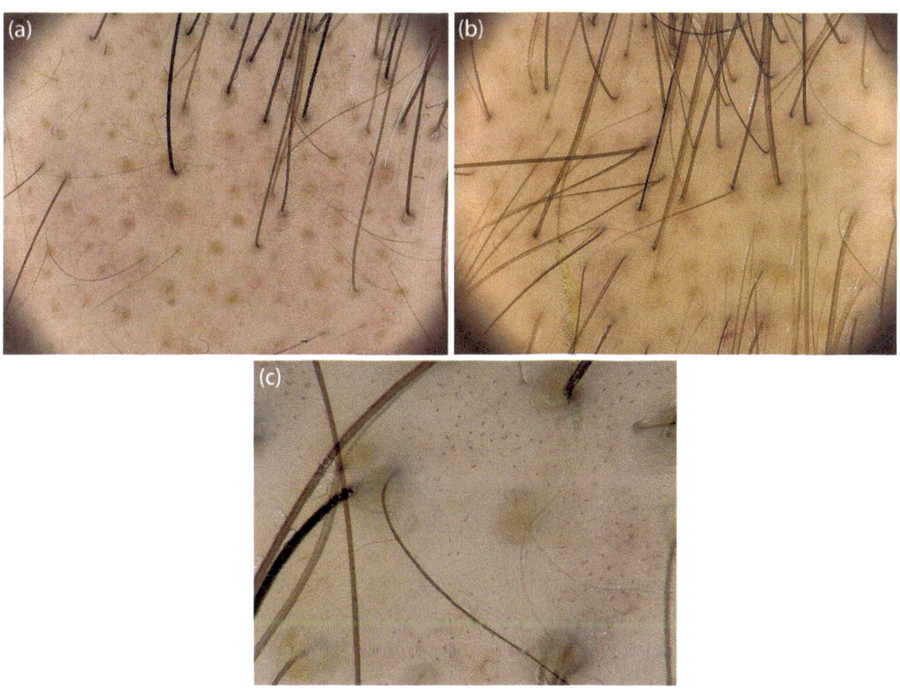

FIGURE 1.2 Yellow dots in androgenetic alopecia. ×20 Numerous yellow dots in the frontal hairline of male pattern hair loss (a); scattered yellow dots in female pattern hair loss (b); ×50 miniaturized hairs within the yellow dot (c).

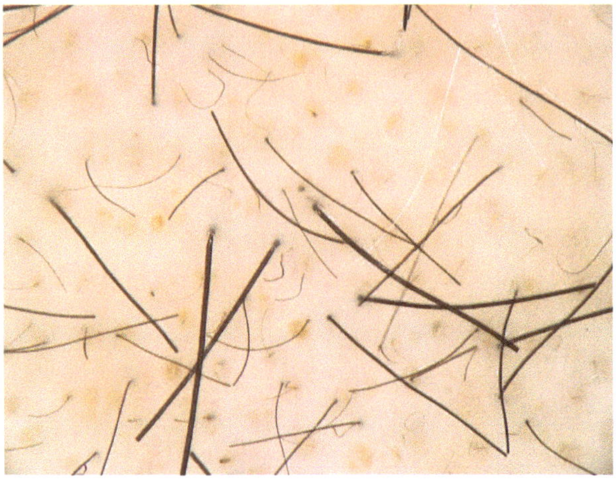

FIGURE 1.3 ×20 yellow dots and broken hairs in trichotillomania.

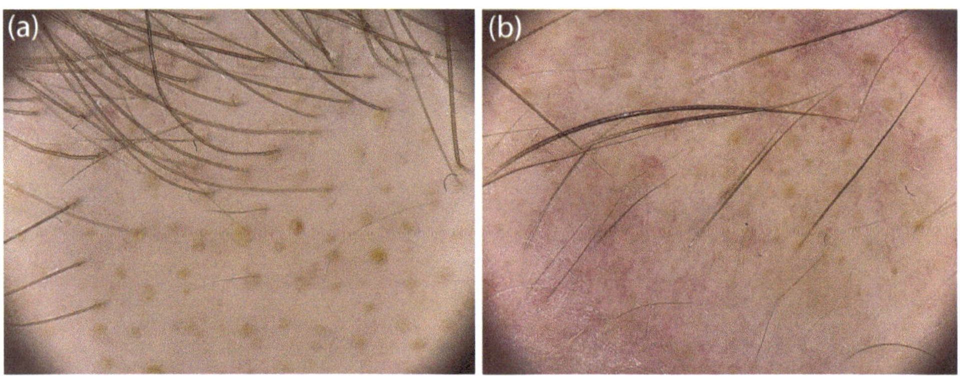

FIGURE 1.4 Frontal fibrosing alopecia. ×20 Yellow dots of the frontal hairline (a) and ×20 eyebrows (b).

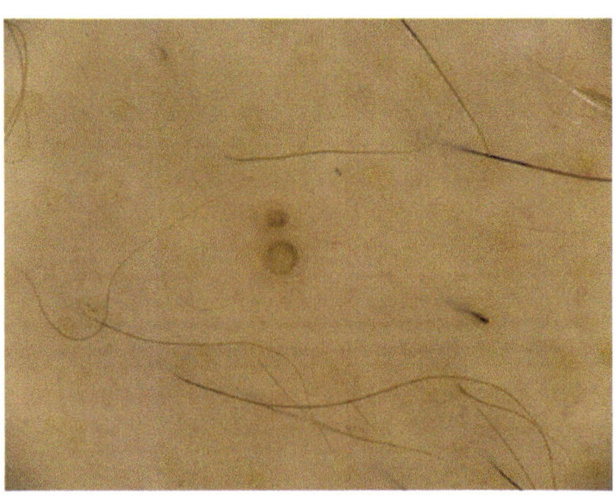

FIGURE 1.5 ×20 3D yellow dot in dissecting cellulitis of the scalp.

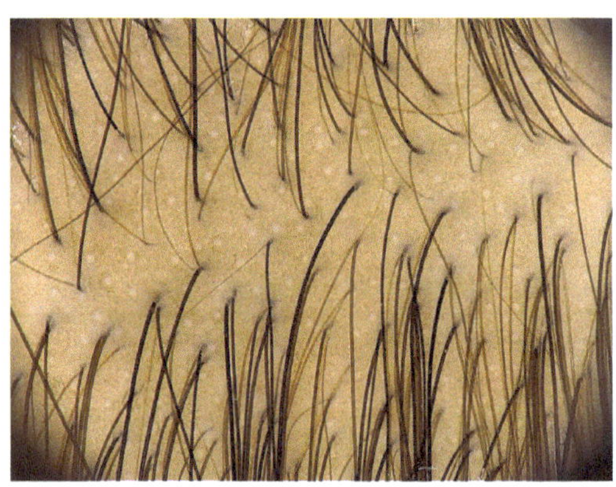

FIGURE 1.6 Androgenetic alopecia. ×20 Regularly distributed pinpoint white dots.

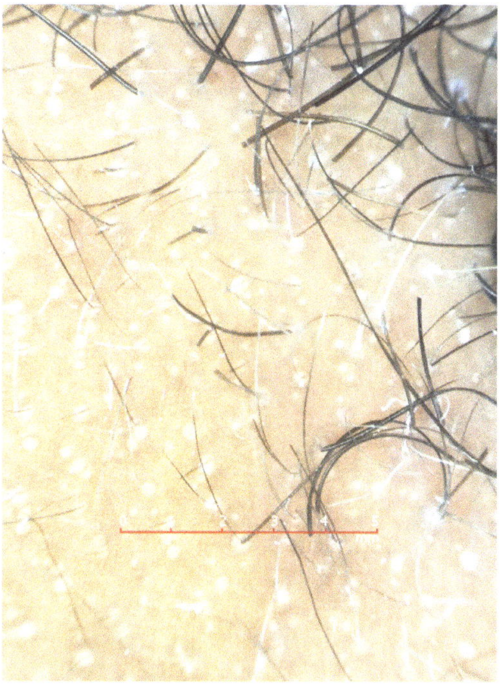

FIGURE 1.7 Alopecia areata. ×20 Regularly distributed pinpoint white dots.

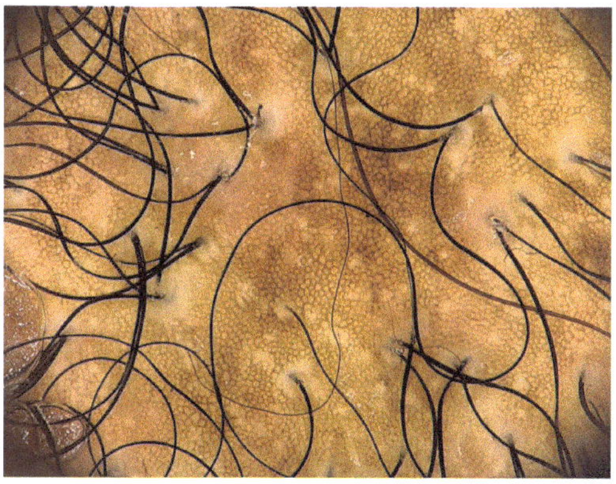

FIGURE 1.8 Scarring alopecia. ×20 Irregularly distributed pinpoint white dots and white patches.

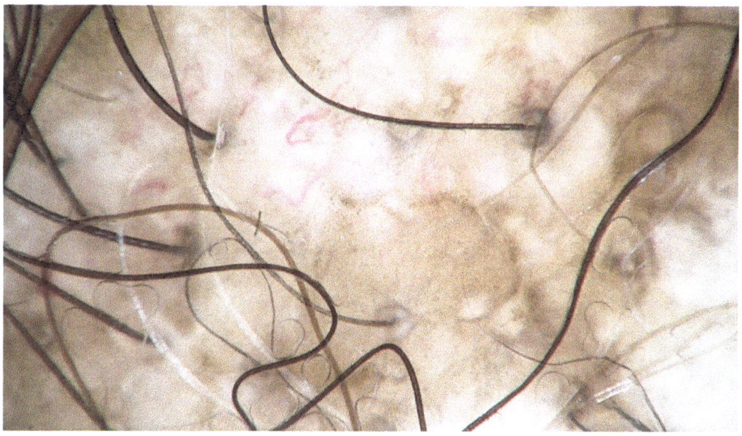

FIGURE 1.9 Discoid lupus erythematosus. ×50 Disappearance of pinpoint white dots, enlarged vessels, and loss of pigment.

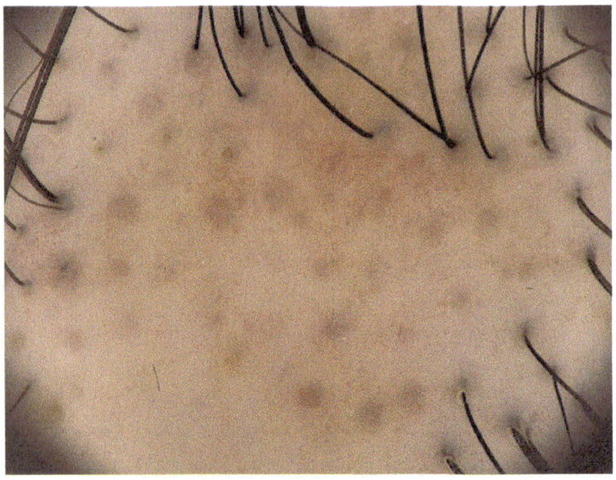

FIGURE 1.10 Discoid lupus erythematosus. ×20 Red dots are typically non-blanchable.

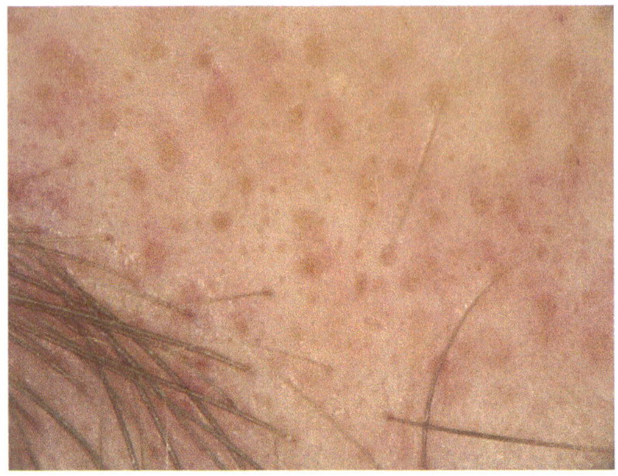

FIGURE 1.11 ×20 Glabellar red dots in frontal fibrosing alopecia.

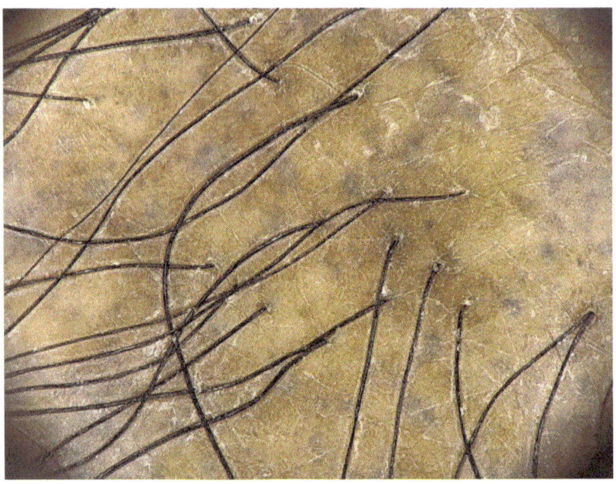

FIGURE 1.12 ×20 Blue-gray dots arranged in a target pattern in lichen planopilaris. The pigmentation spares the interfollicular scalp and corresponds to the previously affected hair follicles.

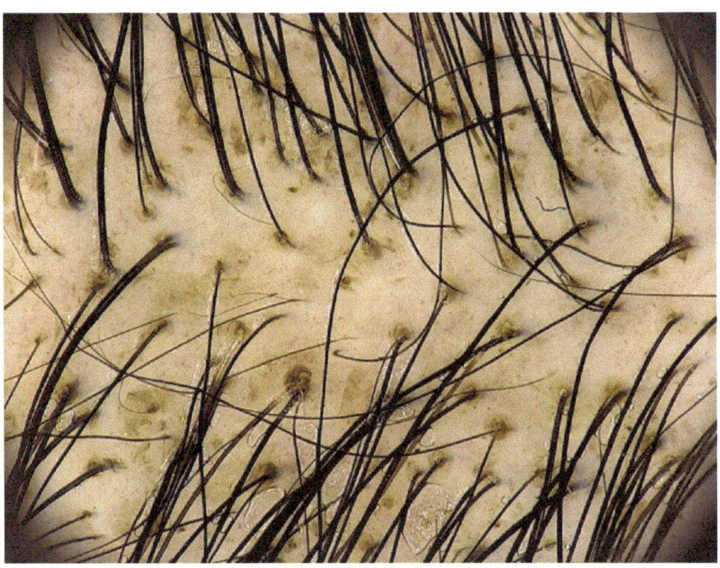

FIGURE 1.13 ×20 Brown/black staining that penetrates the hair follicles due to permanent hair dye.

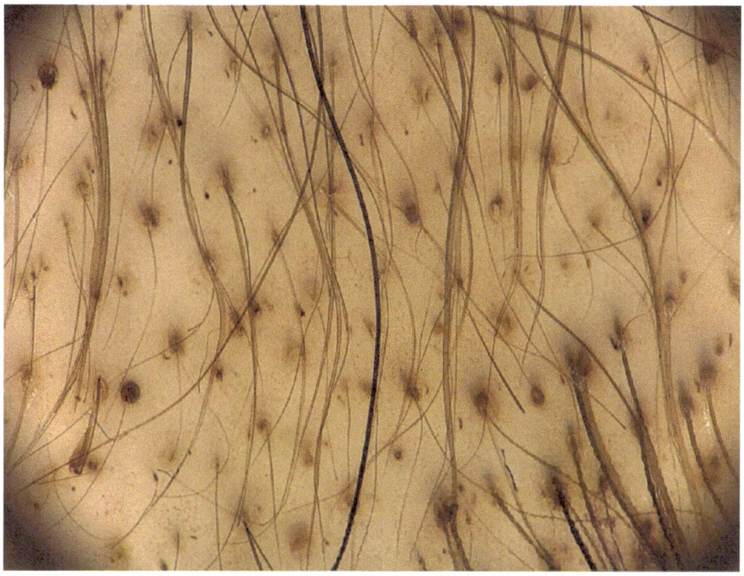

FIGURE 1.14 ×20 Brown/black staining penetrating the hair follicles due to anthralin in a patient affected by alopecia areata.

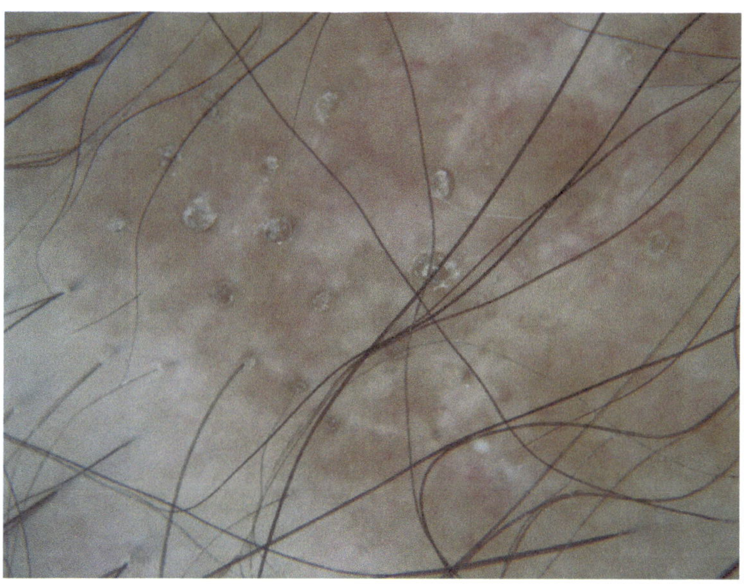

FIGURE 1.15 ×20 Keratotic plugs in discoid lupus erythematosus.

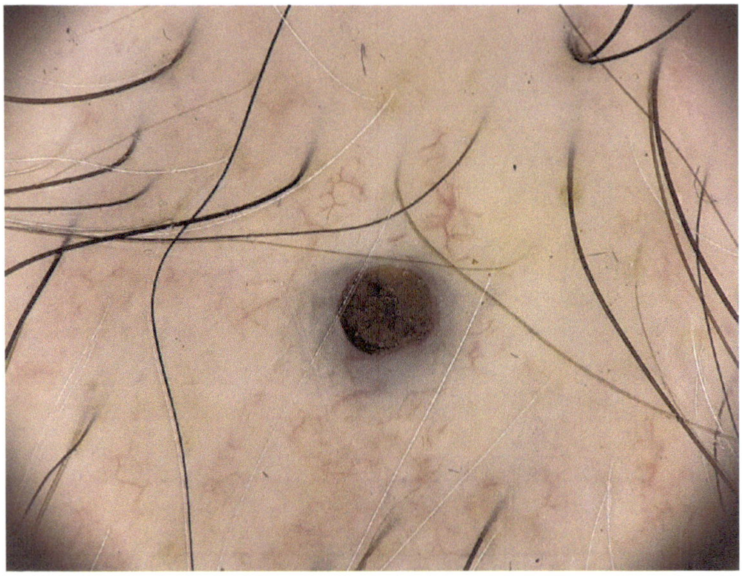

FIGURE 1.16 ×20 Large keratotic plug in dissecting cellulitis of the scalp. The plug is big and dark-colored due to keratin oxidation.

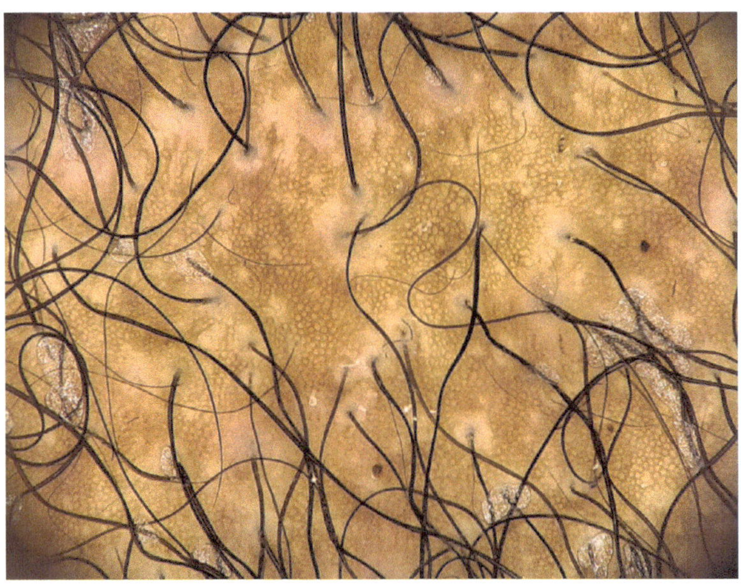

FIGURE 1.17 Gray white halos.

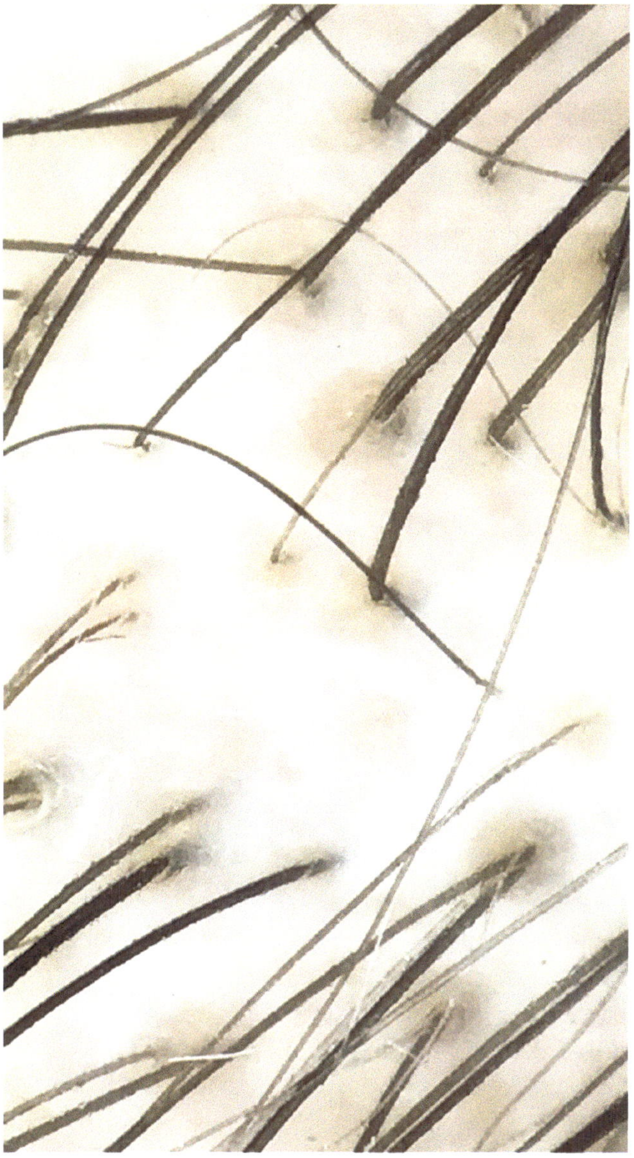

FIGURE 1.18 ×50 Peripilar signs presenting as subtle and depressed yellow-brownish halos around the follicular openings in early-stage androgenetic alopecia.

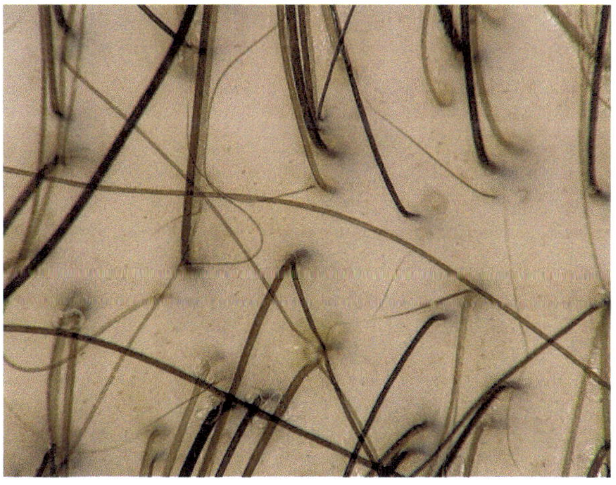

FIGURE 1.19 ×50 Empty follicles in a case of androgenetic alopecia. Note the presence of miniaturized hairs and hair shaft variability.

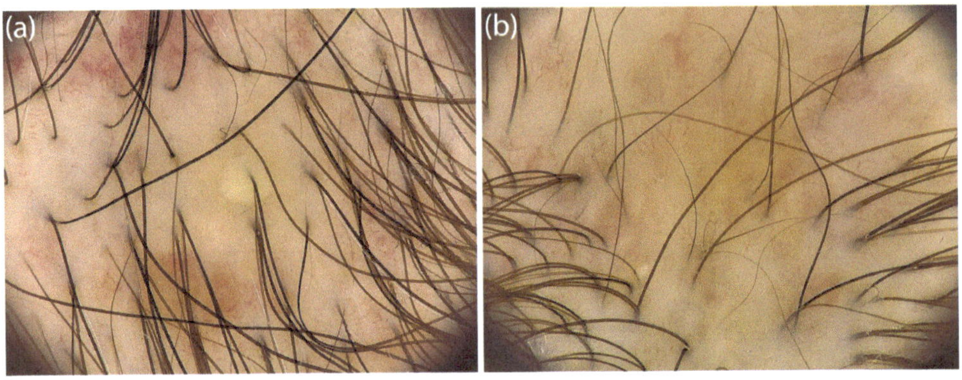

FIGURE 1.20 ×20 Follicular pustules in seborrheic dermatitis, also note the presence of arborizing vessels (a); ×20 follicular pustules in folliculitis decalvans, also note loss of follicular openings and an ingrowing hair (b).

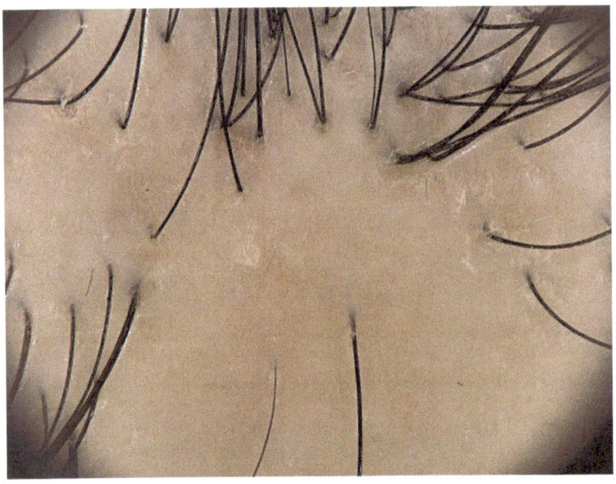

FIGURE 1.21 ×20 Loss of follicular openings in scarring alopecia.

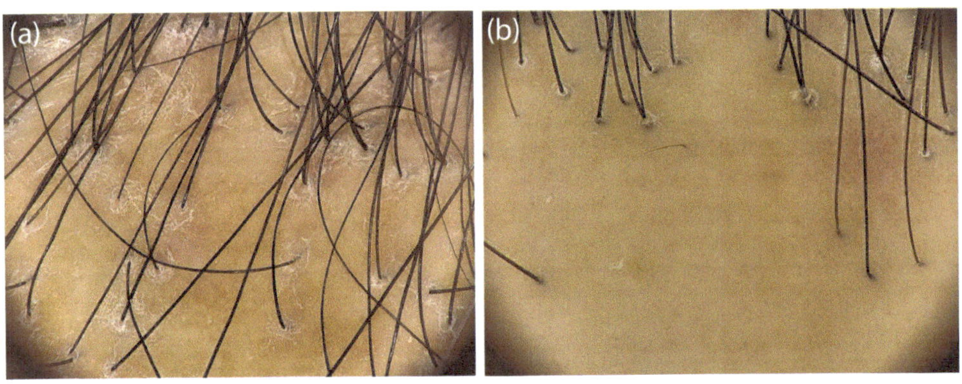

FIGURE 1.22 ×20 Peripilar casts in lichen planopilaris (a); and frontal fibrosing alopecia (b).

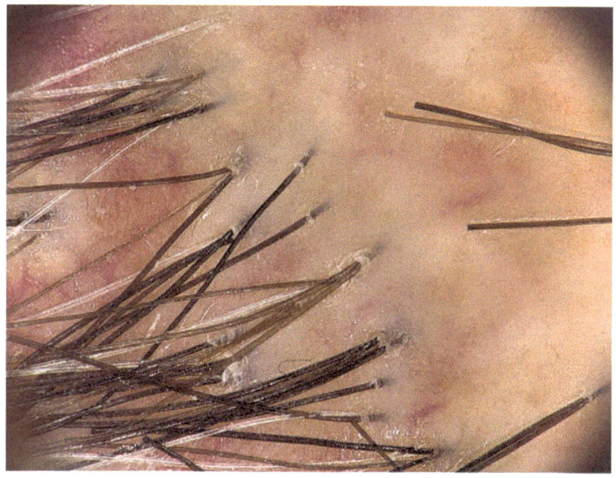

FIGURE 1.23 ×20 Peripilar casts in folliculitis decalvans.

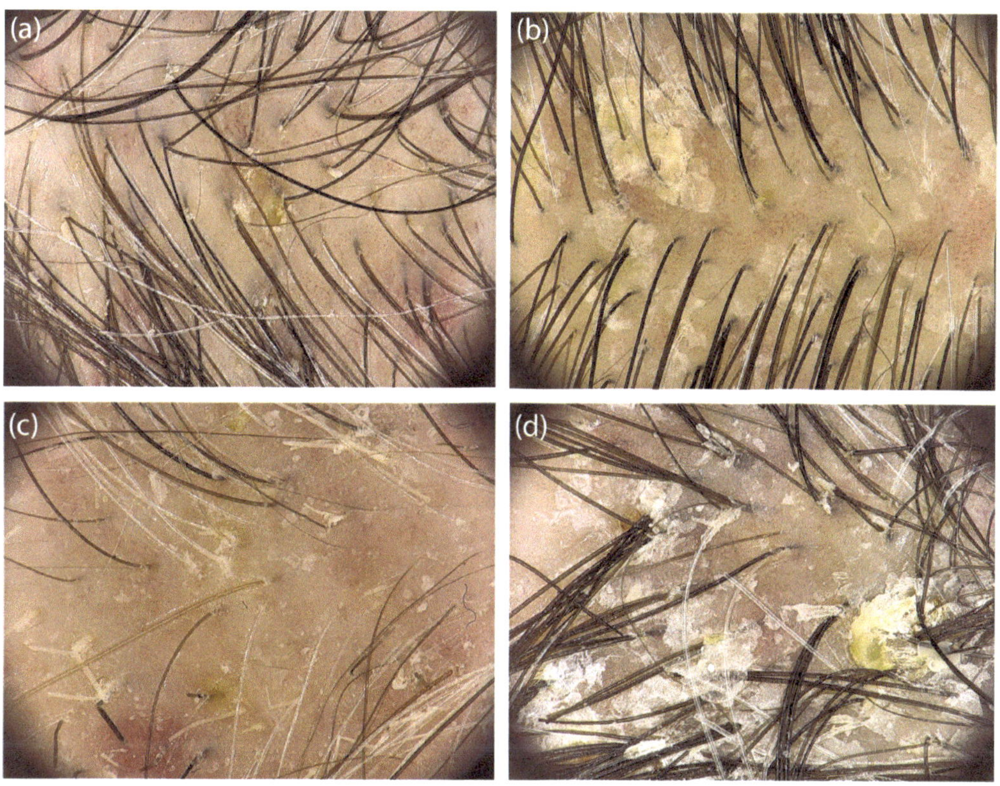

FIGURE 1.24 ×20 Interfollicular yellowish scales in seborrheic dermatitis (a); ×20 inter and perifollicular whitish scales in scalp psoriasis (b); ×40 tinea capitis (c); and ×40 folliculitis decalvans (d). Note typical twisted vessels in (b), comma hair in (c), and hair tufting in (d).

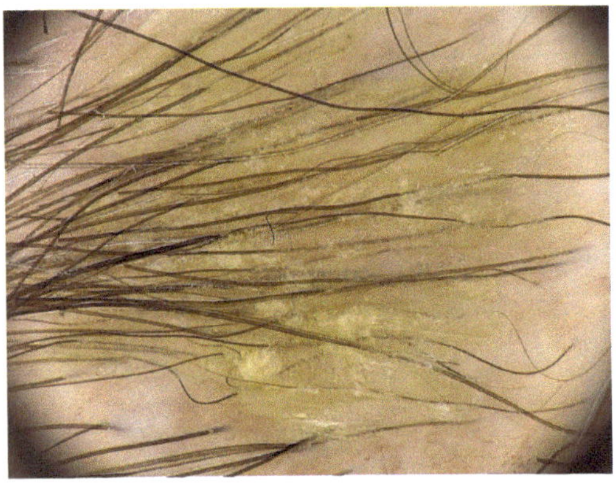

FIGURE 1.25 ×50 Diffuse yellowish crusting and scaling in erosive pustular dermatosis of the scalp.

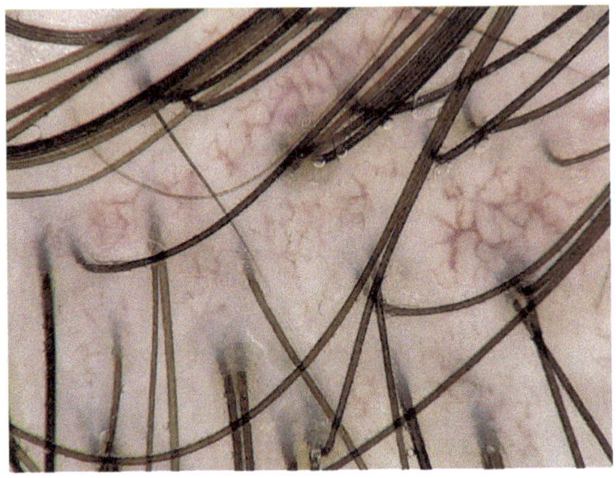

FIGURE 1.26 ×50 Prominent arborizing vessels.

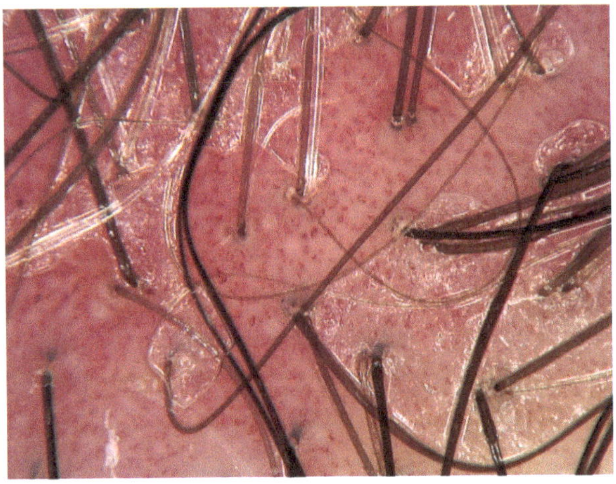

FIGURE 1.27 ×50 Twisted capillary loops in scalp psoriasis.

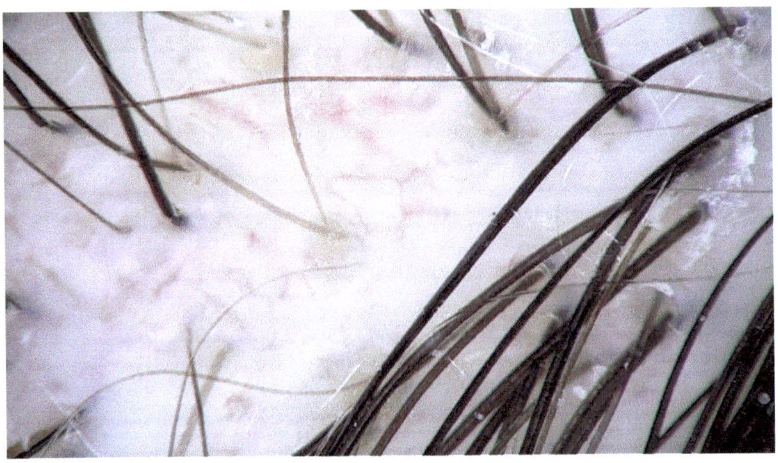

FIGURE 1.28 ×20 Single interspersed enlarged vessels in scalp rosacea.

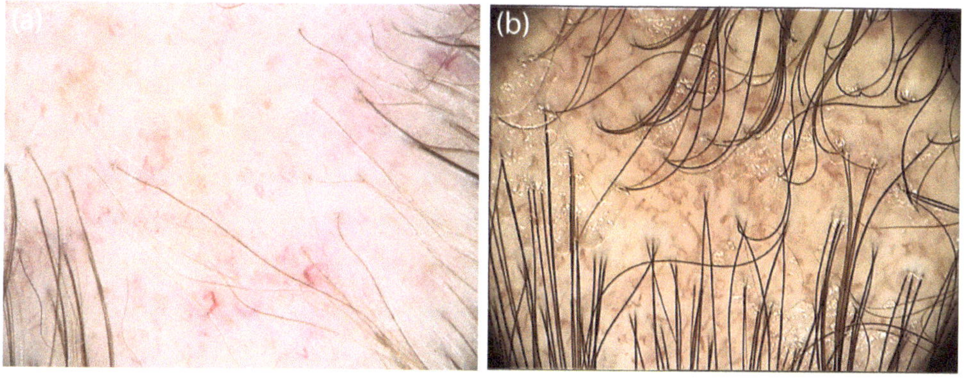

FIGURE 1.29 ×20 Enlarged branching vessels in discoid lupus (a); ×20 enlarged tortuous vessels in dermatomyositis (b).

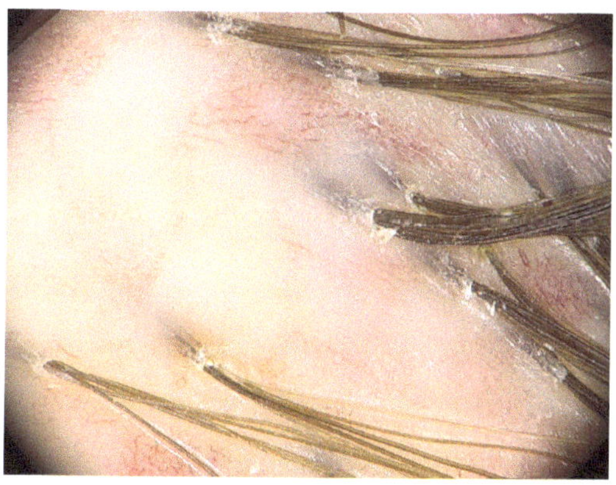

FIGURE 1.30 ×50 Linear radial vessels around the hair follicles in folliculitis decalvans.

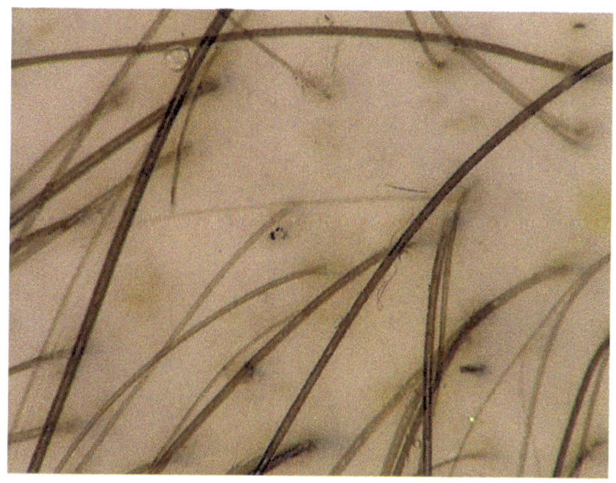

FIGURE 1.31 ×50 Hair powder: The scalp surface presents randomly distributed multiple small dark dots of different shape and size. Also note a broken hair.

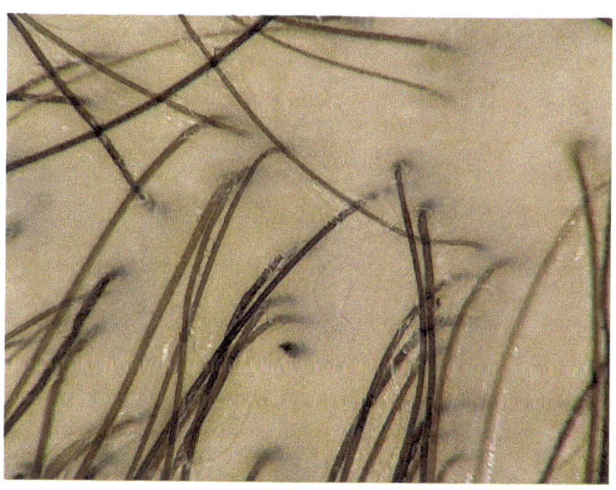

FIGURE 1.32 ×50 Rectangular black structures in the loose anagen hair syndrome.

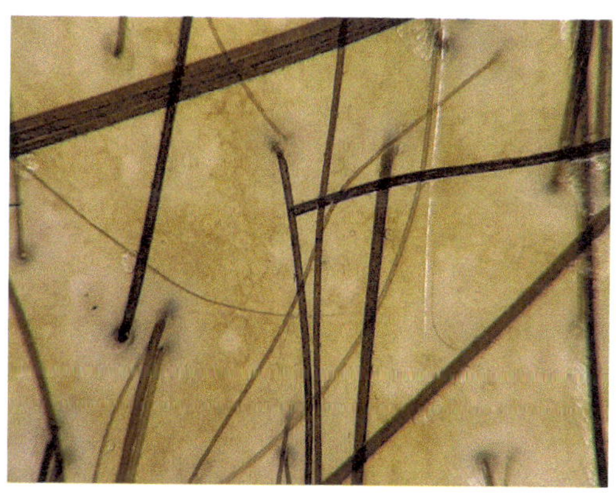

FIGURE 1.33 ×50 Honeycomb network in the sun-exposed scalp of androgenetic alopecia.

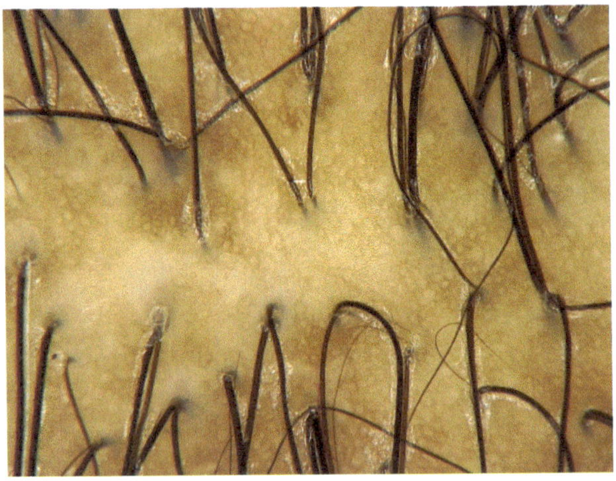

FIGURE 1.34 ×20 Honeycomb network in the pigmented scalp.

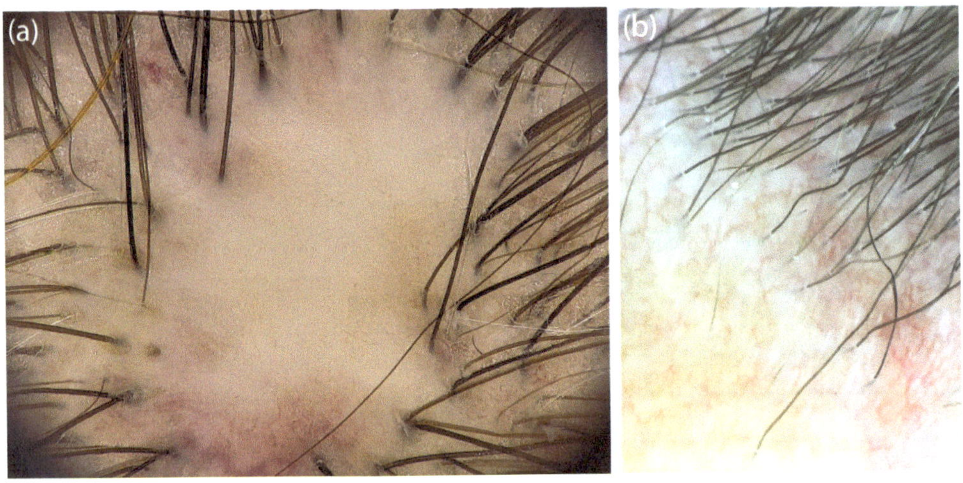

FIGURE 1.35 ×20 White patches devoid of follicular opening in scarring alopecia (a,b).

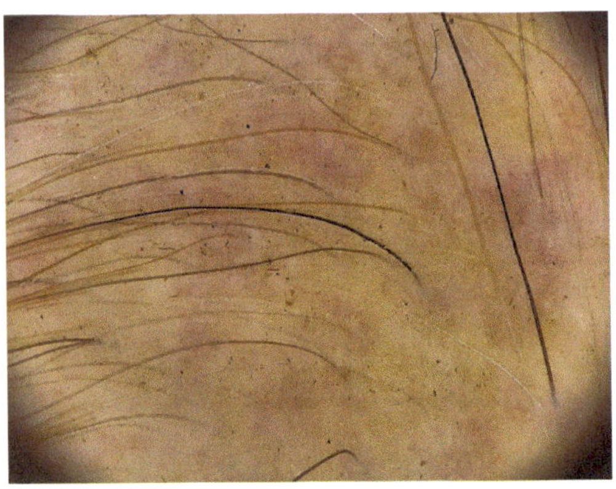

FIGURE 1.36 ×20 Dirty dots in an elderly patient.

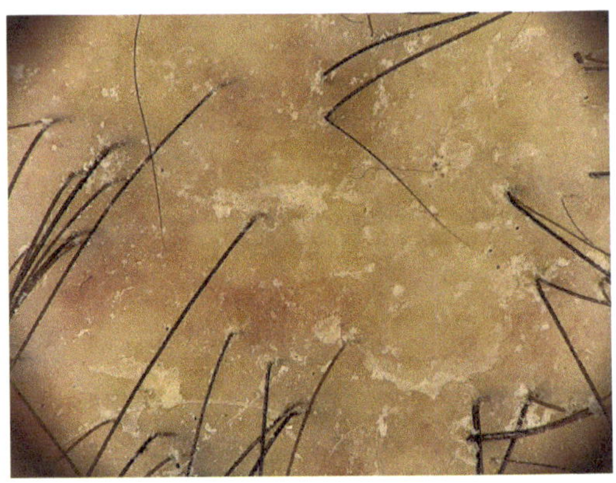

FIGURE 1.37 ×50 Whitish concretions with a granular structure corresponding to residues of topical products, should not be confused with scales.

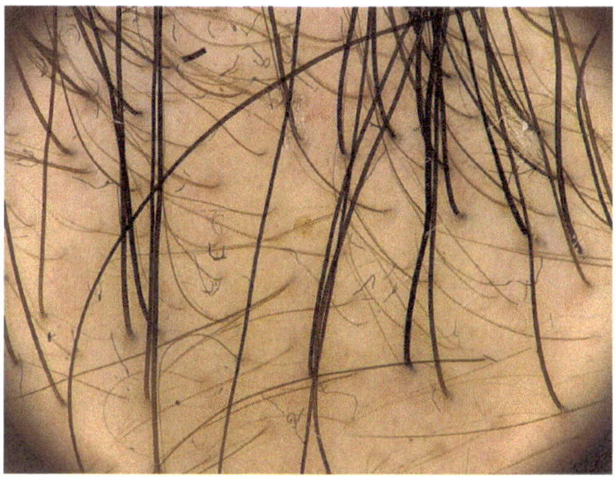

FIGURE 1.38 ×20 Residues of textile fibers in a patient wearing a hat. Also note a hair fragment due to haircut.

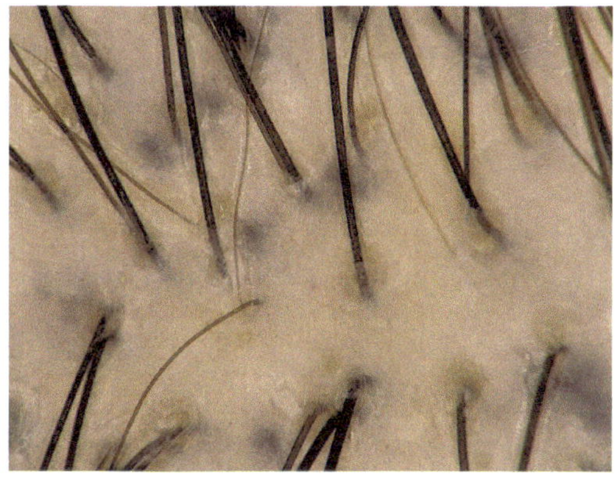

FIGURE 1.39 Micropigmentation. ×50 Multiple pigmented rounded dots.

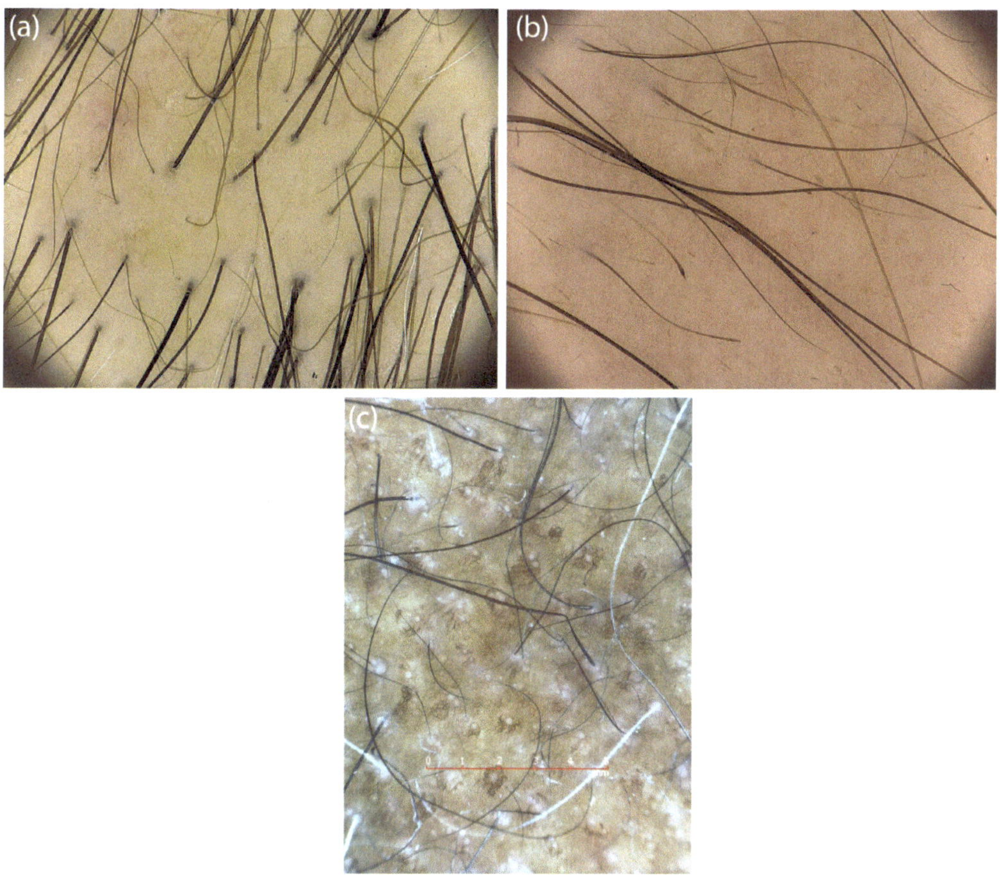

FIGURE 1.40 ×50 Hair diameter diversity in androgenetic alopecia (a); ×50 alopecia areata (b); ×50 central centrifugal cicatricial alopecia (c).

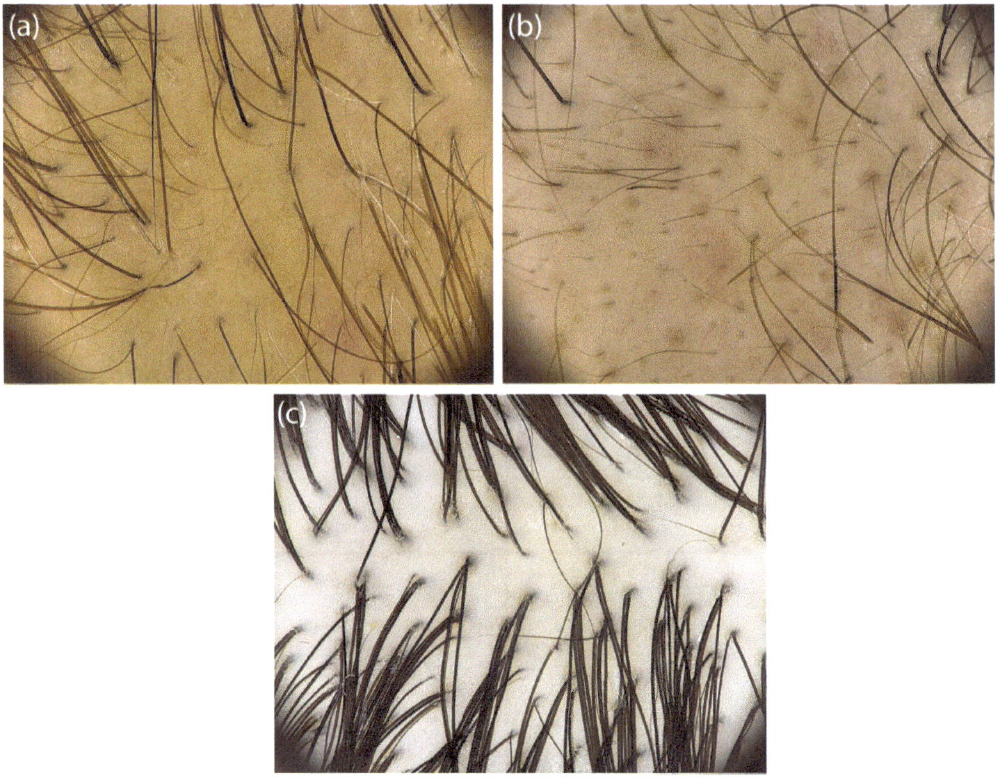

FIGURE 1.41 ×20 Short regrowing hairs in androgenetic alopecia (a), ×20 alopecia areata (b), and ×20 telogen effluvium (c). Note that they are thin (<0.03 mm), hypopigmented, and associated with hair shaft variability in androgenetic alopecia (a); clustered and associated with broken hairs in alopecia areata (b); thick and upright in telogen effluvium (c).

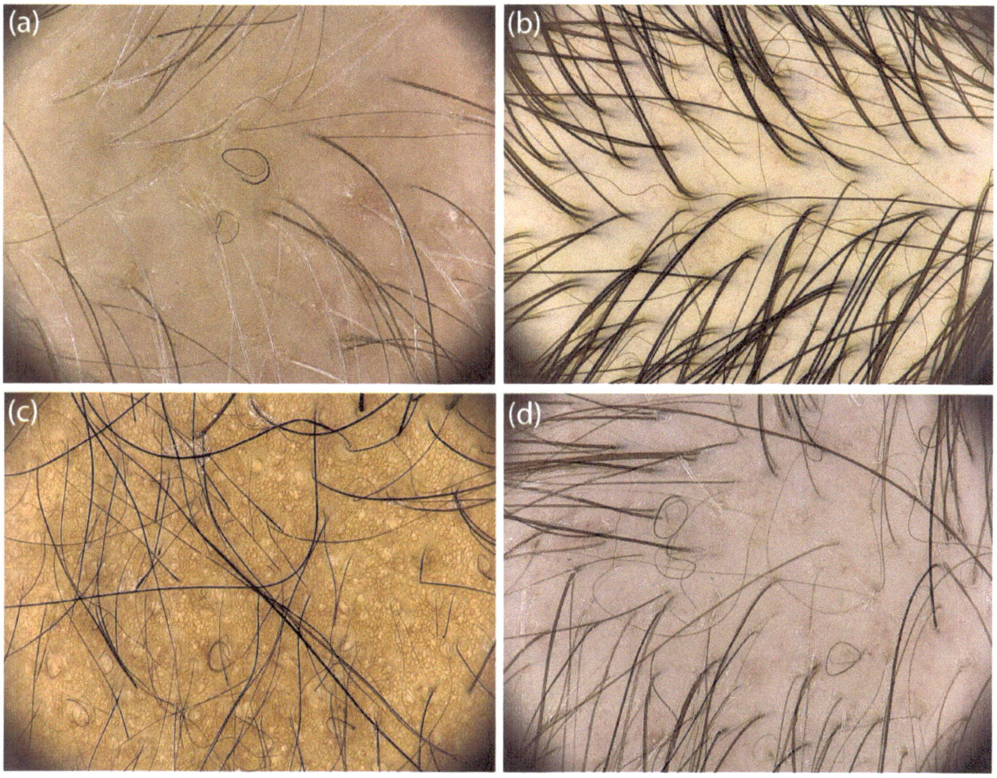

FIGURE 1.42 ×40 Pigtail hairs: The circle hairs are thin with a tapered end (a). Examples of pigtail hairs found in ×20 androgenetic alopecia (b), ×40 alopecia areata (c), and ×40 alopecia areata incognito (d).

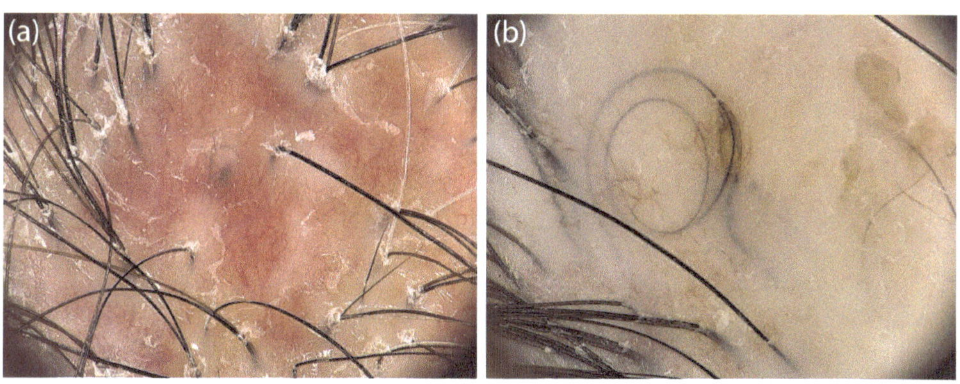

FIGURE 1.43 Embedded thick circle hairs in lichen planopilaris at ×20 (a) and ×50 (b) magnification.

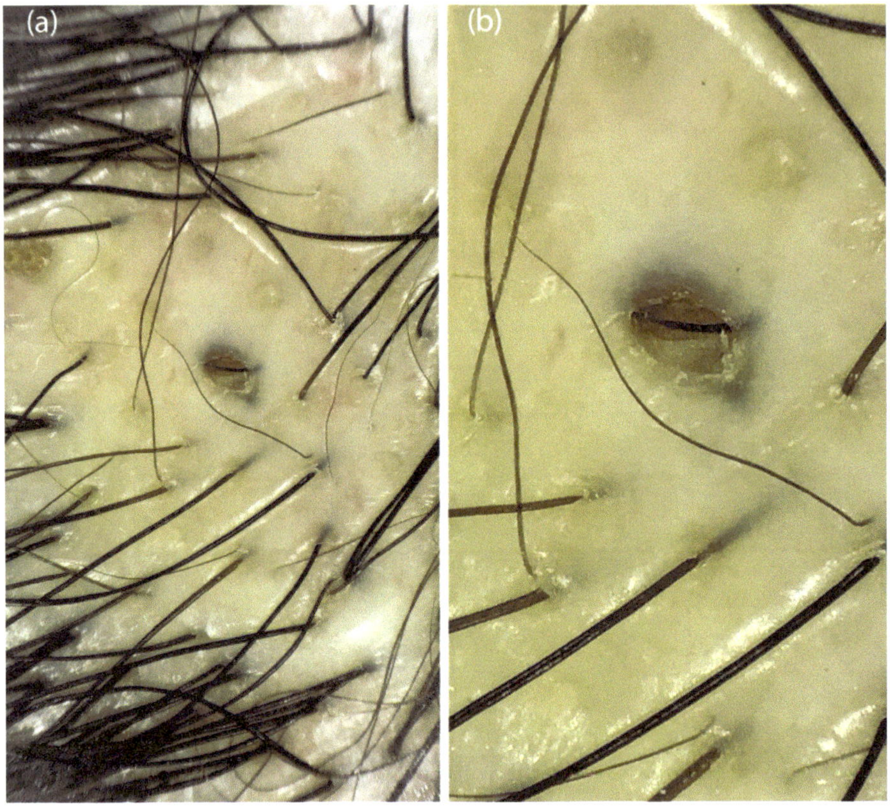

FIGURE 1.44 Embedded thick circle hairs in dissecting cellulitis at ×20 (a) and ×50 (b) magnification.

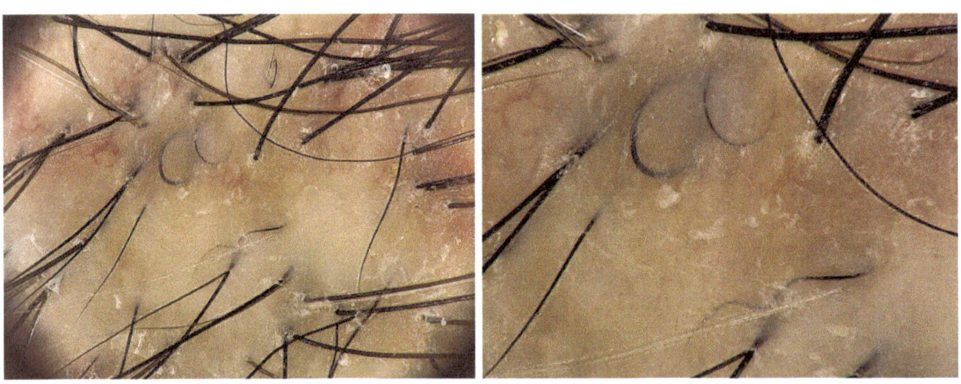

FIGURE 1.45 Double rolled circle hairs at ×20 (a) and ×50 (b) magnification in scarring alopecia.

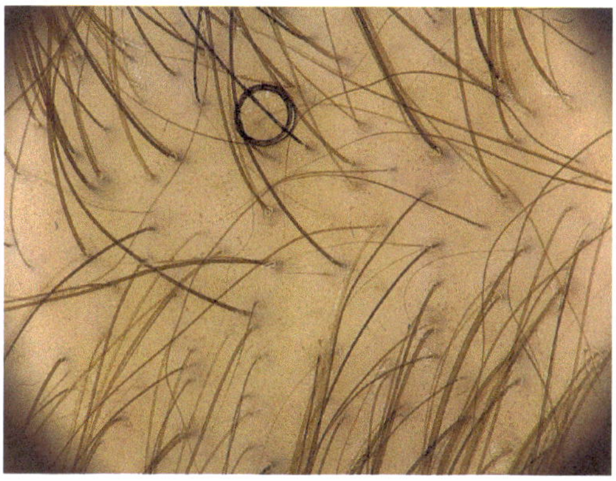

FIGURE 1.46 ×20 Long circle hairs detected in the normal scalp.

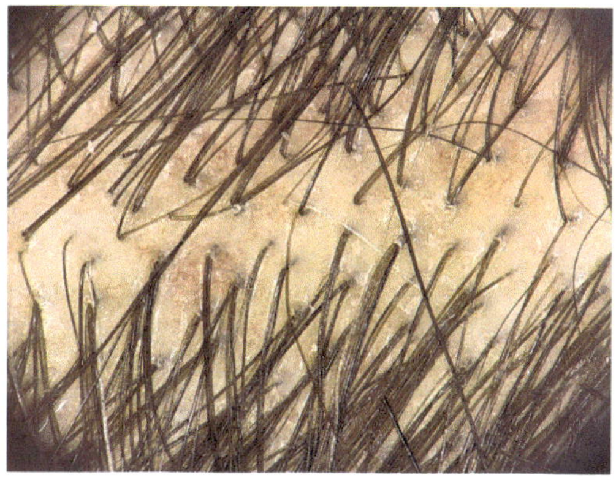

FIGURE 1.47 ×20 Hair tufting with peripilar scales in an apparently normal scalp in a patient with lichen planopilaris.

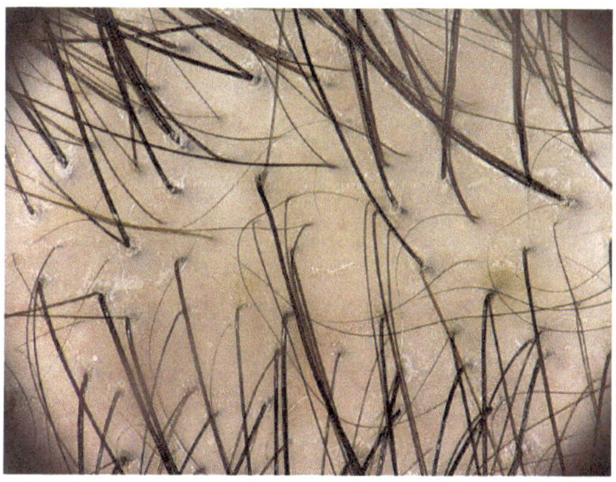

FIGURE 1.48 ×20 Hair tufting with peripilar scales in an apparently normal scalp in a patient with fibrosing alopecia with a pattern distribution.

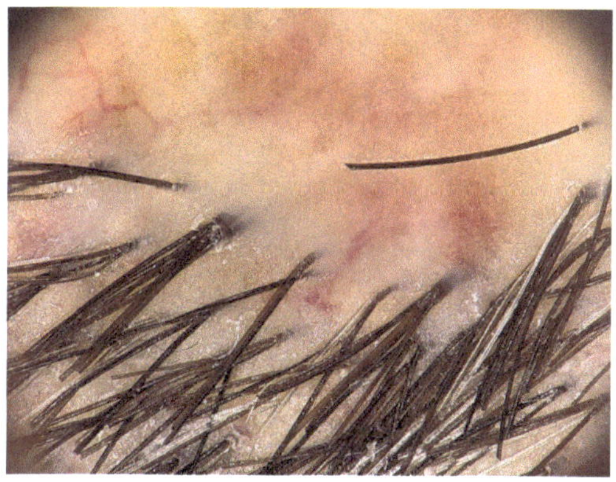

FIGURE 1.49 ×50 Hair tufting with peripilar scales in folliculitis decalvans.

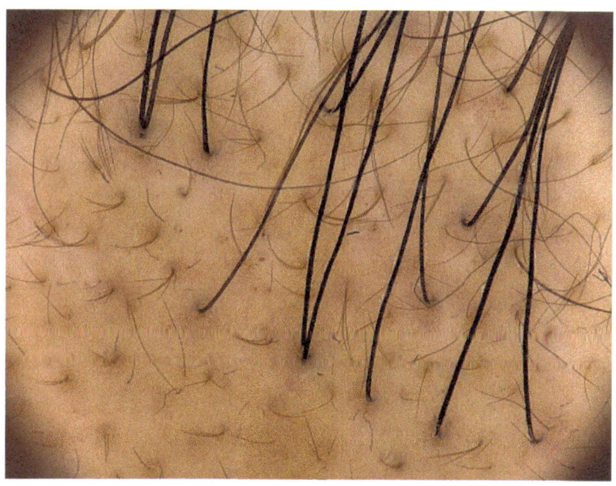

FIGURE 1.50 ×20 Tufting of vellus hairs in a patient with MPHL who underwent hair transplantation.

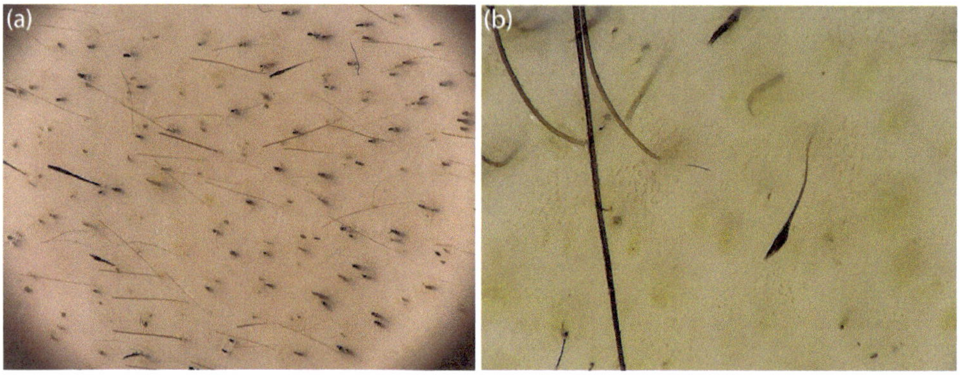

FIGURE 1.51 Exclamation mark hairs in alopecia areata at ×20 (a) and ×50 (b) magnification.

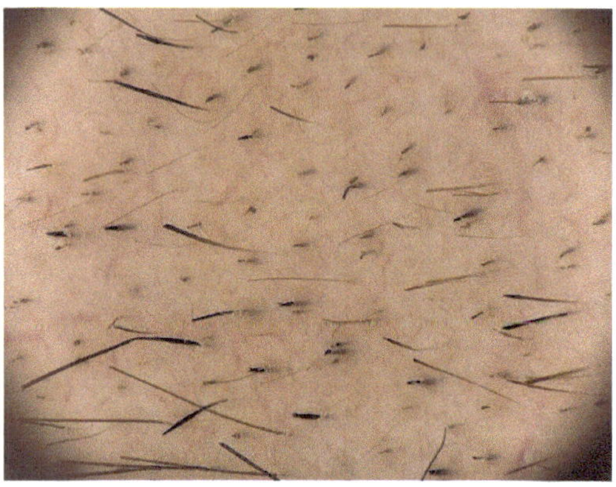

FIGURE 1.52 ×20 Broken hairs at different length seen in alopecia areata

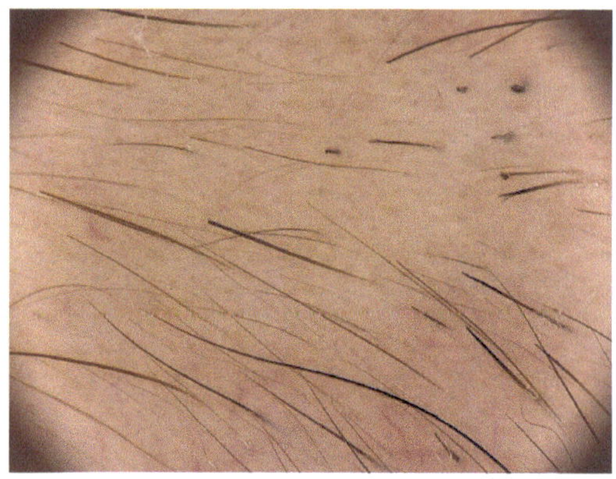

FIGURE 1.53 ×20 Broken hairs in trichotillomania

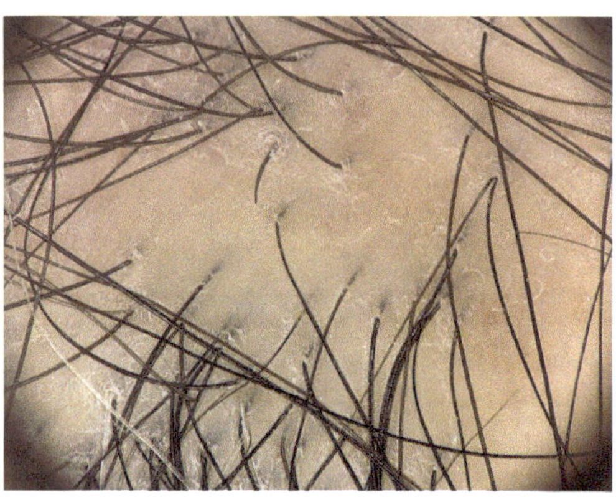

FIGURE 1.54 ×20 Broken hairs surrounded by peripilar casts in lichen planopilaris.

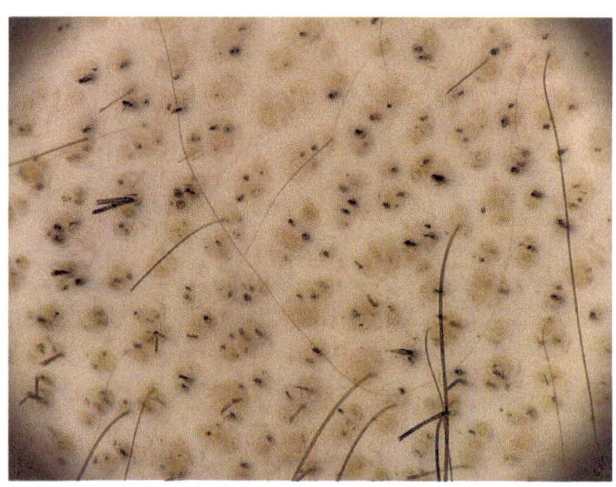

FIGURE 1.55 ×20 Numerous black dots in alopecia areata.

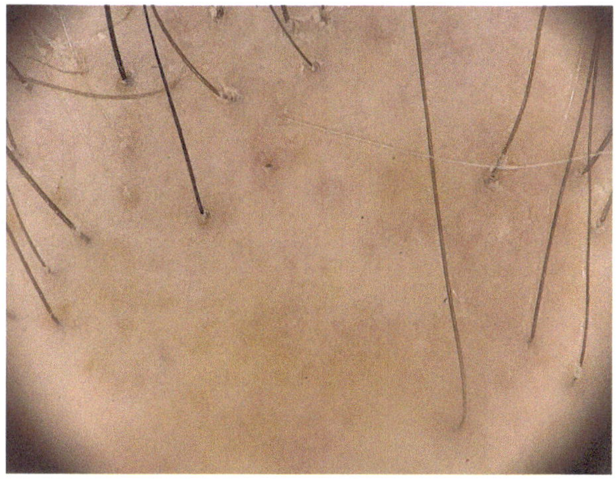

FIGURE 1.56 ×20 Isolated black dot on the hairline of frontal fibrosing alopecia.

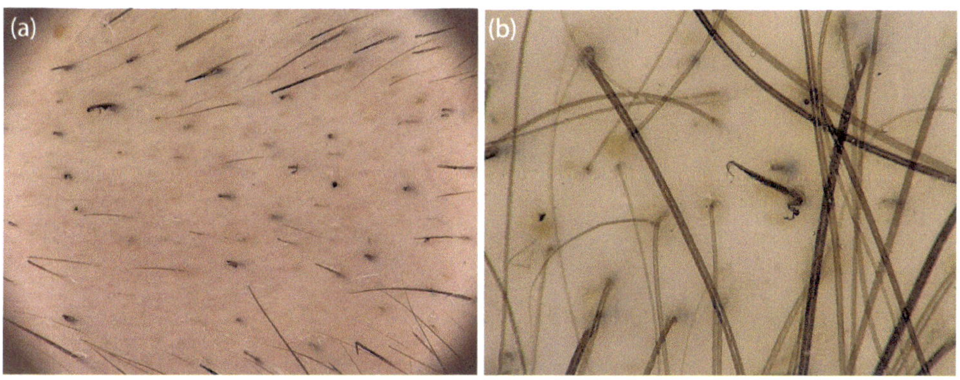

FIGURE 1.57 Question mark hair in trichotillomania seen at ×20 (a) and ×50 (b) magnification.

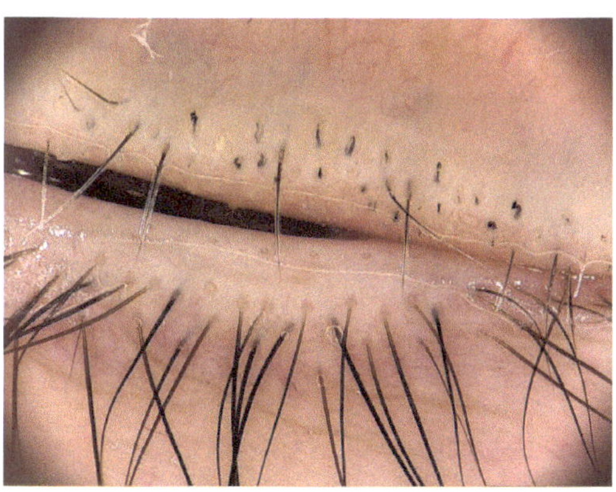

FIGURE 1.58 ×20 Flame hairs in the eyelashes of trichotillomania.

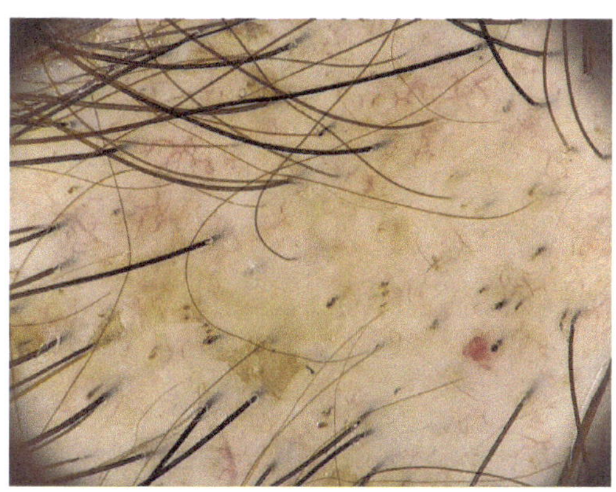

FIGURE 1.59 ×20 Flame hairs in alopecia areata.

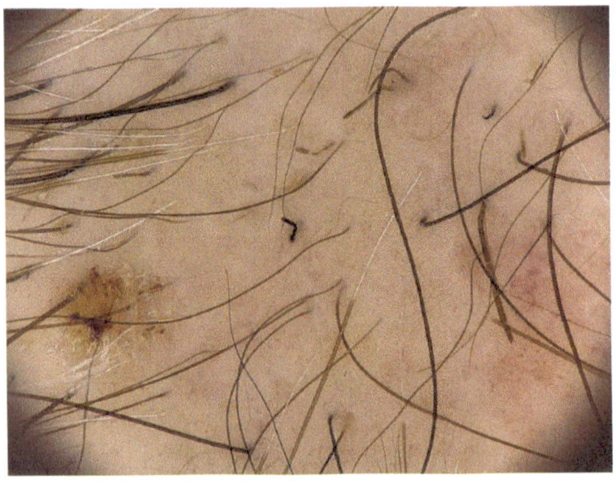

FIGURE 1.60 ×20 Comma hair in tinea capitis.

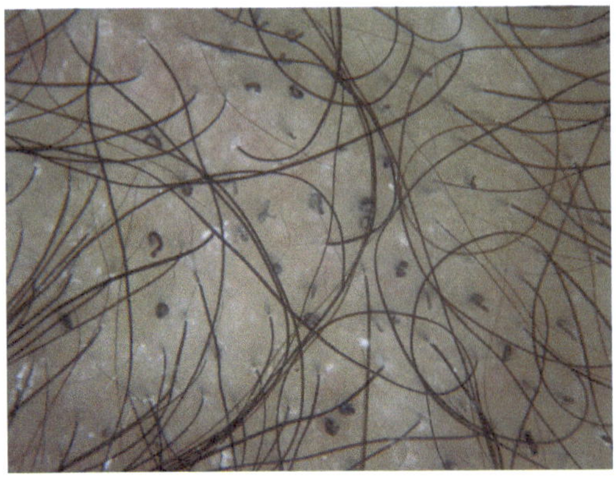

FIGURE 1.61 ×50 Corkscrew hairs in tinea capitis.

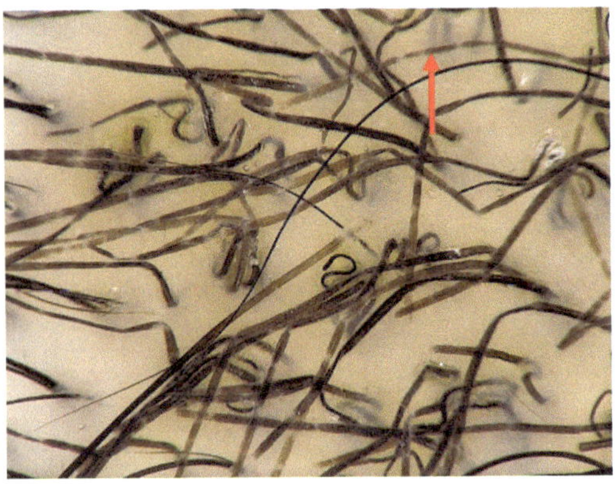

FIGURE 1.62 ×50 Morse-code hairs in tinea capitis.

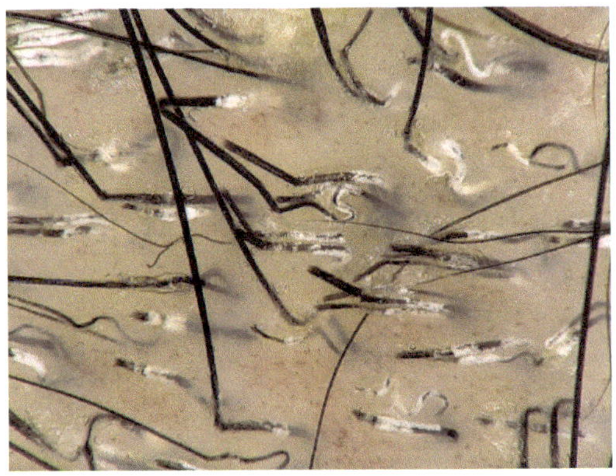

FIGURE 1.63 ×50 Zigzag hair in tinea capitis.

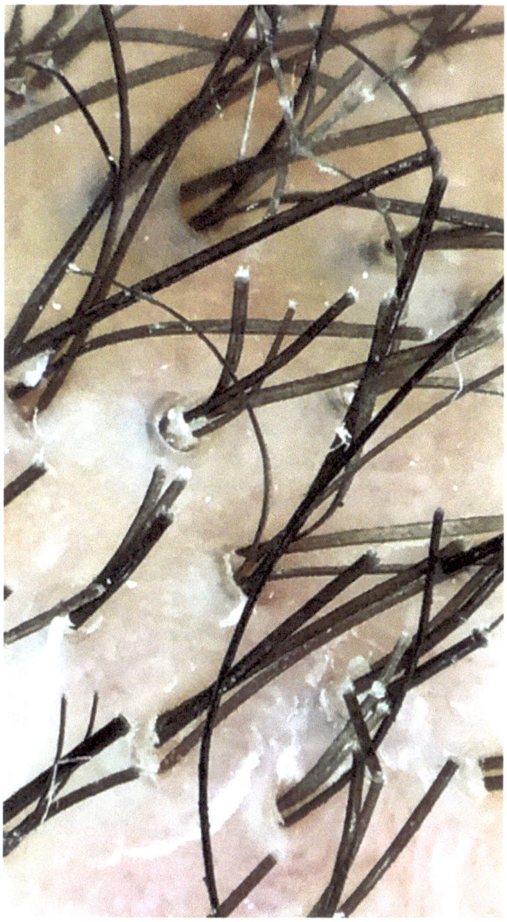

FIGURE 1.64 ×50 Proximal trichorrhexis nodosa.

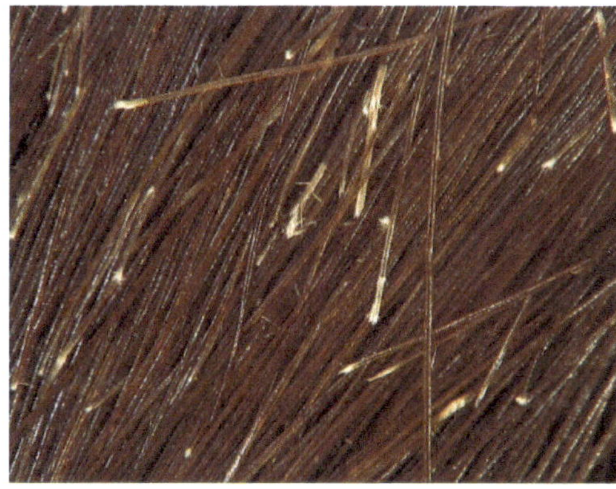

FIGURE 1.65 ×20 Distal trichorrhexis nodosa.

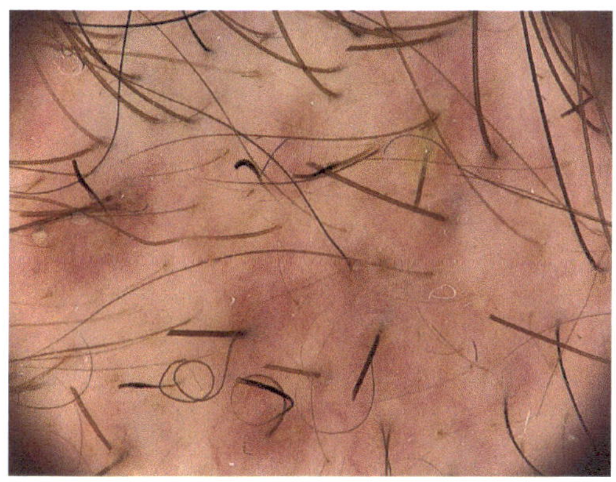

FIGURE 1.66 ×50 Tulip hair after hair transplantation.

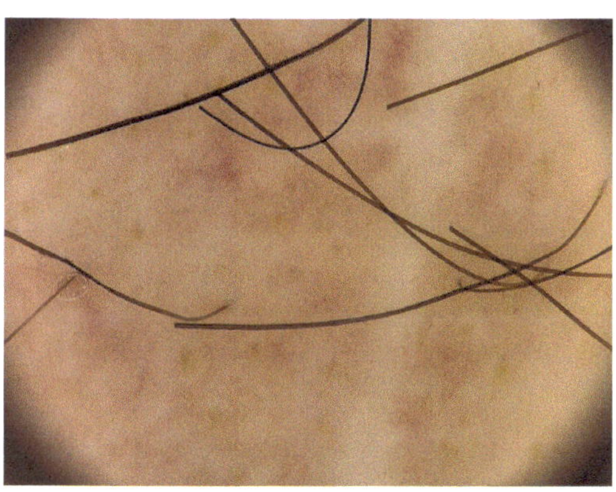

FIGURE 1.67 ×50 Coudability hair in alopecia areata.

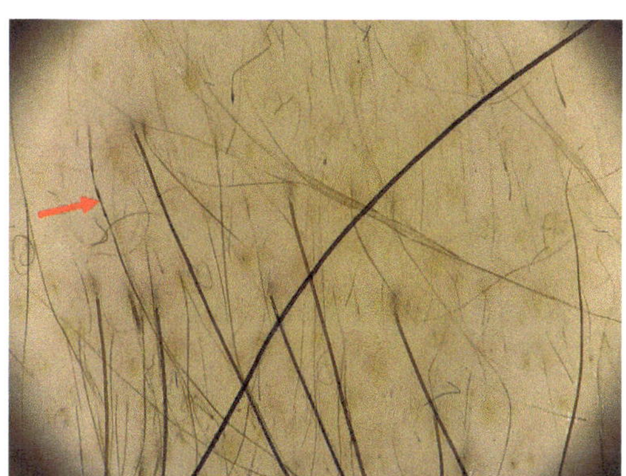

FIGURE 1.68 ×20 Pseudomonilethrix hairs in alopecia areata.

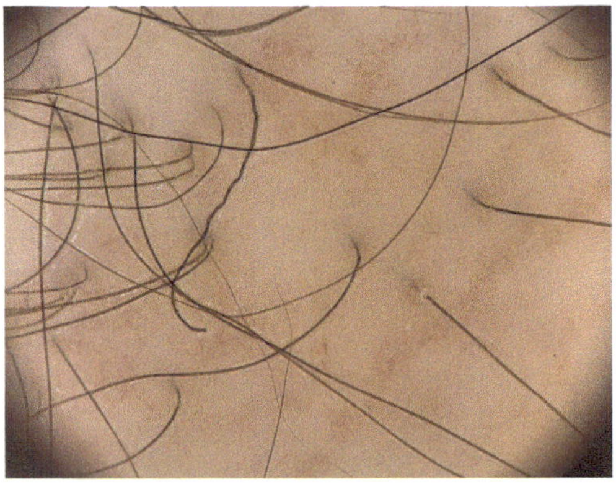

FIGURE 1.69 ×50 Pili torti in scarring alopecia.

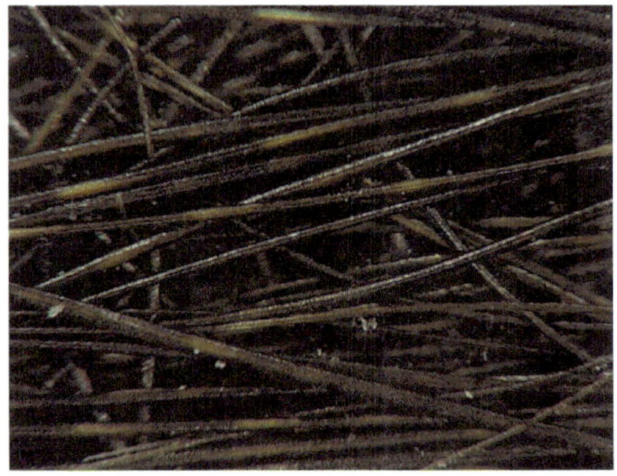

FIGURE 1.70 Pili annulati seen at ×40 magnification.

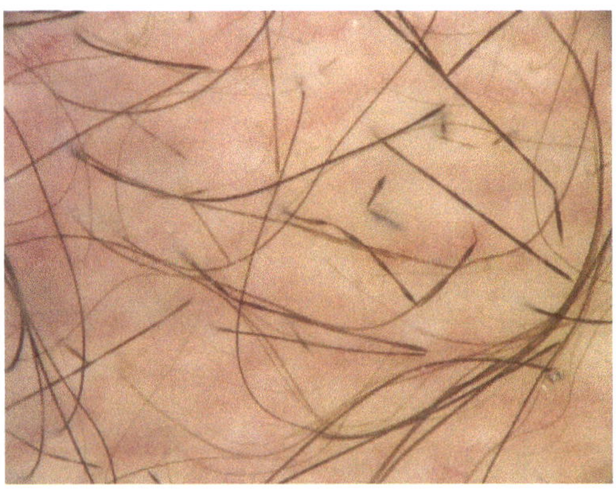

FIGURE 1.71 ×30 Monilethrix hair.

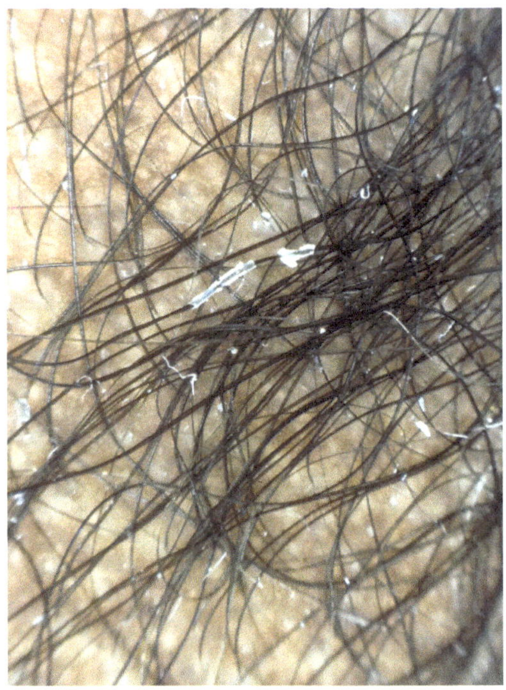

FIGURE 1.72 ×20 Tubular hair casts in traction alopecia. Do not confuse hair casts with nits, which are immobile, oval-shaped, and do not encircle the hair shaft.

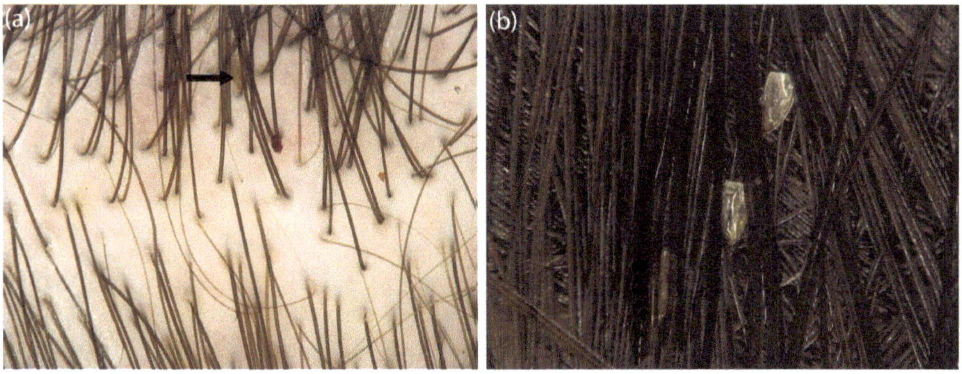

FIGURE 1.73 Viable (a) and empty (b) nits seen at ×20 and ×50 magnification.

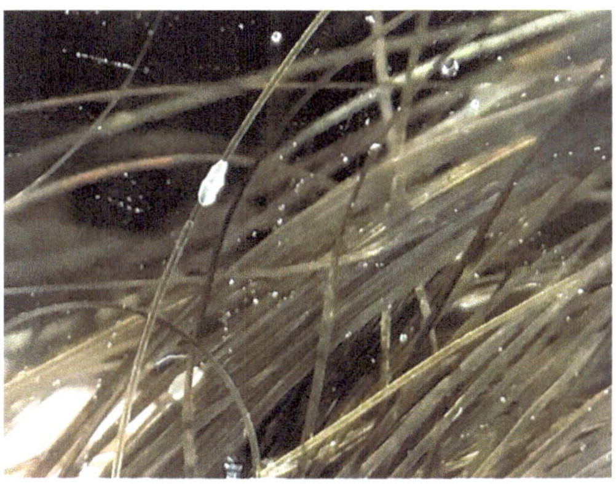

FIGURE 1.74 White Piedra. ×50 The hair shaft is visible through the white nodule.

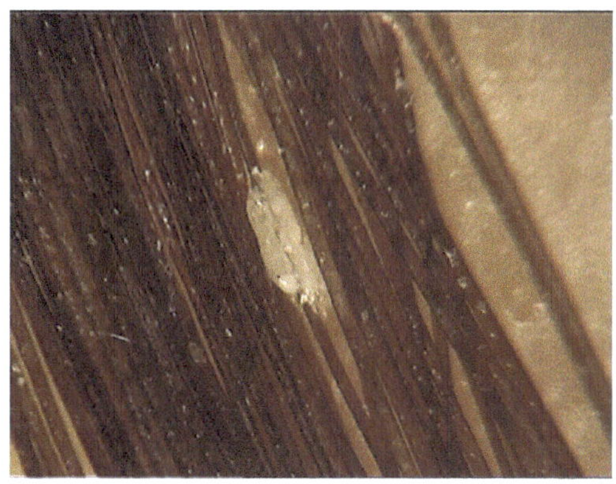

FIGURE 1.75 ×50 Hair spray deposits along the hair shafts.

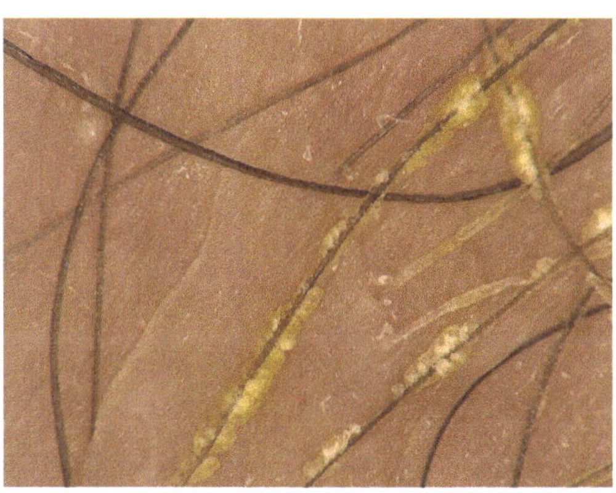

FIGURE 1.76 ×50 Trichomycosis palmellina, white yellow concretions surrounding of the terminal hairs.

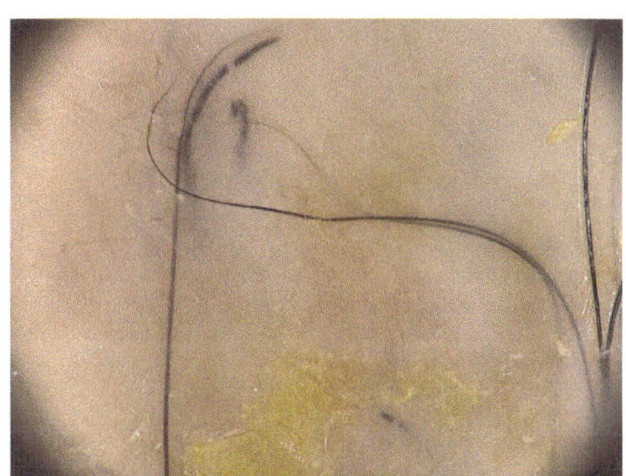

FIGURE 1.77 ×40 Hair roots through the scalp in steroid-induced atrophy.

SUGGESTED READING

Cervantes J, Johr RJ, Tosti A. Dermoscopy of yellow concretions on axillary hair. *Skin Appendage Disord.* 2018;4(2):86–89.

Doche I, Vincenzi C, Tosti A. Casts and pseudocasts. *J Am Acad Dermatol.* 2016;75(4):e147–e148.

Esteves ALV, Serafini NB, Lemes LR, Melo DF. Circular hairs: nomenclature and meanings. *An Bras Dermatol.* 2017;92(6):874–76.

Hoffmann A, Waśkiel-Burnat A, Żółkiewicz J, Blicharz L, Rakowska A, Goldust M, Olszewska M, Rudnicka L. Pili Torti: a feature of numerous congenital and acquired conditions. *J Clin Med.* 2021;10(17):3901.

Kłosowicz A, Alsalhi W, Tosti A. How to optimize trichoscopy for evaluation of scalp vessels. *Skin Appendage Disord.* 2020;6(4):216–19.

Lacarrubba F, Verzì AE, Micali G. Newly described features resulting from high-magnification dermoscopy of tinea capitis. *JAMA Dermatol.* 2015;151(3):308–10.

Lacarrubba F, Verzì AE, Micali G. Trichoscopy in the differential diagnosis of pseudonits. *Skin Appendage Disord.* 2019;5(3):142–45.

Lencastre A, Tosti A. Role of trichoscopy in children's scalp and hair disorders. *Pediatr Dermatol.* 2013;30(6):674–82.

Lima CDS, Lemes LR, Melo DF. Yellow dots in trichoscopy: relevance, clinical significance and peculiarities. *An Bras Dermatol.* 2017;92(5):724–26.

Miteva M, Tosti A. Hair and scalp dermatoscopy. *J Am Acad Dermatol.* 2012;67(5):1040–8.

Miteva M, Tosti A. Dermatoscopy of hair shaft disorders. *J Am Acad Dermatol.* 2013;68(3):473–81.

Mubki T, Rudnicka L, Olszewska M, Shapiro J. Evaluation and diagnosis of the hair loss patient: part II. Trichoscopic and laboratory evaluations. *J Am Acad Dermatol.* 2014;71(3):431.e1–431.e11.

Ocampo-Garza J, Tosti A. Trichoscopy of dark scalp. *Skin Appendage Disord.* 2018;5(1):1–8.

Pirmez R, Piñeiro-Maceira J, Sodré CT. Exclamation marks and other trichoscopic signs of chemotherapy-induced alopecia. *Australas J Dermatol.* 2013; 54:129–32.

Ross EK, Vincenzi C, Tosti A. Videodermoscopy in the evaluation of hair and scalp disorders. *J Am Acad Dermatol.* 2006;55(5):799–806.

Torres F, Tosti A. Trichoscopy: an update. *G Ital Dermatol Venereol.* 2014;149(1):83–91.

Tosti A, Miteva M. Trichoscopy: a new tool for diagnosing hair diseases. *Dermatol Clin.* 2014;32(2):145–51.

Tosti A, Miteva M, Torres F, Vincenzi C, Romanelli P. Hair casts are a dermoscopic clue for the diagnosis of traction alopecia. *Br J Dermatol.* 2010;163(6):1353–5.

Tosti A, Torres F. Dermoscopy in the diagnosis of hair and scalp disorders. *Actas Dermosifiliogr.* 2009;100 Suppl 1:114–9.

2 The Normal Scalp

THE NORMAL WHITE SCALP

- Hair mostly emerging in groups of two to three.
- Simple red loops.
- Arborizing red lines.

In the healthy scalp hair follicles are grouped in follicular units and are seen as groups of two to three hair shafts coming out of the same follicular ostium.

- This ratio varies in physiological conditions influenced by different factors such as scalp area, gender, and age; it is typically higher in the occipital compared to the temporal area.
- Follicular units consist of one primary follicle and two to four secondary follicles.
- Follicular units consisting of only one shaft are also present, and their frequency increases with aging or in hair disorders.
- The temporal regions have the highest proportion of single-hair pilosebaceous units and number of vellus hairs. A potential factor contributing to their lower hair density is the increased spacing between pilosebaceous units.
- There is a natural variability in the thickness of hair shafts within the same follicular unit which does not change in different scalp areas.
- The medulla can be visible as a linear or interrupted white line within the shaft of pigmented and white hair (Figure 2.1).

Normal scalp vessels include interfollicular simple red loops and arborizing red lines. Vessels are best seen using interface solution. Direct pressure on the vessels results in blanching.

Interfollicular simple red loops are multiple fine, red, hairpin-shaped structures that are regularly spaced (Figure 2.2). They correspond to the capillaries in the dermal papillae. Optimal viewing is at ×50 or higher magnification with the camera probe angled tangentially. When viewed from above they appear as pinpoint pale red dots (red dotted vessels). Distribution can be patchy or diffuse.

Arborizing red lines are vessels of larger caliber that correspond to the subpapillary vascular plexus (Figure 2.3). With tangential viewing, they are seen to underlie and articulate with loops to a variable degree in the normal scalp and diseased scalp of all etiologies. They are best viewed at magnifications of ×20 or higher. This pattern is usually focal and more evident on the occipital scalp. These vessels blanch or disappear with pressure.

Presence of scalp deposits can prevent visualization of vessels giving the scalp a cloudy appearance (Figure 2.4).

Dots of irregular size and shape are a normal finding in the interfollicular scalp of prepuberal children and elderly individuals. They represent environmental particles ("dirty dots") and are easily removed after shampooing.

THE NORMAL BLACK SCALP

- Honeycomb-like pigmented network.
- Pinpoint white dots.
- Hair mostly emerging in groups of two in the African scalp.

At dermoscopy the color of the scalp can vary from light brown to dark black and often does not correlate with the skin tone. The whole scalp shows a honeycomb-like pigmented network characterized by pigmented lines, corresponding to rete ridge melanocytes, which surround round hypochromic areas. Perifollicular and interfollicular erythema is also common but size and shape of vessels are not easily seen.

A unique feature of the pigmented scalp is the presence of the pinpoint white dots, which

DOI: 10.1201/9780429351433-2

are small 0.2–0.3 mm white dots regularly distributed between the follicular units (Figure 2.5). They represent follicular and sweat gland openings. Dots corresponding to sweat gland openings are smaller than dots corresponding to empty follicular openings.

The pigmented network is not regular but often shows variable enhancement or fading of pigmentation across the interfollicular scalp with a fingertip pattern (Figure 2.6), and a marked accentuation of pigmentation around the follicular ostia.

Hair density in people of African descent is lower than in Caucasians and the follicular units most commonly consist of a couple of hairs emerging together. Single hair and groups of three hairs are also seen. The hair shafts have a flattened shape and show irregular torsions. The hair shafts extracted with the pull or the tug test frequently present knots and fissures. The scalp commonly presents scales and particles that correspond to residues of leave-on products (Figure 2.7).

The Indian scalp shares the same features described for the black scalp, including the reticular network and the pinpoint white dots. Follicular units are organized in groups of three to four as in the white scalp.

THE ASIAN SCALP

- Increased ratio of thin hairs.
- The peripilar sign is less frequently observed in individuals of Asian descent.

Studies have revealed that healthy individuals of Asian descent tend to have a higher ratio of thin hairs.

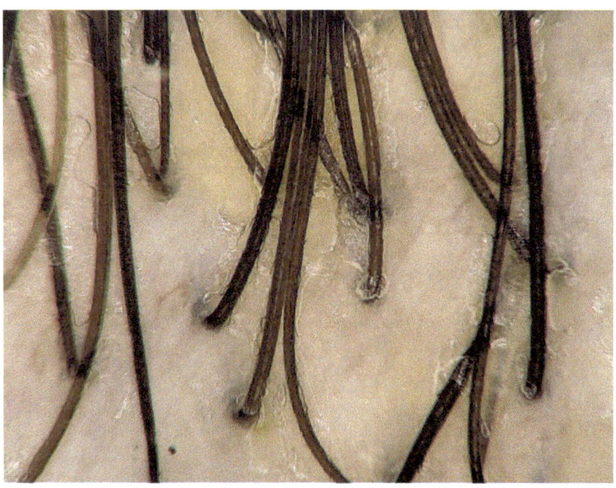

FIGURE 2.1 ×50 Hair shaft medulla is not evident within all hair shafts and can be uninterrupted or interrupted.

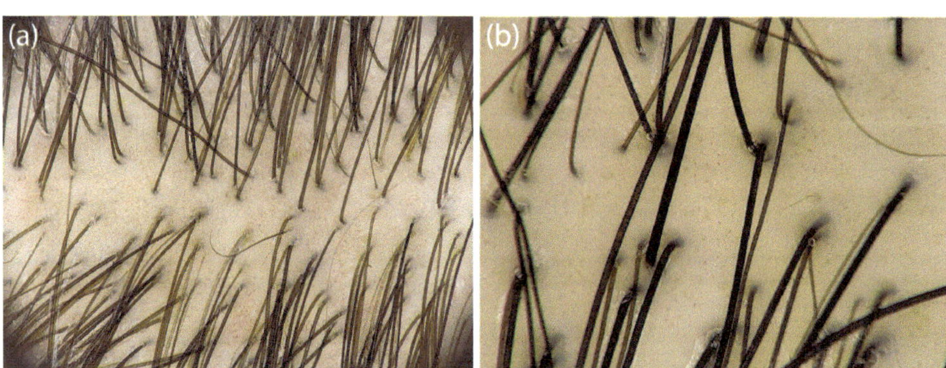

FIGURE 2.2 ×20–×50 Simple loops seen at low (a) and high (b) magnification.

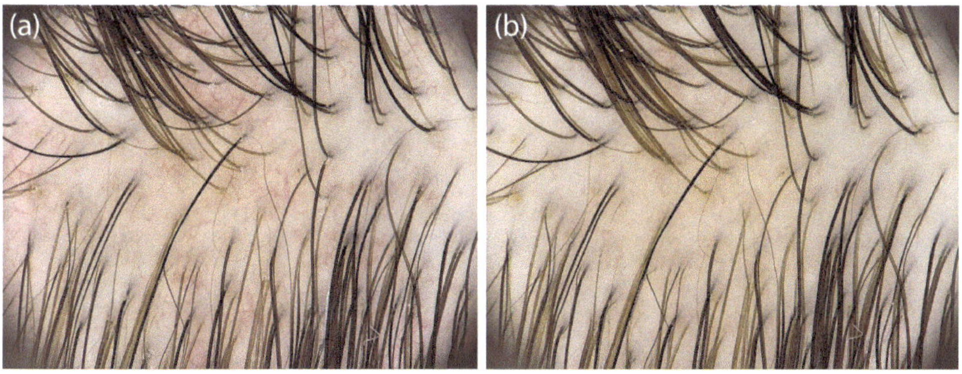

FIGURE 2.3 ×20 Arborizing vessels without pressure (a); ×20 they fade with pressure (b).

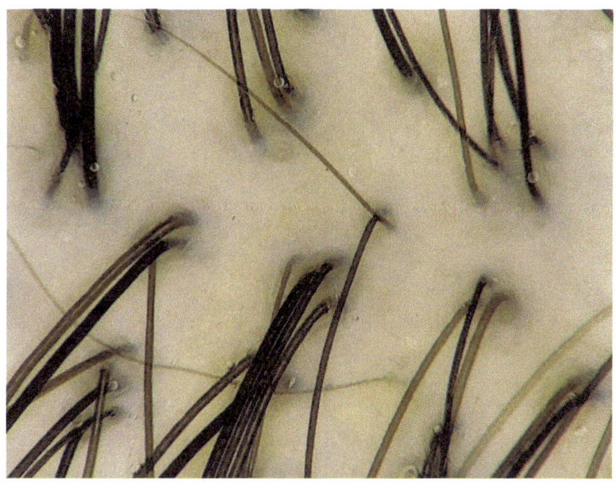

FIGURE 2.4 ×50 Cloudy scalp due to deposits of sebum on the peri- and interfollicular scalp.

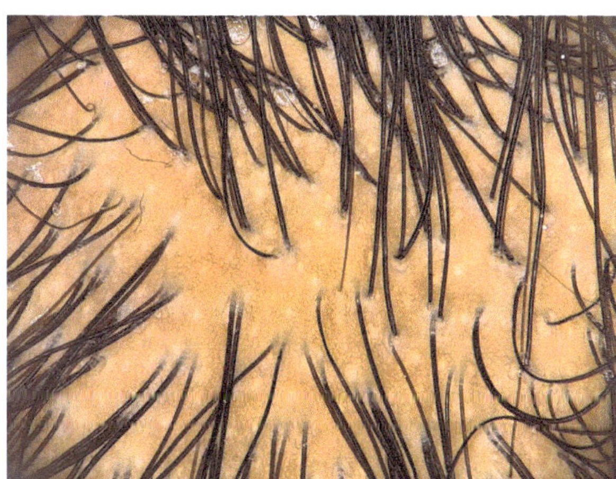

FIGURE 2.5 ×20 Regularly distributed pinpoint white dots.

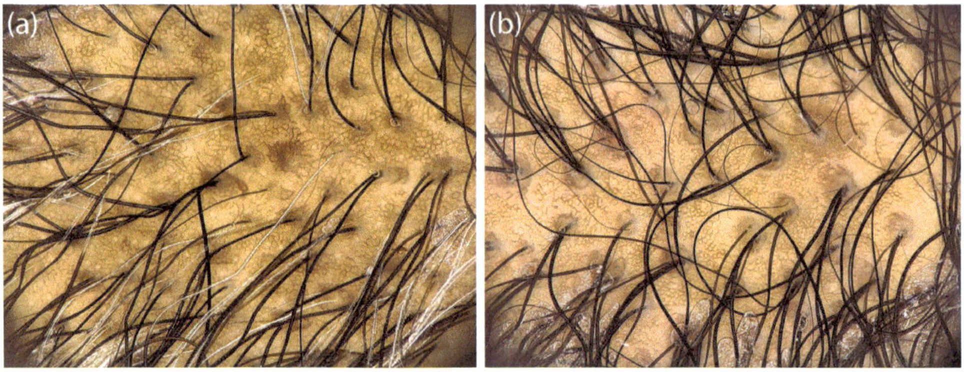

FIGURE 2.6 ×20 Pigmented network with a fingertip pattern is accentuated around the follicular openings: Note that most of the follicular units emerge in groups of two.

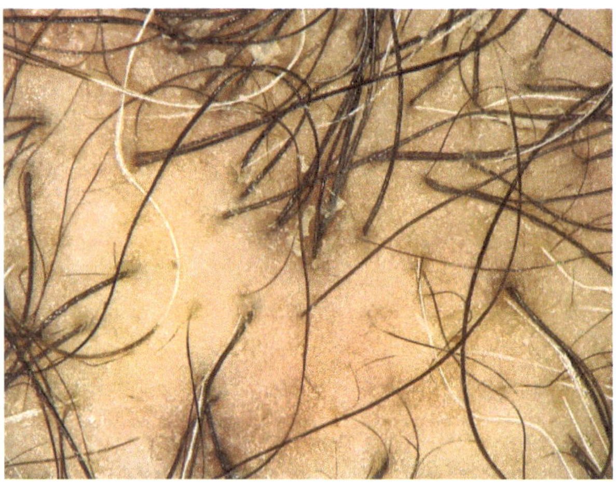

FIGURE 2.7 ×20 Scalp deposits due to hair/scalp products are very common in the black scalp.

SUGGESTED READING

Abraham LS, Piñeiro-Maceira J, Duque-Estrada B, Barcaui CB, Sodré CT. Pinpoint white dots in the scalp: dermoscopic and histopathologic correlation. *J Am Acad Dermatol.* 2010;63(4):721–2.

Ocampo-Garza J, Tosti A. Trichoscopy of dark scalp. Skin Rakowska A. Trichoscopy (hair and scalp videodermoscopy) in the healthy female. Method standardization and norms for measurable parameters. *J Dermatol Case Rep.* 2009;3(1):14–9.

Ross EK, Vincenzi C, Tosti A. Videodermoscopy in the evaluation of hair and scalp disorders. *J Am Acad Dermatol.* 2006;55(5):799–806.

Yin NC, Tosti A. A systematic approach to Afro-textured hair disorders: dermatoscopy and when to biopsy. *Dermatol Clin.* 2014;32(2):145–51.

3 Instruments for Scalp Dermoscopy

Scalp dermoscopy (also known as trichoscopy) is the examination of the scalp with a dermatoscope. This traditionally consists of a magnifier (typically ×10), a non-polarized light source, a transparent plate, and the use of a liquid medium between the instrument and the scalp. Modern dermatoscopes use polarized light instead of a liquid medium to eliminate skin surface reflections.

Some instruments digitally capture and process the images that can be stored and compared with follow-up pictures.

Instruments for digital dermatoscopy reach magnifications ranging from ×20 to ×140. Most studies on scalp dermoscopy have been done with magnifications ranging from ×20 to ×70. Some instruments are equipped with software to measure relevant trichological parameters, including hair shaft diameter, hair density, and number of hairs per follicular unit.

INSTRUMENTS FOR SCALP DERMOSCOPY

Require a Smartphone Camera

Mechanical Connections

- DermLite® connection kits

Magnetic Connections

- Handyscope®
- DermLite Foto X
- proVEOS with HairMetrix®

Attach Directly to the Smartphone

Low-cost lenses

Require a Laptop (Cable Connection)

- Low-cost instruments (microscopes)

Complete System That Includes the Photocamera/Camera

- FotoFinder Videodermatoscope
- Casio DZ-D100 Dermocamera®
- HairMetrix

Handyscope (FotoFinder Systems GmbH, Bad Birnbach, Germany) is a mobile-connected dermatoscope. The old model was attached to the smartphone with a special cover that encased the smartphone. The new model attaches to the smartphone through a magnetic adaptor. It allows for taking polarized and non-polarized images with magnification of ×20. Images can be enlarged utilizing the smartphone or the camera.

DermLite Foto X® (3 Gen LLC., San Juan Capistrano, CA, USA) is a dermoscopy lens that attaches to virtually any digital camera, including smartphones. It provides both polarized, non-polarized and UV lighting and is attached to the camera or smartphone magnetically (using special adaptors sold by the company MagnetiConnect®) or via a standard threaded connection with the computer.

proVEOS® is a dermatoscope that magnetically attaches to mobile phones and captures polarized, non-polarized, UV, and 3D surface images. The proVEOS takes images at ×12.5 magnification and integrates directly with Canfield's HairMetrix software.

FotoFinder Videodermatoscope® (FotoFinder Systems GmbH, Bad Birnbach, Germany) is an immersion non-polarized and polarized dermoscopy system with a video-camera equipped with lenses providing optical magnification ranging from ×20 to ×140. The images obtained

DOI: 10.1201/9780429351433-3

are visualized on a monitor and stored on a computer.

HairMetrix D200 is a digital dermatoscope with a magnification range from ×15 to ×200 and 5MP image quality capturing polarized and non-polarized images.

The Casio DZ-D100 Dermocamera is a camera combined with a dermatoscope able to take both global images and polarized, non-polarized, and UV mode-dermoscopy images.

LOW-COST INSTRUMENTS

Several low-cost instruments can be acquired online and attached to the smartphone or the computer. Micali et al. evaluated inexpensive handheld videomicroscopes for trichoscopy and determined they could identify hair shaft variations but struggled to identify other features such as yellow dots, white dots, and perifollicular scales when compared to medical videodermatoscopes. However, improved technology and new instruments can detect yellow dots, perifollicular scales, and casts among other features. Instrument magnification ranges from ×50 to ×1000, with ×50 recommended for trichoscopy.

Hair Measurement

Hair measurements can be important for patient follow-up and to evaluate drug efficacy in clinical trials. Hair measurements were traditionally performed after shaving and tattooing a target area of the scalp (hair count). This technique, however, is often not acceptable for patients and several companies developed alternative systems that can measure thickness and density without shaving. Although tattooing is still required for perfect measures, some experts utilize templates that avoid tattooing. Measures without tattooing, however, are not perfect, as they are obtained on a small scalp area that cannot be perfectly relocated.

Virtual tattooing has recently been developed and can overcome the problem.

Instruments for Hair Measurement

- Folliscope®
- HairMetrix
- Tricholab®
- FotoFinder with TrichoScale® AI

The FotoFinder technology can be integrated with the TrichoScale DX to provide a detailed assessment of hair measures and works with clipped and non-clipped hair. The TrichoScale DX analysis includes measurements of hair count, density, the proportion of terminal and vellus hair, and the anagen and telogen phases of hair growth. Data are captured and reported in real time.

The Tricholab camera is an advanced compact digital trichoscope utilized in conjunction with FotoFinder systems. Tricholab offers a patented technology called Virtual Tattoo™, which aids in ensuring consistency across examinations by using a pattern matching technique to identify the same area of the scalp in subsequent reviews. Furthermore, Tricholab employs AI to optimize the Field of View based on hair density and thickness, adjusting it to the most appropriate size for accurate measurements.

For clinical research, Tricholab provides a suite called TrichoLAB studio, which includes a FotoFinder portrait stand optimized for scalp photography, equipped with a high-resolution digital camera and polarized flash light system, enabling reproducible images of various scalp areas.

HairMetrix is a fully automated system for hair analysis. Utilizing advanced artificial intelligence algorithms, HairMetrix is designed to deliver real-time consultations. With a magnification range from ×15 to ×200 and 5MP image quality, this system can analyze follicular details without the need for hair cutting. The system has user-friendly ergonomics and includes a live image display during examinations and the capability for direct image acquisition, magnification, and analysis without peripheral devices.

The quality of images varies depending on instruments; videodermatoscopes usually provide the best images. The possible magnification varies depending on instruments.

See further Tables 3.1 and 3.2 and Figure 3.1.

TABLE 3.1
Characteristics of Different Instruments Utilized for Trichoscopy

Device	Magnification
Handyscope	×20
DermLite	×10
HairMetrix	×15–×200
HairMetrix with proVEOS	Up to ×12.5
FotoFinder with TrichoScale	Up to ×120 optical
FotoFinder Medicam 1000s®	×20–×140 optical
Casio DZ-D100 Dermocamera	×8 Digital zoom
Tricholab Camera	×20–×70
Folliscope	×50–×100

TABLE 3.2
Characteristics of Different Instruments Utilized for Hair Measures

Instrument	Immediate Result	Manual Measurement Required	High-Cost Instrument
Derma Reader/Folliscope	Yes	Yes	No
Folliscope 5.0	Yes	Yes	No
HairMetrix	Yes	No	Yes
FotoFinder with TrichoScale DX	Yes	No	Yes
Tricholab	No	No	No (price is for consultation)

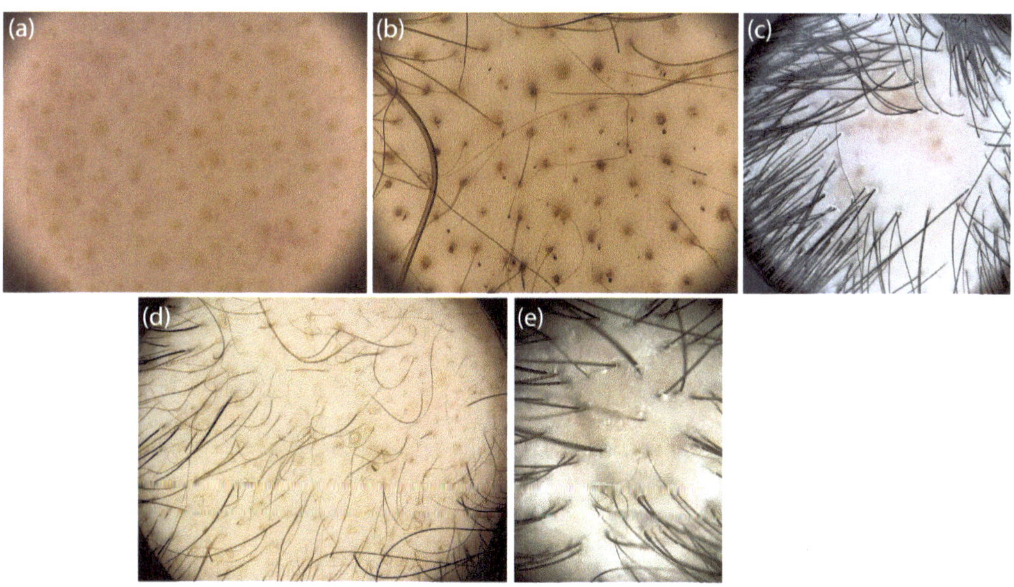

FIGURE 3.1 Images taken by: ×20 the FotoFinder videodermatoscope (a); ×20 the Handyscope (b); ×20 the Veox Dermscope® (c); ×8 the Casio dermatoscope (d); and ×50 a low-cost dermatoscope (e).

SUGGESTED READING

Bokhari L, Cottle P, Grimalt R, Kasprzak M, Sicińska J, Sinclair R, Tosti A. Efficiency of hair detection in hair-to-hair matched trichoscopy. *Skin Appendage Disord*. 2022;8(5):382–88.

Verzì AE, Lacarrubba F, Micali G. Use of low-cost videomicroscopy versus standard videodermatoscopy in trichoscopy: a controlled, blinded noninferiority trial. *Skin Appendage Disord*. 2015;1(4):172–4.

4 Non-Scarring Alopecias

Patterned

- Male pattern hair loss (MPHL)
- Female pattern hair loss (FPHL)
- Endocrine alopecia
- Lipedematous alopecia

Diffuse

- Telogen effluvium (acute or chronic)
- Chemotherapy alopecia
- Permanent/persistent alopecia after chemotherapy
- Alopecia areata incognita

Patchy

- Alopecia areata
- Trichotillomania
- Traction alopecia
- Friction alopecia
- Dissecting cellulitis
- Pressure alopecia
- Lupus profundus (panniculitis)
- Radiotherapy alopecia
- Traumatic alopecia

PATTERNED

Male Pattern Hair Loss/Androgenetic Alopecia (Figures 4.1–4.4)

- Hair diameter diversity: Presence of hairs with different thickness reflects progressive miniaturization. This has also been described as "anisotrichosis" and is better assessed using high magnification (×40–×50). A diversity >20% is diagnostic.
- Miniaturization does not affect all the hairs in the follicular units until final stages of the disease. It initially involves secondary follicles and it is quite typical to find follicular units with hairs of different thickness.
- Short thin vellus hairs: Sign of severe miniaturization. Are more numerous on the vertex, temporal, and frontal areas.
- Peripilar signs: Characterized by the presence of a light-brown depressed halo, roughly 1 mm in diameter at the follicular ostium around the emergent hair shaft. Most commonly found in early androgenetic alopecia and is linked to perifollicular inflammation. In patients with dark phototypes the peripilar sign has a dark-brown color.
- Yellow dots: These are a sign of severe miniaturization and are numerous in patients with severe baldness. They correspond to follicular ostia filled with keratin and sebum and often contain a thin short regrowing hair.
- Pinpoint white dots: Detected in patients with skin of color or in the sun-exposed scalp of patients with severe MPHL. They correspond to empty follicular ostia and sweat gland openings.
- Scalp pigmentation: This is commonly observed on the scalp of patients with androgenetic alopecia as a consequence of sun exposure. Pigmentation has a typical honeycomb-like pattern.
- Increased number of single hair follicular units.

Female Pattern Hair Loss/Androgenetic Alopecia (Figures 4.5–4.9)

- Hair diameter diversity: A diversity >20% is diagnostic. In women with severe FPHL the majority of follicular units in the frontal area contain a single hair shaft.
- Short vellus hairs (<0.03 mm): Are hypopigmented, short hairs and might have a wavy/bent shape. The detection of >10% or more than six vellus hairs in the frontal scalp using a ×20 magnification is a major criterion for diagnosis.
- Pigtail circle hairs: They are thin and usually scattered.

DOI: 10.1201/9780429351433-4

- In women with diffuse FPHL dermoscopy can show the presence of terminal hairs and diffusely distributed short thin hairs, without evidence of hairs of intermediate diameter. This might represent a sign of acute miniaturization.
- Peripilar signs: More common in patients with early FPHL.
- Yellow dots: These are a sign of severe miniaturization and are more numerous in patients with severe FPHL. More than four yellow dots in four images from the frontal scalp at high magnification is considered a major criterion for diagnosis.
- Pinpoint white dots: These are detected in patients with skin of color and in the sun-exposed scalp of severe FPHL.
- Scalp pigmentation: The honeycomb-like pattern is seen in sun-exposed areas and in patients of color.
- Focal atrichia: Is seen in postmenopausal women who present small bald areas that look cicatricial to the naked eye; dermoscopy shows miniaturization of contiguous follicular units with yellow dots and short vellus hairs.
- Increased number of single hair follicular units corresponds to disease severity.

Endocrine Alopecia (Figure 4.10)

- The main trichoscopic features of endocrine therapy-induced alopecia are hair shaft variability and thin short regrowing hairs.

Lipedematous Alopecia (Figure 4.11)

- Trichoscopy shows linear vessels possibly caused by compression of the superficial plexus, and hair shaft miniaturization.

DIFFUSE

Acute Telogen Effluvium (Figures 4.12–4.15)

- Hairs extracted with a pull test show telogen roots.
- Short regrowing hairs of normal thickness usually upright.
- Absence of shaft variability.
- In acute cases telogen roots can be found on the scalp surface.
- In telogen effluvium associated with COVID-19 infection the scalp can present dilated capillaries.
- Presence of hair shaft variability indicates associated androgenetic alopecia.

Chronic Telogen Effluvium

Dermoscopy:

- Short regrowing hairs
- Absence of variability

Chemotherapy Alopecia (Figure 4.16)

- Since patients usually shave many signs are often not present.
- Dermoscopy: Black dots, broken hairs of different lengths, flame hairs, pseudomonilethrix, coudability hairs. Yellow dots and pinpoint white dots are not numerous as the process is acute.
- Dermoscopic signs may persist for several months after treatment cessation.

Permanent/Persistent Alopecia after Chemotherapy (Figure 4.17)

- Dermoscopy: Hair shaft diameter variability, yellow dots, increased vellus hairs, pigtail hairs, marked predominance of single-hair follicular units.

Alopecia Areata Incognita (Figure 4.18)

- Dermoscopy: Yellow dots, pigtail hairs (numerous), short miniaturized regrowing hairs.
- A specific trichoscopic is the "color-transition sign": The proximal hair shaft is lighter in color.
- Presence of hair shaft variability indicates associated androgenetic alopecia.

PATCHY

Alopecia Areata

- Yellow dots: Round or polycyclic yellow to yellow-pink dots, which may be devoid of hair or contain black dots, exclamation mark hairs, or broken hairs.
- Correspond to dilated infundibula filled with sebum, varying in color and size. They appear brighter in children and are less visible on darker skin (Fitzpatrick skin phototypes IV–V).
- Absence of yellow dots does not exclude the diagnosis of alopecia areata; this feature is common in children or long-lasting disease.
- White dots: Pigmented scalp shows pinpoint white dots instead of yellow dots. These may be empty or contain broken hairs or black dots.
- Exclamation mark hairs: Broken hairs with a thick hyperpigmented distal tip and a thinner, hypopigmented proximal end. The broken tip is the result of the hair breakage during the keratinization. The presence of multiple exclamation mark hairs is diagnostic of alopecia areata. They are mainly found at the active lesion margins and indicate disease activity. Their formation requires at least 2–3 weeks. If plucked, they reveal a telogen root.
- Broken hairs: May have different lengths and predominate in acute alopecia areata, where there are negative prognostic markers.
- Black dots: Dark brown to black debris of different size inside empty follicular openings/yellow dots. They correspond to hair shaft remains after hair breakage before scalp emergence. They can be very diffuse or sparse. Numerous diffuse black dots are typical of acute disease.
- Coudability hair: Progressive narrowing of the proximal hair shaft. They are usually few and seen in the scalp surrounding the patches.
- Pseudo-monilethrix: Irregular multiple restrictions of the hair shaft. Usually affects a few hairs surrounding the patches. It corresponds to the Pohl-Pinkus constrictions described at microscopy.
- Short regrowing hairs of normal thickness: Most often have a light color, an upright tip, and are seen in clusters.
- Thin regrowing hairs: Hypopigmented, short, thin hairs that are commonly seen in chronic disease. Not indicative of hair regrowth.
- Pigtail hairs (circle thin hairs): Short, coiled hairs with tapered ends. When numerous, they are diagnostic of alopecia areata. They are often seen in acute disease in association with broken hairs and exclamation mark hairs. More common in children.
- Classic dermoscopic signs are difficult to be detected in the beard area or in the shaved scalp (see Chapter 21).
- Typical signs cannot always be detected in the eyebrows and eyelashes.

Acute vs. Chronic Alopecia Areata (Figures 4.19–4.26)

Dermoscopy is useful to establish disease activity and to distinguish between acute vs. chronic stages

- Signs of acute alopecia areata: Black dots, exclamation mark hairs and other types of broken hairs, circle hairs.
- Signs of chronic alopecia areata: Yellow dots and short regrowing hairs.

Trichotillomania (Figures 4.27, 4.28)

- Question mark hairs: Broken hairs with a coiled tip. Are diagnostic but not numerous and need to be searched.
- Short hairs with a longitudinal split (hamburger sign).
- Flame hairs and hair powder are not specific in the author's experience

as can be seen in alopecia areata and other types of anagen effluvium.

- Broken hairs, black dots, yellow dots, pinpoint white dots, crusts, erosions are not specific.
- Differential diagnosis with alopecia areata can be challenging, but exclamation mark hairs are not detected.

Traction Alopecia (Figures 4.29, 4.30)

- Broken hairs and black dots: These are usually sparse and should be searched.
- Presence of vellus hairs.
- Tubular hair casts: Should be searched at the margin of the patch to establish if the hairstyle is still causing traction.

Friction Alopecia (Figures 4.31, 4.32)

- Short broken hairs with frayed ends (proximal trichorrexis nodosa/broom hairs).
- Broken hairs with multiple irregular transverse white bands.
- Prominence of follicular openings, epidermal thickening, and post-inflammatory hyperpigmentation.

Dissecting Cellulitis—Early Non-Scarring Phase (Figure 4.33)

- Dermoscopy of early disease shows typical signs of anagen effluvium, including yellow dots, black dots, pigtail hairs.
- 3D yellow dots/keratotic plugs enlarged follicular openings filled by a big keratin plug that might cover underlying distorted hair shafts.
- Follicular clefts due to the fibrotic remodeling around the hair follicle.
- Scalp erythema, exudate, arborizing vessels and giant capillaries.
- Subtle changes may also be present in individuals with hidradenitis suppurativa, even when there are no apparent scalp lesions or symptoms.

Pressure Alopecia (Figures 4.34, 4.35)

- Dermoscopy shows typical features of anagen effluvium, including black dots, broken hairs, yellow dots, circle hairs, short regrowing hairs.

Lupus Profundus (Panniculitis) (Figure 4.36)

- Yellow dots, black dots, broken hairs, short regrowing hairs.
- Enlarged tortuous convoluted vessels.
- Alopecia areata is the primary differential diagnosis: Presence of enlarged tortuous vessels is the clue for distinction.

Radiotherapy Alopecia (Figures 4.37, 4.38)

Dermoscopy depends on radiation dose:

- Temporary epilation from single short-term exposure to 300–600 Gy of irradiation shows features of anagen effluvium with yellow dots, broken hairs, black dots, and flame hair.
- Higher radiation doses cause features of both anagen effluvium and cicatricial alopecia depending on dosages and duration.

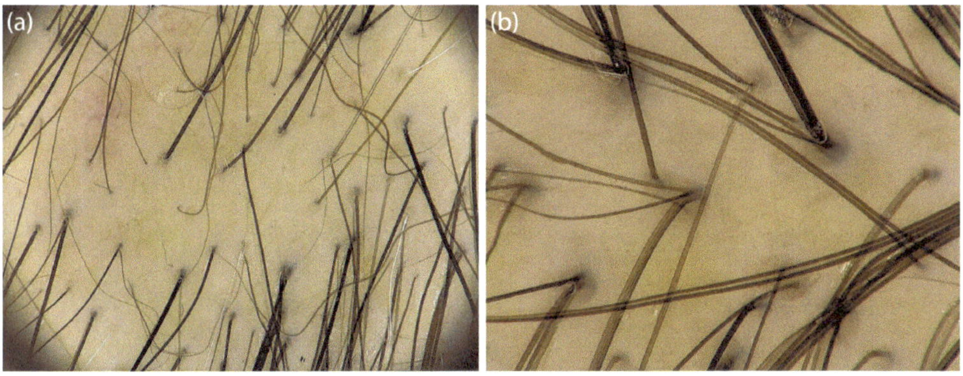

FIGURE 4.1 ×20 Hair shaft variability in MPHL, note involvement of secondary follicles (a); ×50 this is better detected at high magnification (b).

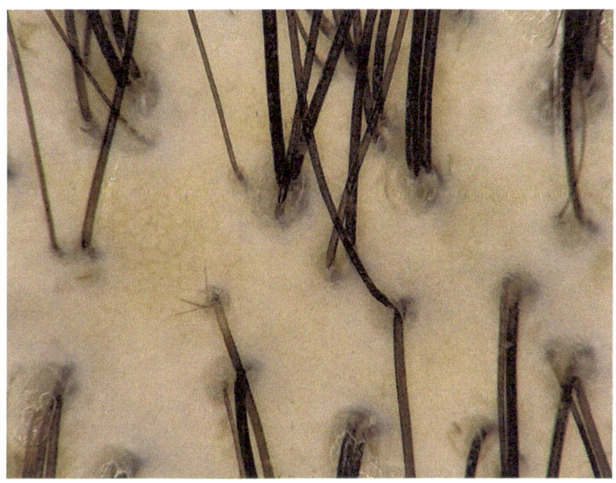

FIGURE 4.2 ×50 The secondary follicles of a follicular unit are severely miniaturized, also note peripilar sign.

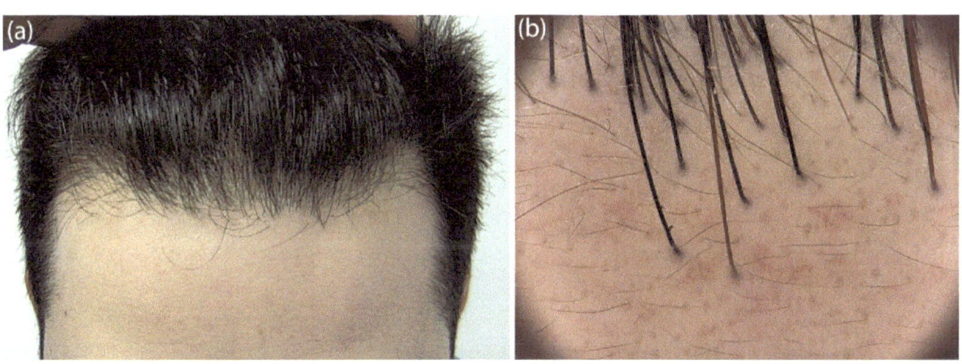

FIGURE 4.3 Clinical presentation of MPHL that may resemble frontal fibrosing alopecia (a); ×20 trichoscopy shows the presence of vellus hairs at the hairline and confirms the diagnosis of MPHL (b).

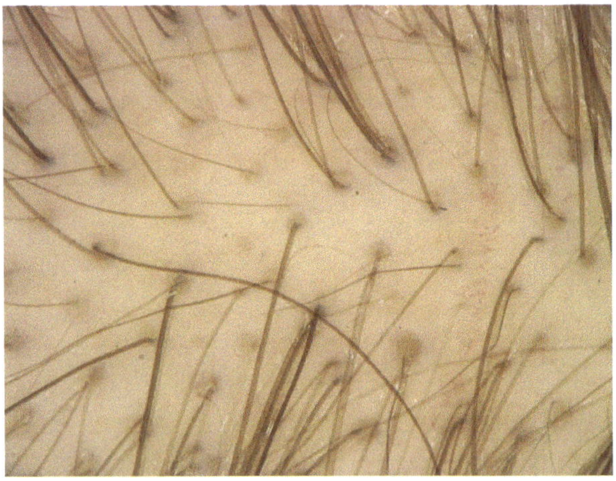

FIGURE 4.4 ×40 Peripilar sign.

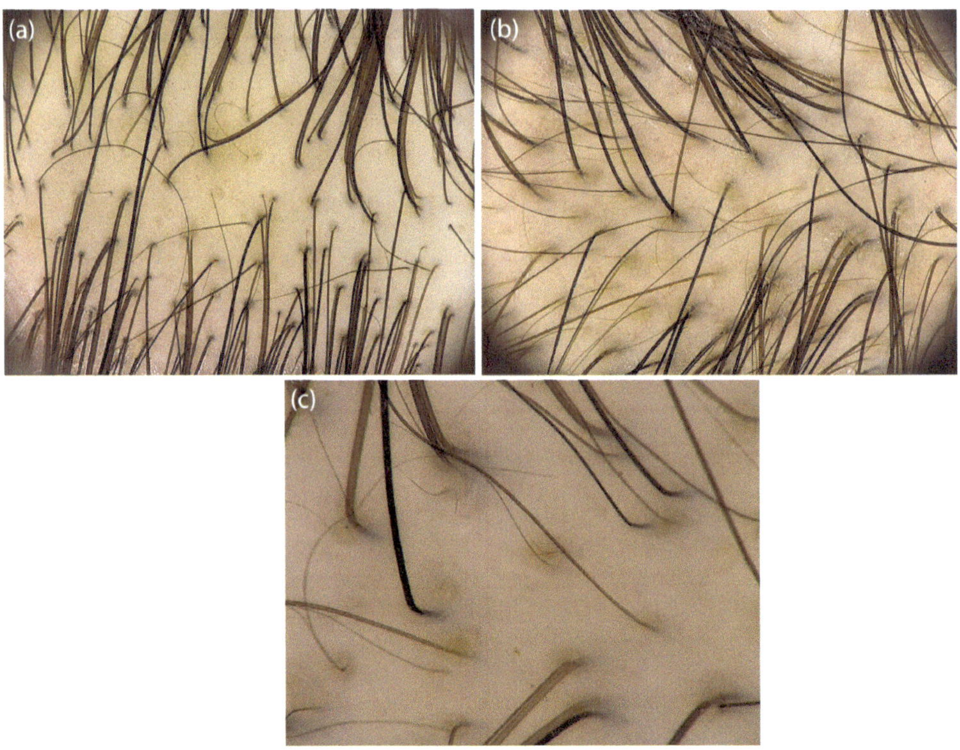

FIGURE 4.5 FPHL. ×20 Hair shaft variability and empty follicles (a); hair shaft variability and thin short regrowing hairs (b); ×50 miniaturized hairs and yellow dots (c).

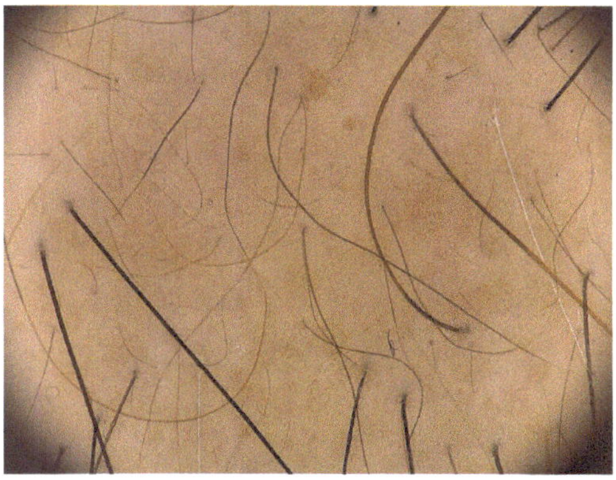

FIGURE 4.6 ×20 FPHL with numerous short regrowing hairs in the frontal scalp; follicular units consist of a single hair.

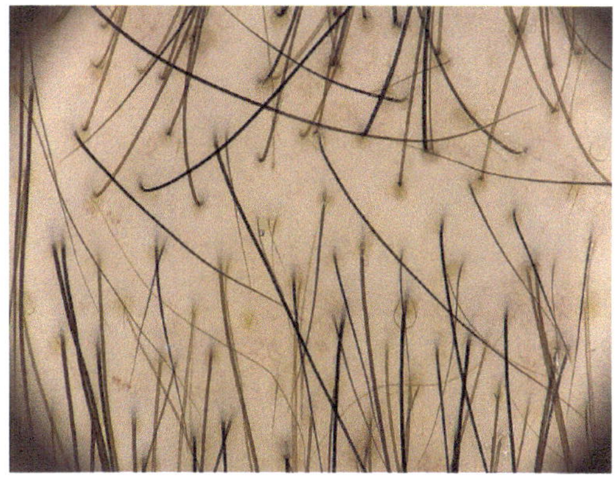

FIGURE 4.7 ×40 Hair shaft variability, thin short regrowing hair, pigtail hair, and short regrowing hair of normal thickness in FPHL associated with acute telogen effluvium.

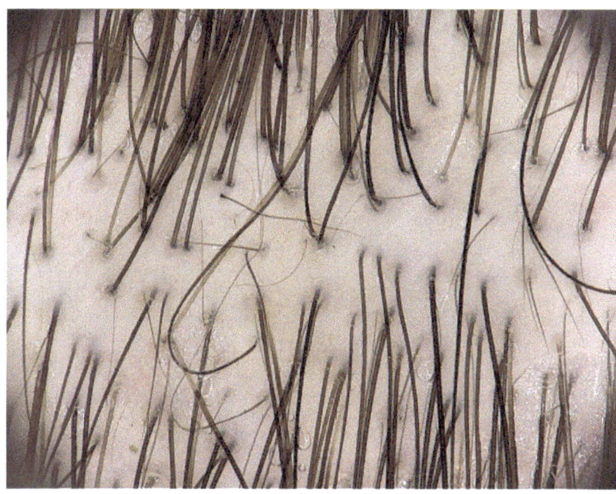

FIGURE 4.8 ×20 FPHL and acute telogen effluvium; note the presence of short regrowing hairs of normal thickness and thin short regrowing hairs.

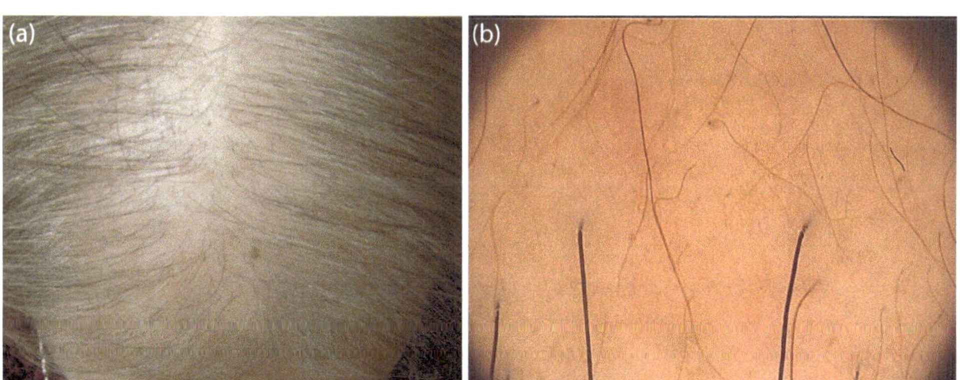

FIGURE 4.9 Focal atrichia in FPHL (a); the area shows diffuse miniaturization ×20 (b).

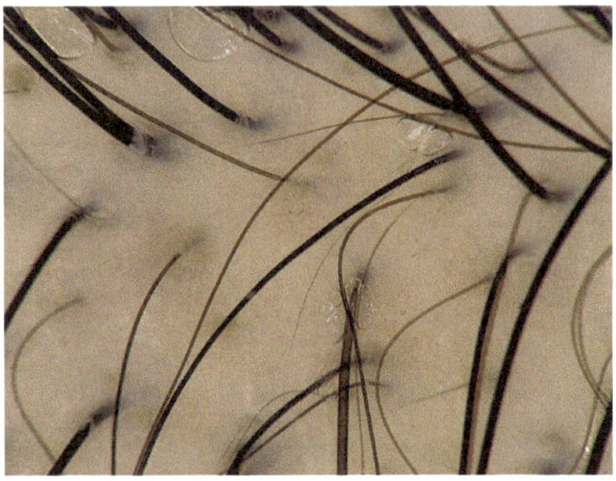

FIGURE 4.10 ×50 Hair shaft variability in endocrine therapy-induced alopecia.

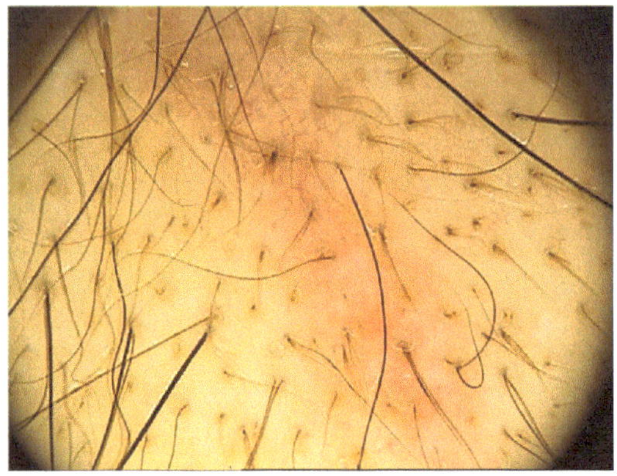

FIGURE 4.11 ×20 Hair shaft variability and telangiectatic thin vessels in lipedematous alopecia.

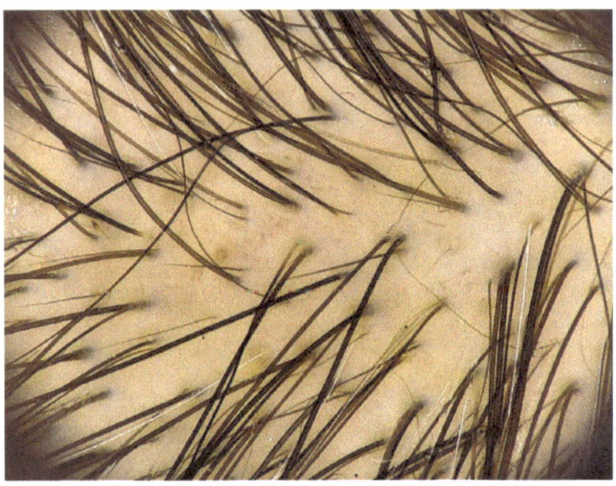

FIGURE 4.12 ×20 Acute telogen effluvium; note short regrowing hairs of normal thickness.

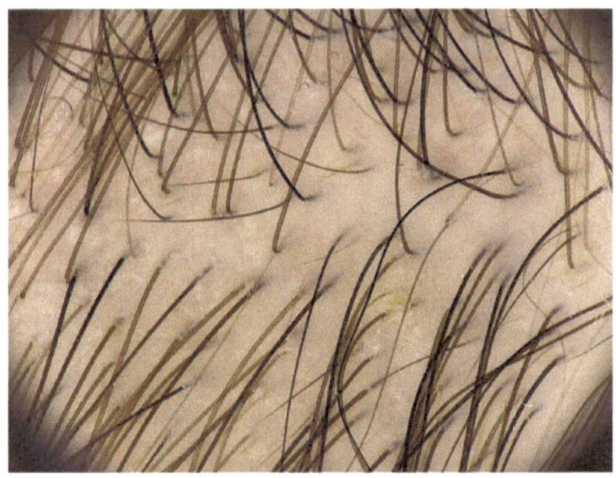

FIGURE 4.13 ×20 Acute telogen effluvium in scalp psoriasis.

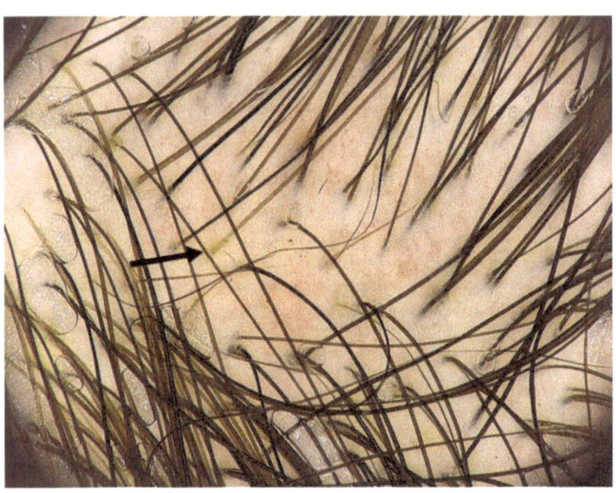

FIGURE 4.14 ×20 Acute telogen effluvium after COVID-19 infection; note a telogen root on the surface of the scalp and dilated capillaries.

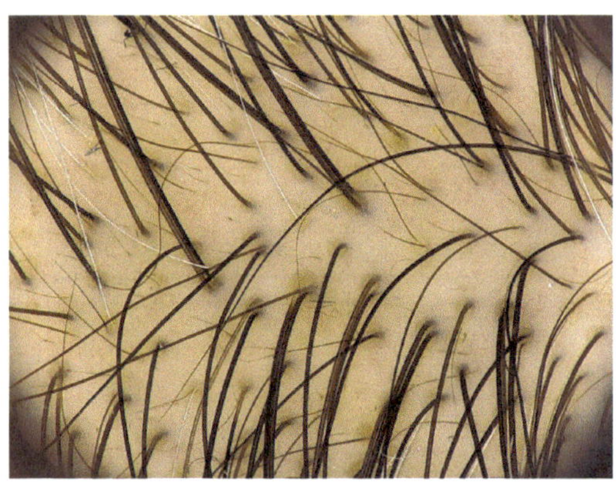

FIGURE 4.15 ×20 Acute telogen effluvium in androgenetic alopecia; note the presence of hair shaft variability and thin short regrowing hairs.

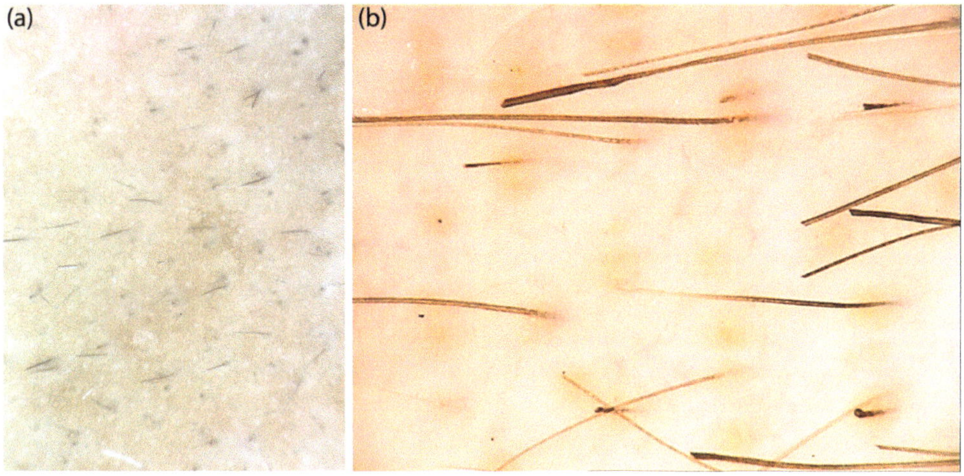

FIGURE 4.16 Chemotherapy alopecia. ×20 Pinpoint white dots and black dots in a patient of color. Note that the long, broken hairs have a sharp tip due to shaving (a); ×50 yellow dots, black dots, broken hair, and short hairs with sharp tip in non-pigmented scalp.

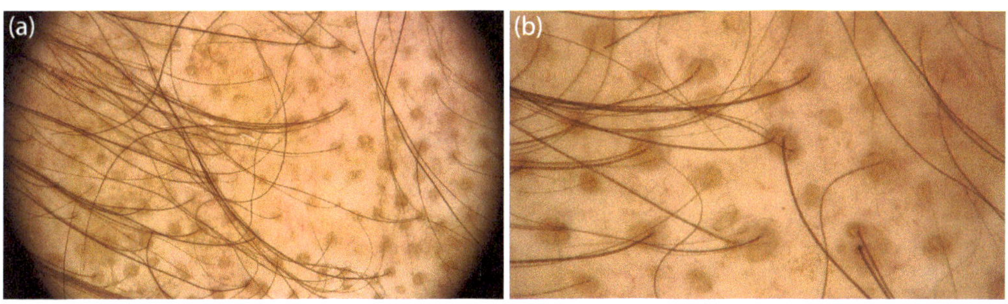

FIGURE 4.17 Permanent/persistent alopecia after chemotherapy at ×20 (a) and ×50 (b) magnifications showing hair shaft variability, numerous yellow dots, and a pigtail hair.

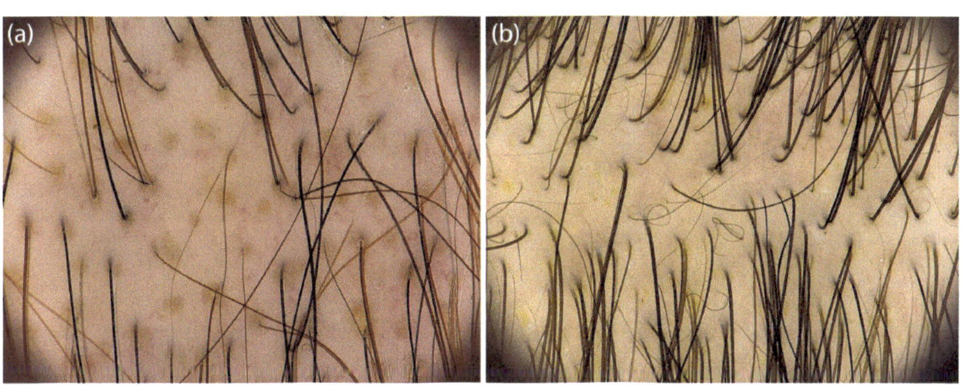

FIGURE 4.18 Alopecia areata incognita. ×40 Numerous yellow dots and short regrowing hairs (a); ×20 yellow dots and numerous pigtail hairs (b).

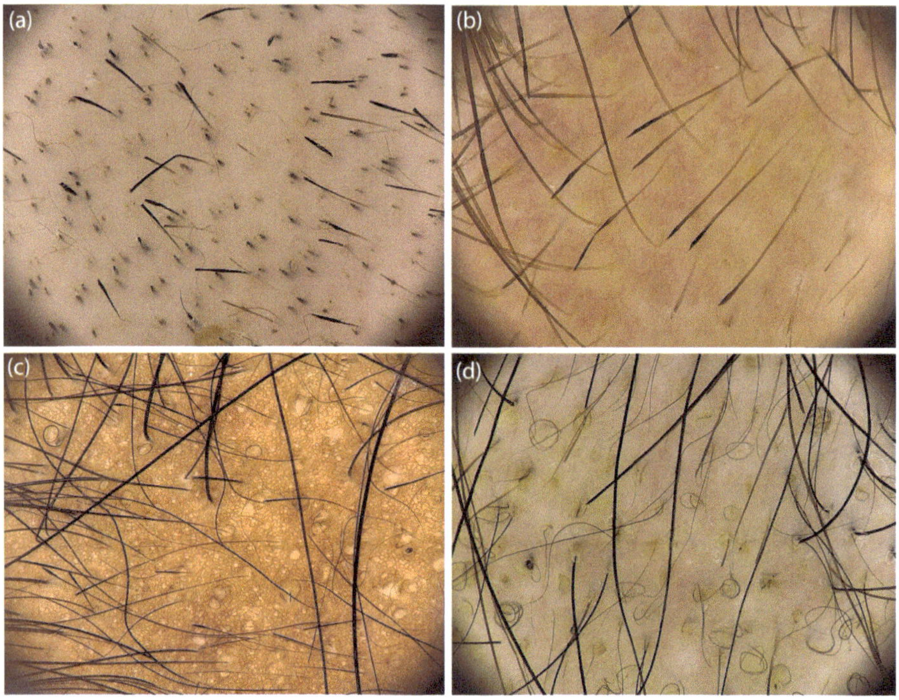

FIGURE 4.19 Acute alopecia areata. ×20 Broken hairs, exclamation mark hairs, and black dots (a); ×50 exclamation mark hairs at higher magnification (b); ×20 exclamation mark hairs and circle hairs in pigmented scalp (c); ×50 broken hairs and thin circle hairs (pigtail hairs) (d).

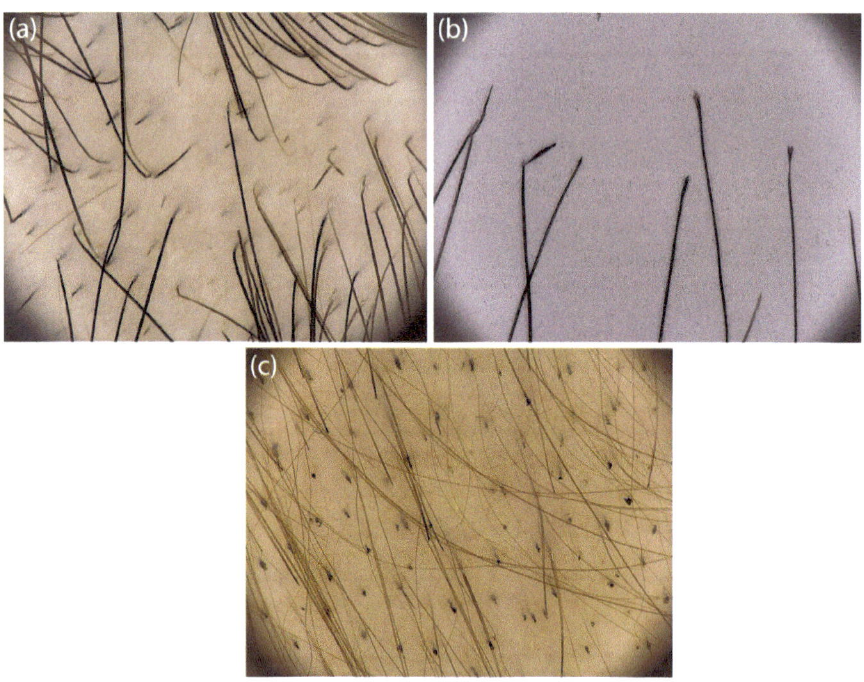

FIGURE 4.20 Acute alopecia areata. ×20 Broken hairs and exclamation mark hairs (a); ×20 pull test shows dystrophic anagen roots (b); ×20 follow-up after few weeks showing diffuse black dots (c).

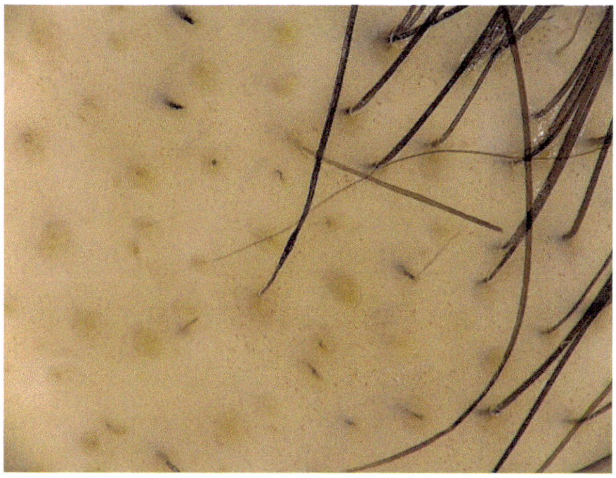

FIGURE 4.21 Acute alopecia areata. ×50 coudability hair.

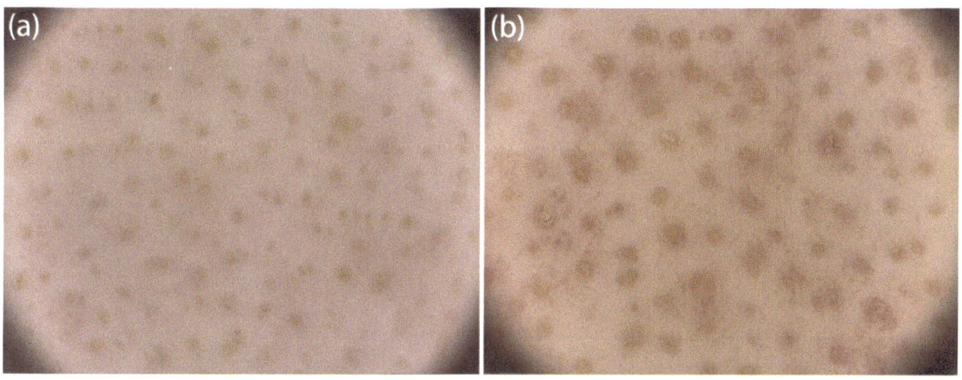

FIGURE 4.22 Chronic alopecia areata. ×50 Yellow dots in alopecia areata are regularly distributed and have a variable size (a); ×50 yellow dots with a keratotic component (b).

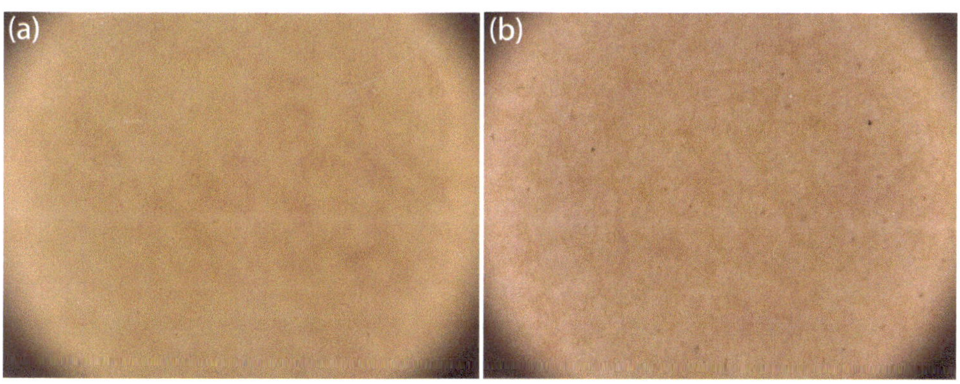

FIGURE 4.23 ×40 Yellow dots are not evident in chronic longstanding alopecia areata in an adult (a) and ×50 in a pediatric patient (b).

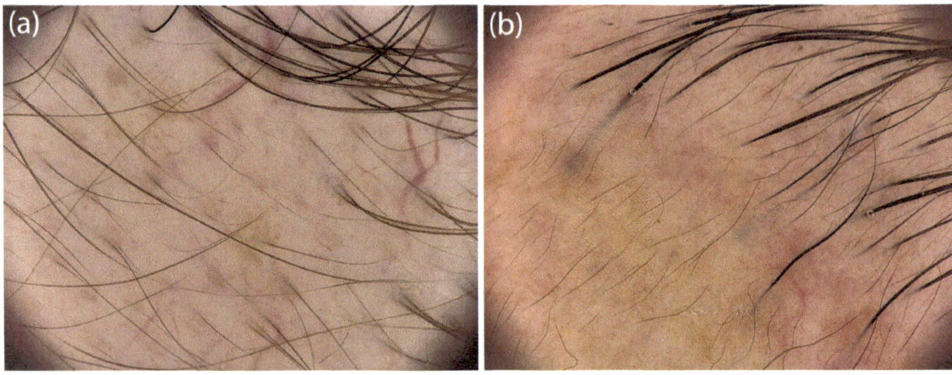

FIGURE 4.24 ×20 Clustered short regrowing hairs in alopecia areata (a); ×50 note scalp atrophy with visible anagen bulbs due to steroid injections (b).

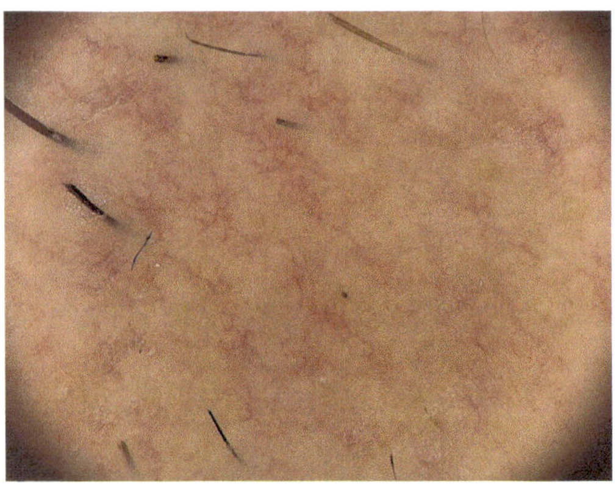

FIGURE 4.25 ×50 Beard alopecia areata showing black dots, and not evident yellow dots.

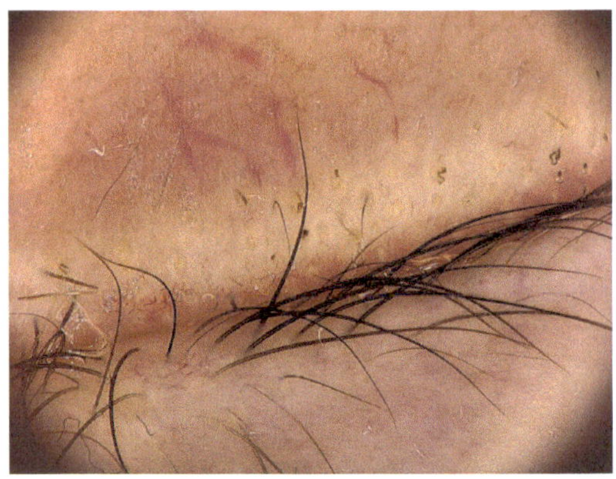

FIGURE 4.26 ×50 Alopecia areata of the eyelashes showing multiple broken hairs and flame hairs.

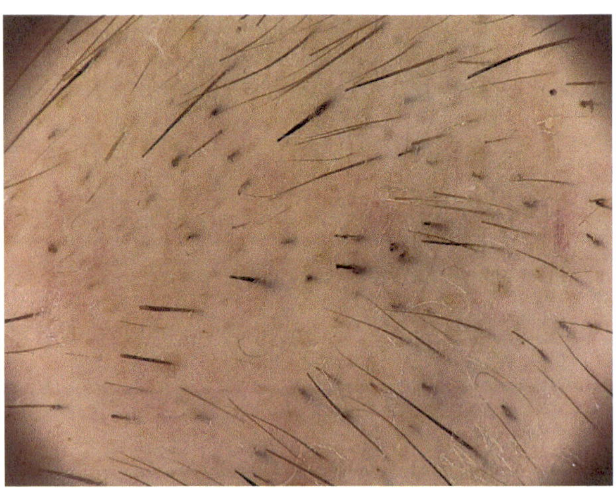

FIGURE 4.27 Trichotillomania. ×20 Broken hairs and black dots

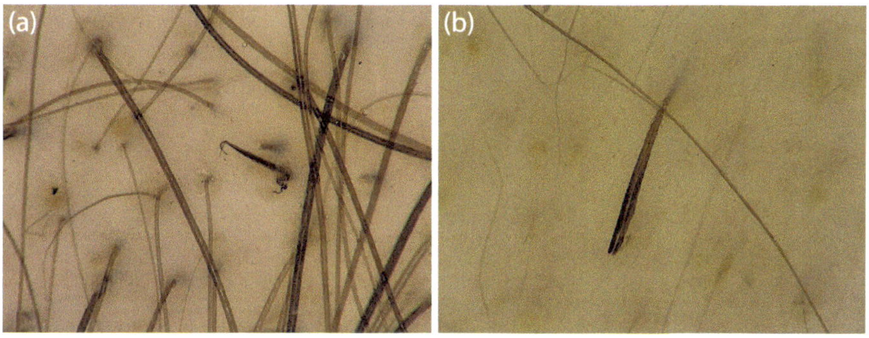

FIGURE 4.28 Trichotillomania. ×50 Question mark hair (a) and hamburger sign (b).

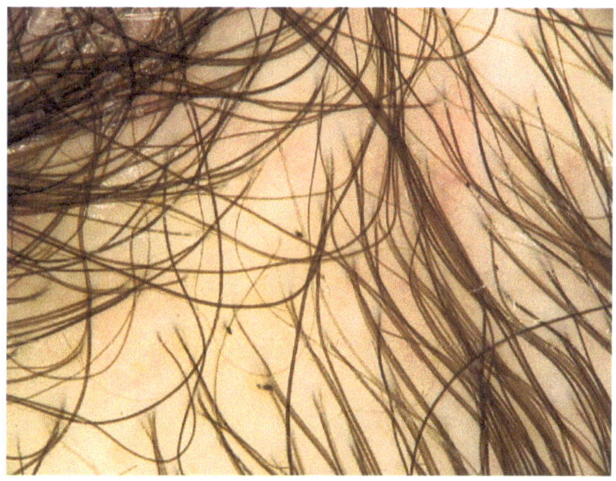

FIGURE 4.29 ×20 Traction alopecia due to hair extensions showing broken hairs and black dots.

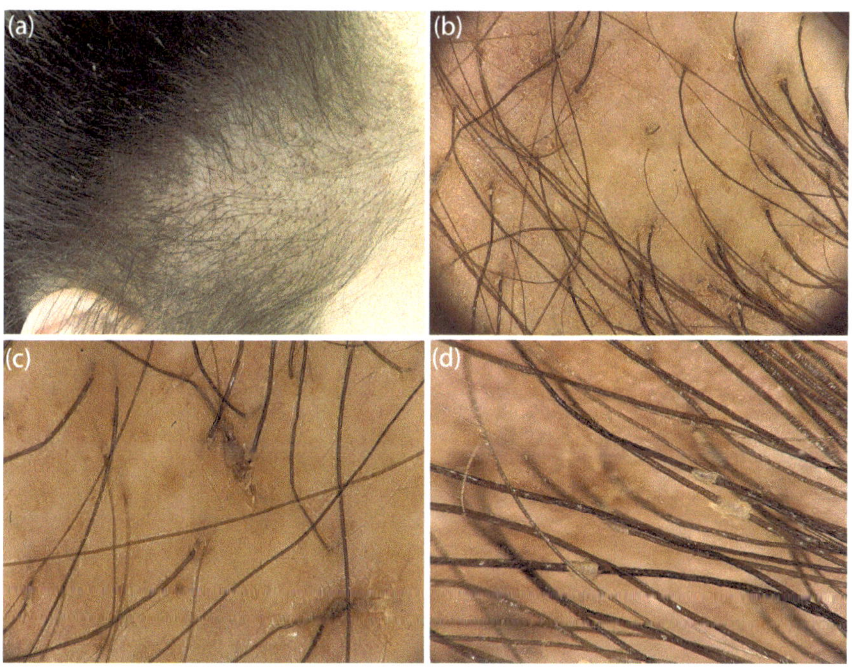

FIGURE 4.30 Marginal traction alopecia (a); ×20 broken hair, pili torti, and peripilar casts (b); ×50 exposure of the hair root due to severe traction (c); and ×50 tubular structures encircling the hair shafts at the margin of the patch (d).

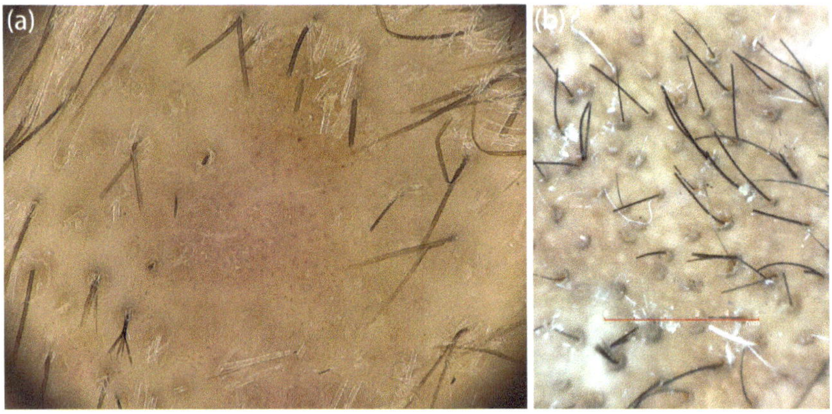

FIGURE 4.31 Lichen simplex chronicus of the scalp. ×20 Broom hairs, broken hairs, and trichorrhexis nodosa (a); ×50 prominence of follicular ostia (b).

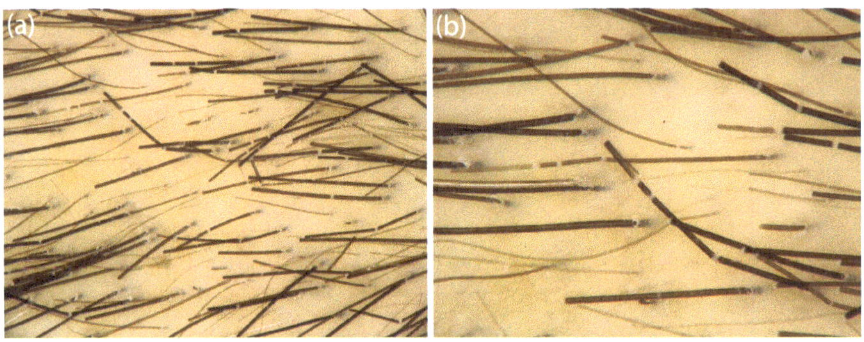

FIGURE 4.32 Friction alopecia. ×20 Trichorrhexis nodosa affecting the hair shaft at multiple levels (a); ×50 the pattern can resemble the Morse-code hairs of tinea capitis (b).

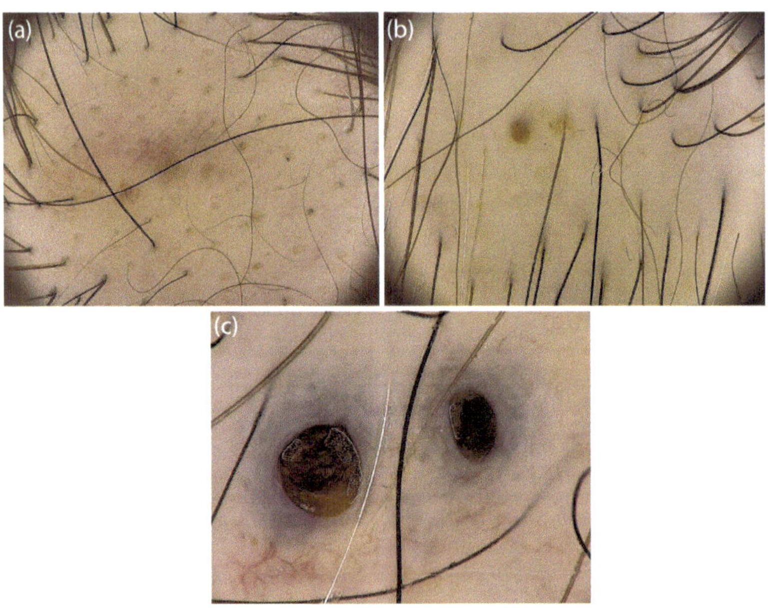

FIGURE 4.33 Dissecting cellulitis. ×20 Yellow dots and telangiectatic vessels (a); ×40 3D yellow dots (b); and ×60 keratotic plugs (c).

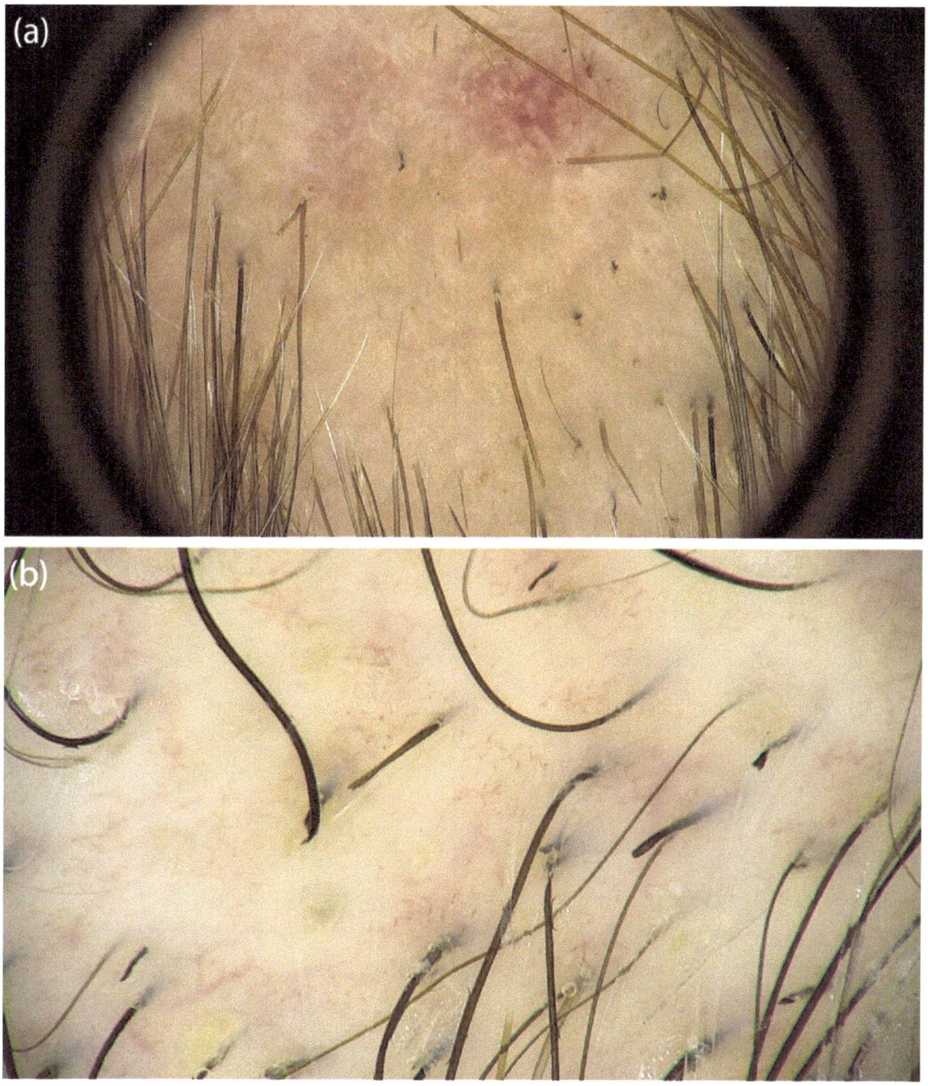

FIGURE 4.34 Pressure alopecia. ×20 Black dots, broken hairs, and patchy erythema (a); ×50 broken hairs of different length (b).

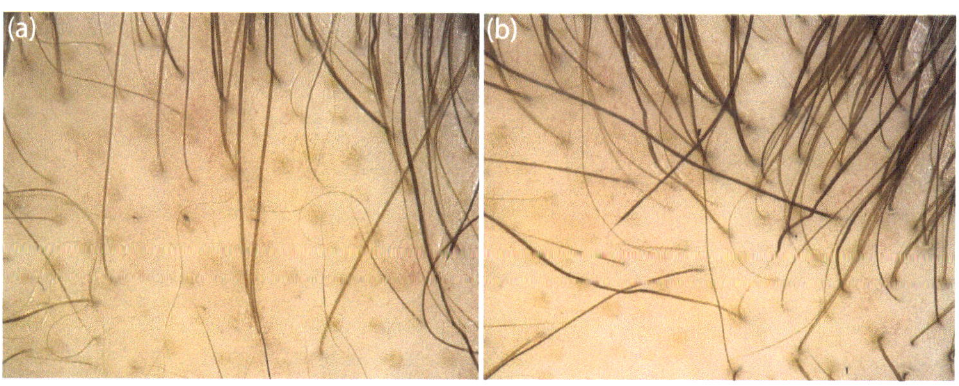

FIGURE 4.35 Patchy pressure alopecia due to mesotherapy. ×20 Yellow dots and black dots (a); ×50 coudability with irregular torsion of the affected hair shafts (b).

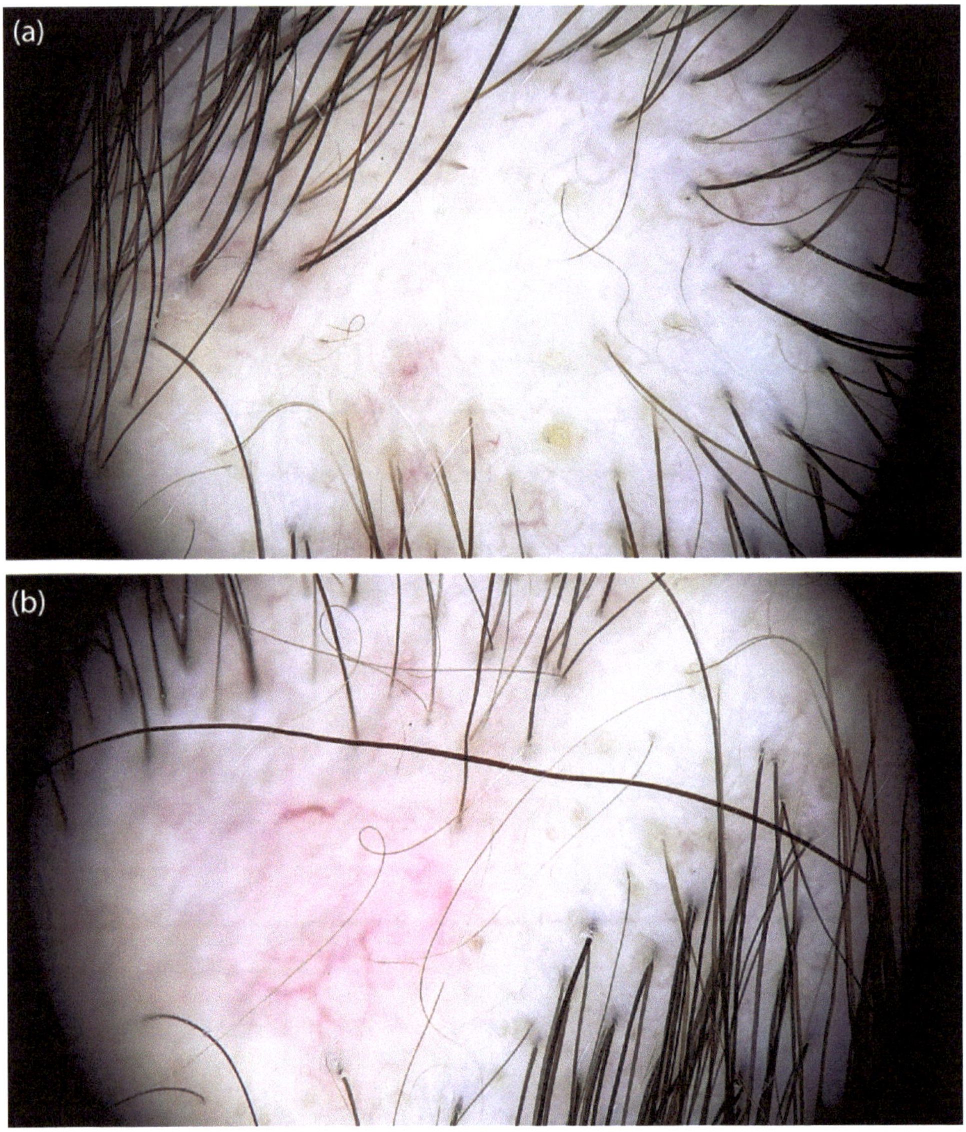

FIGURE 4.36 Lupus profundus. ×20 Yellow dots, circle hairs, short regrowing hairs (a); ×40 enlarged convoluted vessels (b).

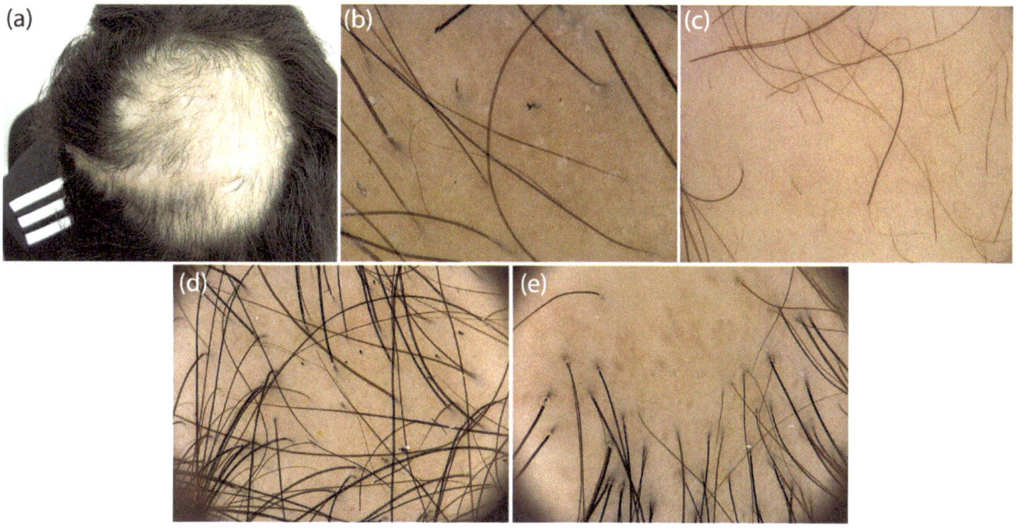

FIGURE 4.37 Radiotherapy alopecia. Note that the patch contains tufts of terminal hairs that were in telogen at the time of radiotherapy (a); ×50 flame hairs (b); ×50 broken hairs (c); ×20 black dots (d); ×20 loss of follicular opening in the scarring areas (e).

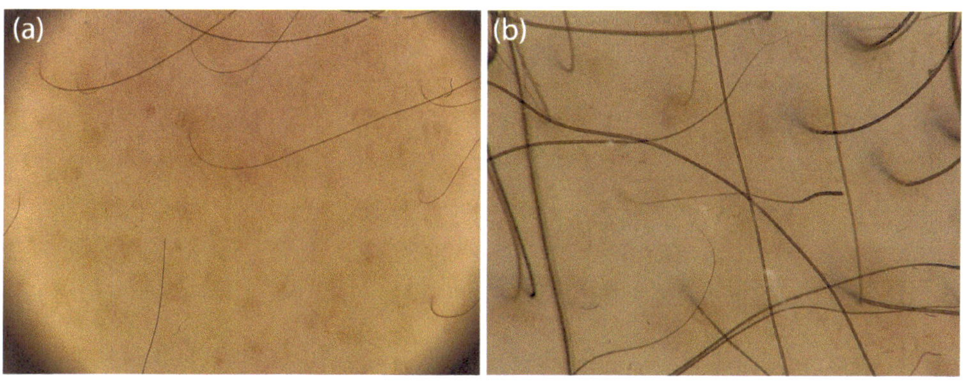

FIGURE 4.38 ×20 Loss of follicular openings may not be completely evident (a); ×50 dystrophic/broken hairs can be found years after the end of radiotherapy (b).

SUGGESTED READING

Ardigò M, Tosti A, Cameli N, Vincenzi C, Misciali C, Berardesca E. Reflectance confocal microscopy of the yellow dot pattern in alopecia areata. *Arch Dermatol*. 2011;147(1):61–4.

de Lacharrière O, Deloche C, Misciali C, Piraccini BM, Vincenzi C, Bastien P, Tardy I, Bernard BA, Tosti A. Hair diameter diversity: a clinical sign reflecting the follicle miniaturization. *Arch Dermatol*. 2001;137(5):641–6.

de Moura LH, Duque-Estrada B, Abraham LS, Barcaui CB, Sodre CT. Dermoscopy findings of alopecia areata in an African-American patient. *J Dermatol Case Rep*. 2008;2(4):52–4.

Doche I, Miotto I, Rivitti-Machado MC, Melo DF, Larrondo J, Cabrera R, Rajabi-Estarabadi A, Tosti A. Trichoscopic and imaging study of lipedematous alopecia: report of five cases. *J Eur Acad Dermatol Venereol*. 2020;34(10):e599–e602.

Duque-Estrada B, Vincenzi C, Misciali C, Tosti A. Alopecia secondary to mesotherapy. *J Am Acad Dermatol*. 2009;61(4):707–9.

Fowler E, Tosti A. A Case of friction alopecia in a healthy 15-year-old girl. *Skin Appendage Disord*. 2019;5(2):97–99.

Guerrero-Putz MD, Flores-Dominguez AC, Castillo-de la Garza RJ, Figueroa-Sanchez JA, Tosti A, Garza-Rodríguez V. Anagen effluvium after neurointerventional radiation: trichoscopy as a diagnostic ally. *Skin Appendage Disord.* 2022;8(2):102–7.

Herskovitz I, de Sousa IC, Tosti A. Vellus hairs in the frontal scalp in early female pattern hair loss. *Int J Trichology.* 2013;5(3):118–20.

Inui S, Nakajima T, Itami S. Coudability hairs: a revisited sign of alopecia areata assessed by trichoscopy. *Clin Exp Dermatol.* 2010;35(4):361–5.

Kinoshita-Ise M, Fukuyama M, Ohyama M. Color-transition sign: a useful trichoscopic finding for differentiating alopecia areata incognita from telogen effluvium. *J Dermatol.* 2018;45(8):e224.

Lacarrubba F, Micali G, Tosti A. Scalp dermoscopy or trichoscopy. *Curr Probl Dermatol.* 2015;47:21–32.

Malakar SS, Mehta PR, Malakar SS. Tulipoid hair: anagen effluvium marker! *Int J Trichology.* 201810(4):188–90.

May Lee M, Naldi L, Piraccini BM, Starace M, Alessandrini A, Sechi A. Trichoscopy as a tool to evaluate early dissecting cellulitis in patients affected by hidradenitis suppurativa: a prospective monocentric observational study. *Skin Appendage Disord.* 2023;9(4):275–79.

Piraccini BM, Voudouris S, Pazzaglia M, Rech G, Vicenzi C, Tosti A. Lipedematous alopecia of the scalp. *Dermatol Online J.* 2006;12(2):6.

Rakowska A, Slowinska M, Kowalska-Oledzka E, Olszewska M, Rudnicka L. Dermoscopy in female androgenic alopecia: method standardization and diagnostic criteria. *Int J Trichology.* 2009;1(2):123–30.

Rakowska A, Slowinska M, Olszewska M, Rudnicka L. New trichoscopy findings in trichotillomania: flame hairs, V-sign, hook hairs, hair powder, tulip hairs. *Acta Derm Venereol.* 2014;94(3):303–6.

Ross EK, Vincenzi C, Tosti A. Videodermoscopy in the evaluation of hair and scalp disorders. *J Am Acad Dermatol.* 2006;55(5):799–806.

Sinclair R, Torkamani N, Jones L. Androgenetic alopecia: new insights into the pathogenesis and mechanism of hair loss. *F1000Res.* 2015;4:585.

Tosti A, Torres F, Miteva M. Dermoscopy of early dissecting cellulitis of the scalp simulates alopecia areata. *Actas Dermosifiliogr.* 2013;104(1):92–3.

Tosti A, Whiting D, Iorizzo M, Pazzaglia M, Misciali C, Vincenzi C, Micali G. The role of scalp dermoscopy in the diagnosis of alopecia areata incognita. *J Am Acad Dermatol.* 2008;59(1):64–7.

Udompanich S, Chanprapaph K, Suchonwanit P. Linear and annular lupus panniculitis of the scalp: case report with emphasis on trichoscopic findings and review of the literature. *Case Rep Dermatol.* 2019;11(2):157–65.

5 Primary Scarring Alopecias

- Loss of follicular openings is the marker of scarring alopecia in the non-pigmented scalp (Figure 5.1).
- Irregular pinpoint white dots and white patches are the marker of scarring alopecia in the pigmented scalp (Figure 5.1).
- Dermoscopy is very useful for:

a) distinguishing scarring from non-scarring alopecias
b) differential diagnosis of different primary scarring alopecias
c) selecting optimal biopsy site in all scarring alopecias
d) detecting signs of disease activity

LICHEN PLANOPILARIS (LPP) (FIGURES 5.2–5.5)

Clinical Variants

- Frontal fibrosing alopecia (FFA) causing a receding frontal hairline, loss of eyebrows, and facial lesions
- Fibrosing alopecia in a pattern distribution (FAPD): affecting the central scalp, resembling androgenetic alopecia with scalp itching, follicular erythema, and hyperkeratosis

Dermoscopy

- Loss of follicular openings (non-pigmented scalp).
- Irregular distributed pinpoint white dots and white patches (pigmented scalp).
- Peripilar casts/scales: Silvery-white collar-like scale rings encircling the hair follicles at their emergence.
- Tufted hairs: Presence of multiple hairs (typically two to three) emerging from a single follicular opening, surrounded by a common peripilar cast.
- Absence of vellus hairs at the hairline (FFA).
- Peri- and interfollicular erythema: Corresponding to vasodilation secondary to tissue ischemia.
- Broken hairs at different lengths, often surrounded by peripilar casts (few).
- Pili torti: irregular twisted hair shaft along their longitudinal axis, distorted by the perifollicular fibrosis (few).
- White patches on an erythematous background (strawberry ice cream color), corresponding to early onset fibrosis in the non-pigmented scalp.
- White patches/structureless area: End-stage fibrosis.
- Blue-gray dots: With a targetoid pattern in a follicular distribution, are occasionally seen in pigmented scalp where follicles have been destroyed.
- Tubular casts: Concentric, semi-transparent, white to grayish scales encircling the proximal hair shaft.
- Trichoscopy of the hairs that are lost or pulled show anagen hair roots with sheaths.

FRONTAL FIBROSING ALOPECIA (FIGURES 5.6–5.16)

Dermoscopy

Scalp

- Absence of follicular openings.
- Yellow dots and short regrowing hairs may be present.
- Absence of vellus hairs, this is typical and occurs in most of the cases.
- Peripilar casts with strong correlation between thickness of peripilar casts and degree of lymphocytic infiltrate.

DOI: 10.1201/9780429351433-5

- Transparent emergences of the proximal hair shafts in the temporal scalp.
- Broken hairs, black dots, pili torti (few).

Facial Lesions

- Facial papules appear as white-yellowish round homogeneous well-defined structures.
- Lichen pigmentosus: Dots, globules, and blotches (black/ brown/violet).

Eyelashes/Eyebrows

Dermoscopy of eyebrows and eyelashes can be tricky as it often shows features of non-scarring alopecia (see Chapter 13).

Eyelashes

- Loss of follicular openings (follicular atrichia)
- Broken hairs and black dots
- Hair bulbs visibility in the upper eyelashes
- Ingrown hairs (few)

Eyebrows

- Yellow dots.
- Multiple pinpoint white dots (dark-skin phototypes).
- Short thin/vellus hairs.
- Black dots.
- Dystrophic hairs: Misshapen or structurally abnormal hairs.
- Tapering hairs: Can lead to a misdiagnosis of alopecia areata.
- Broken hairs.
- Eyebrows growing in different directions.
- Pili torti.
- The "lonely hair sign" is distinctive for FFA, where one or a few isolated terminal hairs persist in the middle of the forehead. These may be affected or unaffected by the peripilar casts.
- Absence/presence of vellus hairs in the frontal hairline allows to distinguish frontal fibrosing alopecia from MPHL/FPHL that sometimes share similar clinical presentations.

FIBROSING ALOPECIA IN A PATTERN DISTRIBUTION (FAPD) (FIGURES 5.17–5.20)

Dermoscopy

- Hair shaft diameter variability
- Loss of follicular openings, may be subtle
- Hair tufting with peripilar casts surrounding 2 (V sign) or more hairs emerging from the same follicular unit
- Perifollicular erythema

DISCOID LUPUS ERYTHEMATOSUS (DLE) (FIGURES 5.21–5.28)

Dermoscopy

- Enlarged branched vessels: These are typical and very important to distinguish lupus from other conditions including lichen planopilaris.
- Loss of follicular openings in non-pigmented scalp.
- Loss/disruption of pigmented network in pigmented scalp: This is an important feature in the pigmented scalp to distinguish DLE from lichen planopilaris, where the network is preserved.
- Loss of pinpoint white dots in the pigmented scalp: This is exclusive of DLE in the pigmented scalp and is a consequence of the involvement of interfollicular structures.
- Patches of dark brown heterogeneous staining at borders and within the patch.
- Keratotic plugs: Hyperkeratosis obstructing follicular openings.
- Red dots (red spider on yellow dots): Blanch only partially after pressure and are indicative of active disease. Red dots are considered a favorable prognostic sign, suggesting potential for hair regrowth.
- Peripilar casts are identical to those seen in lichen planopilaris; the differential diagnosis is based on the vessels' architecture.
- Inter- and perifollicular scaling.

- Blue-gray dots in a speckled pattern are occasionally seen in the pigmented scalp and correspond to melanin incontinence affecting both the follicular and interfollicular structures. They are different from the blue-gray dots arranged in a target pattern in lichen planopilaris where the incontinentia pigmenti only affects the hair follicles.
- White patches: Are shiny-white and differ from the "strawberry ice cream" color seen in lichen planopilaris.

Lupus profundus (tumidus) may occasionally affect the scalp and produce alopecia. The disease usually presents in patches where erythema and edema are prominent features. Scarring is not the rule (see Chapter 4).

FOLLICULITIS DECALVANS (FD) (FIGURES 5.29–5.35)

Dermoscopy

- Loss of follicular openings.
- Follicular and interfollicular pustules and crusting: Yellowish deposits due to exudations are more common than typical pustules.
- Perifollicular hemorrhages and crusting.
- Hair tufting: Tufts are composed of more than six hairs, and sometimes hundreds of hairs, emerging from a single dilated opening. Although tufting in LPP usually contains less than six hairs, an overlap of these two conditions can occur. Normal scalp can also show dermoscopy signs.
- Thick peripilar casts: White-yellowish scales encircling the hair shafts at their base with tapering toward the distal end.
- Tubular scales: White-yellowish scales encircling the hair shafts after their emergence. If the yellow color is prevalent, it indicates ongoing exudation and is a hallmark of disease activity.
- Perifollicular scaling: It can be mild (thinner than the hair shaft), moderate (thicker than the hair shaft), or severe.
- Starburst hyperplasia: Radiating fibrotic strands around the hair follicle.
- Abnormal vascular pattern includes coiled/twisted dilated capillaries (similar to psoriasis), giant capillaries, and/or stretched linear vessels radially arranged around the compounded follicles. The vascular pattern is important to distinguish FD from LPP.
- White and milky-red areas: White and milky-red areas where follicular openings are absent, indicating areas of scarring in the inactive or burnt-out stages of FD.

Dermoscopy features vary depending on disease activity: Perifollicular erythema, follicular pustules, yellow tubular scaling, and yellow crusts are associated with active disease.

ACNE KELOIDALIS NUCHAE

Figure 5.36; see Chapter 8.

CENTRAL CENTRIFUGAL CICATRICIAL ALOPECIA

See Chapter 8.

SECONDARY SCARRING ALOPECIAS

Figures 5.37–5.39.

- Alopecia is a feature of numerous conditions that involve the dermis and secondarily destroy the hair follicles.

Dermoscopic features are not specific:

- Loss of follicular openings.
- White structureless areas.
- The hairs surrounding the scar often show hair tufting and peripilar casts.
- Embedded ingrown hairs.
- Pili torti.
- Erythema and telangiectasia.

EROSIVE PUSTULAR DERMATOSIS OF THE SCALP (EPDS) (FIGURE 5.40)

Dermoscopy features are quite aspecific:

- Extensive yellowish crusts.
- Peripheral pustules.
- White patches.
- Evident on-focus dermal vessels: Branching and dilated vessels are easily detectable due to the thinning of the epidermis.
- Hair roots through the scalp: Clue for diagnosis but often not very numerous. The severe atrophy of the skin allows for the hair follicle bulbs to be visible through the surface.
- Pili torti.

Overall, erosive pustular dermatosis of the scalp presents trichoscopic features that necessitate careful differentiation from other scalp conditions with similar appearances, including tinea capitis, folliculitis decalvans, and pemphigus vulgaris and foliaceus.

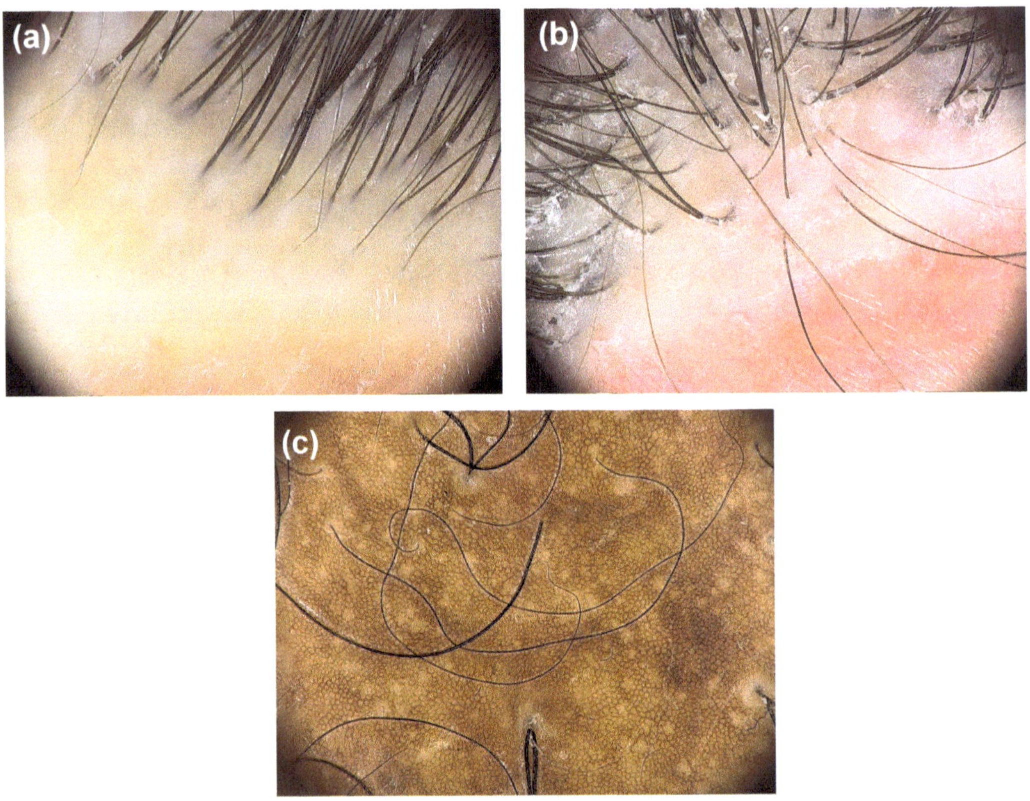

FIGURE 5.1 Scarring alopecia in non pigmented (a,b) and pigmented scalp (c). ×20 Loss of follicular openings and whitish structureless areas in long-standing scarring alopecia; the absence of inflammatory signs indicates that the disease is not active (a). In active scarring alopecias the absence of follicular openings is associated with signs of inflammation (b). Irregularly distributed pinpoint white dots, white patches, and reduced hair density (c).

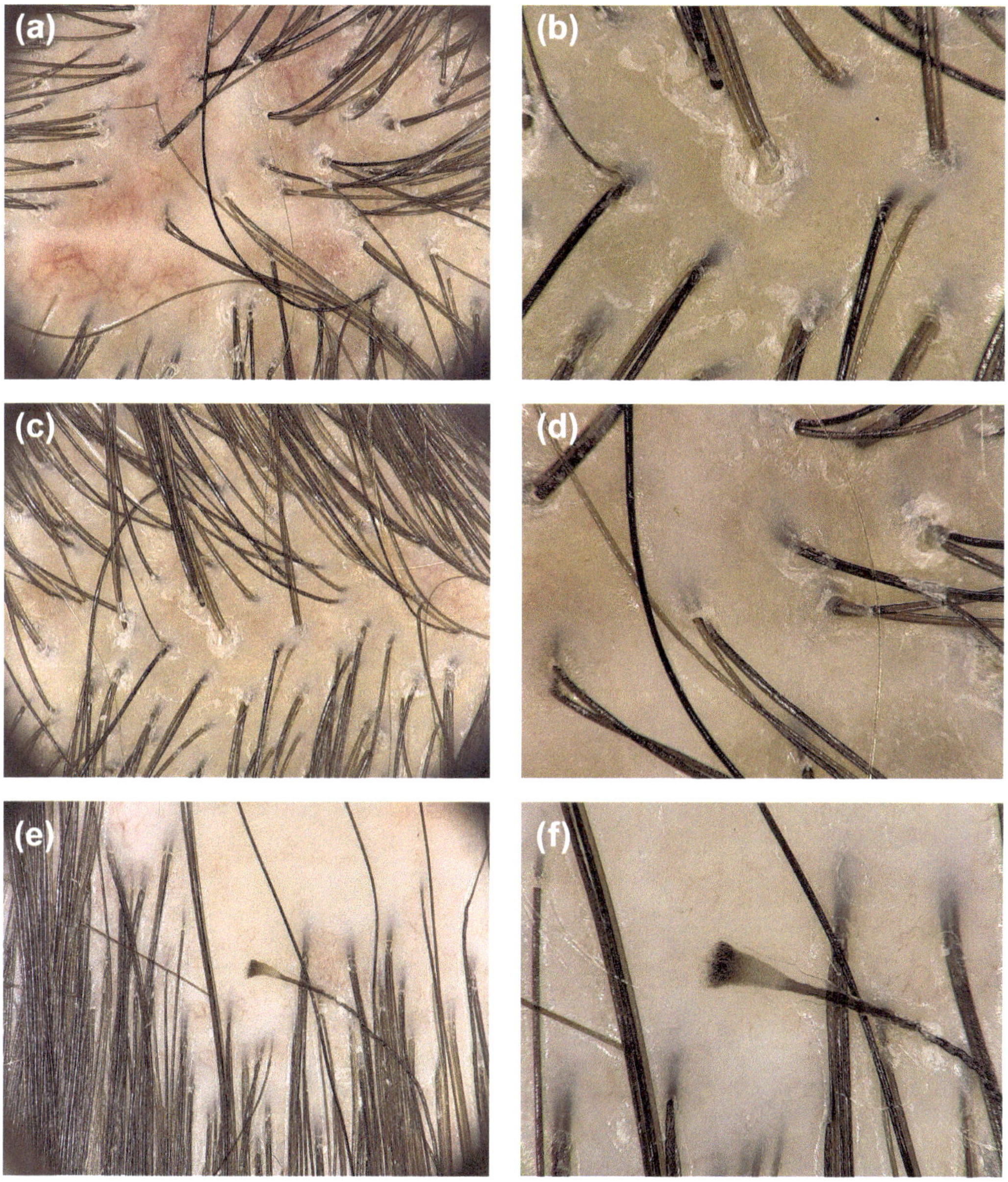

FIGURE 5.2 Lichen planopilaris. ×20 Peripilar casts and loss of follicular openings (a). ×50 Higher magnification of the casts; note also tufting (b). ×20 Peripilar casts and encircling tubular structures; loss of follicular openings is not very evident (c). ×50 Close-up view showing tufting with peripilar casts and tubular structures (d). ×20 Loss of follicular openings and an anagen root with a pili torti shaft (e). ×50 Higher magnification of the anagen root (f).

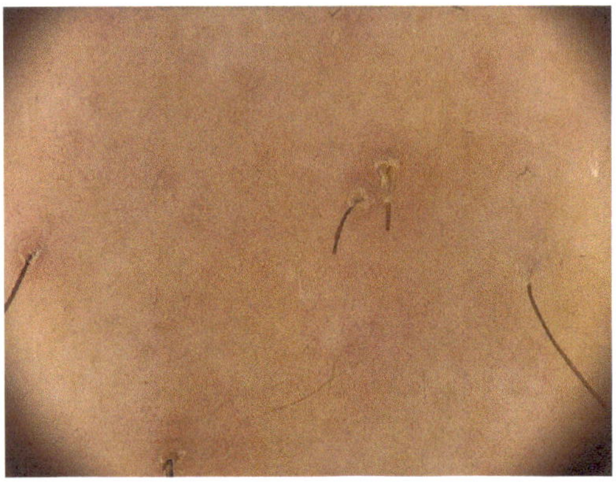

FIGURE 5.3 Lichen planopilaris. ×20 Loss of follicular openings and broken hairs surrounded by peripilar casts.

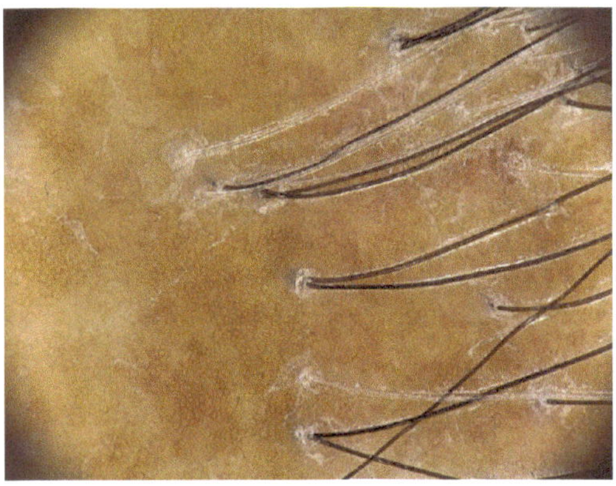

FIGURE 5.4 Lichen planopilaris. ×20 V sign characterized by a peripilar cast surrounding a tuft consisting of two hairs.

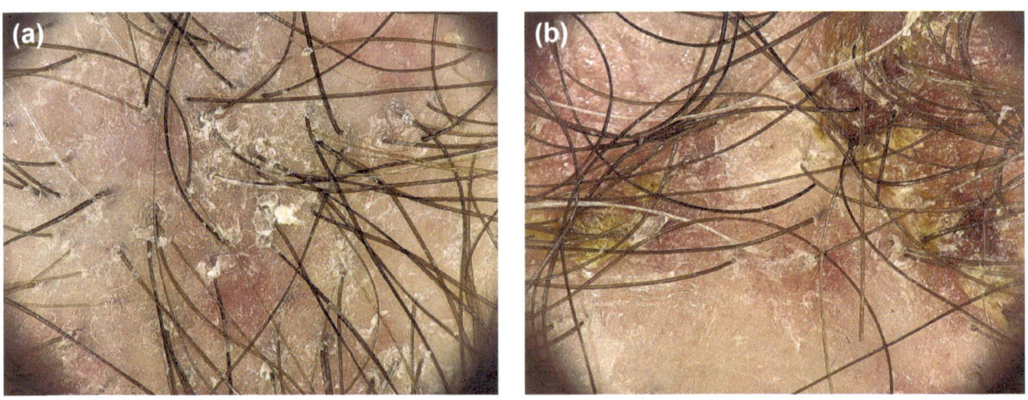

FIGURE 5.5 Lichen planopilaris overlap with folliculitis decalvans: ×50 Pronounced peripilar casts and interfollicular scaling (a). ×50 Interfollicular exudation and crusting in the same patient (b).

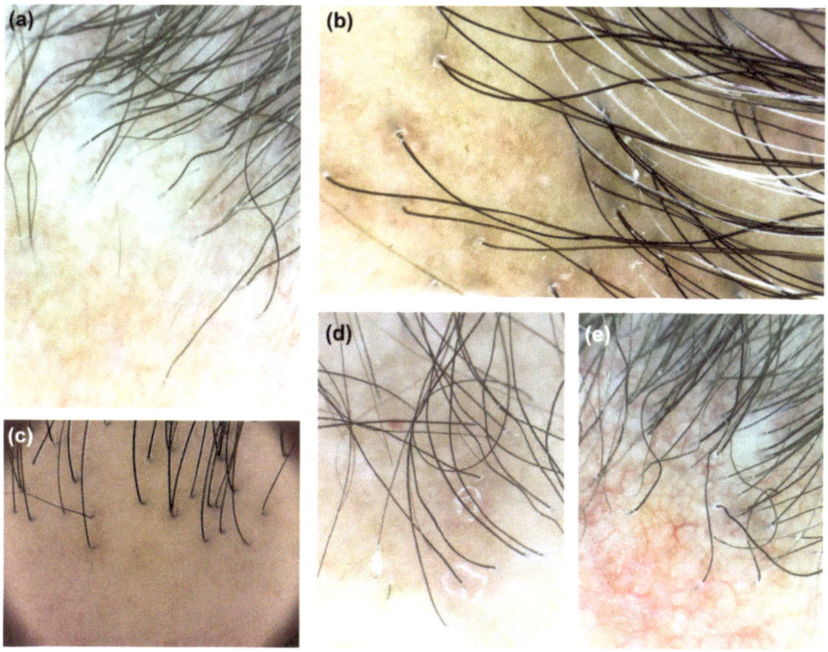

FIGURE 5.6 Frontal fibrosing alopecia. ×20 Loss of follicular openings and of vellus hairs in the hairline, erythema, subtle peripilar casts, pili torti, and hair tufting (a); ×20 loss of vellus hairs, peripilar casts, irregularly distributed pinpoint white dots and white patches (b); ×50 peripilar casts and V sign (c); ×50 encircling tubular structure (d); ×20 pili torti and prominent arborizing vessels (e).

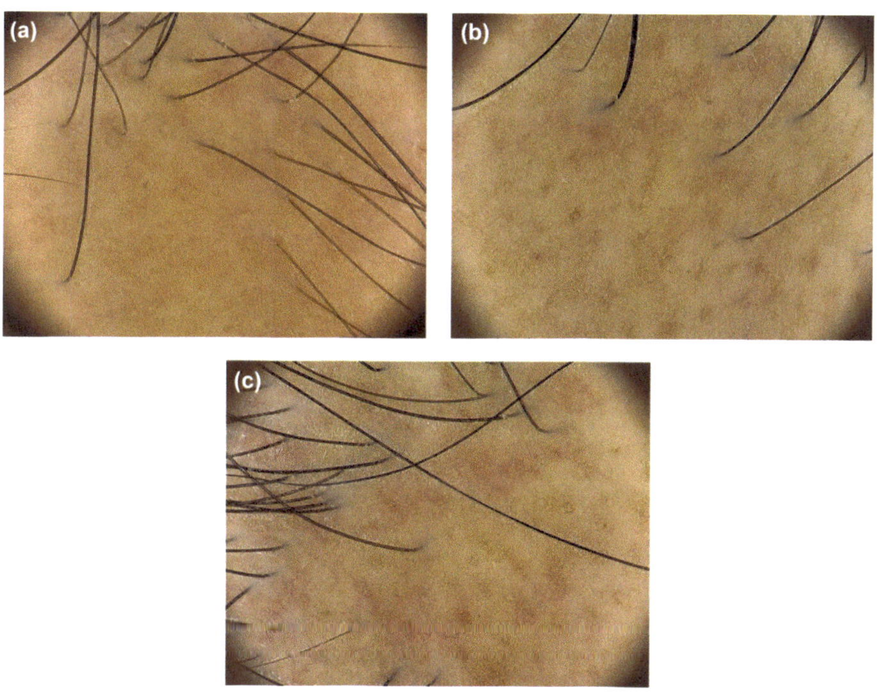

FIGURE 5.7 Frontal fibrosing alopecia. ×40 Transparent emergences of the proximal hair shafts on the parietal scalp (a,b); whitish peripilar halos representing perifollicular fibrosis surrounding the emergences of the affected hair shafts (c).

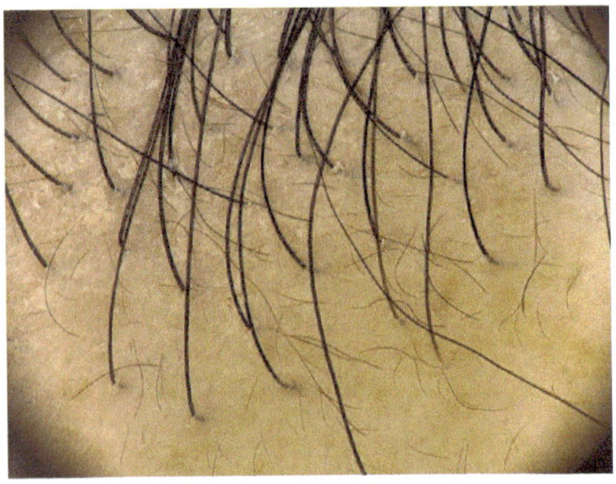

FIGURE 5.8 Frontal fibrosing alopecia. ×20 Presence of vellus hairs does not totally exclude the diagnosis of FFA, since they can be preserved in rare cases. In this case, the presence of peripilar casts is a clue for diagnosis.

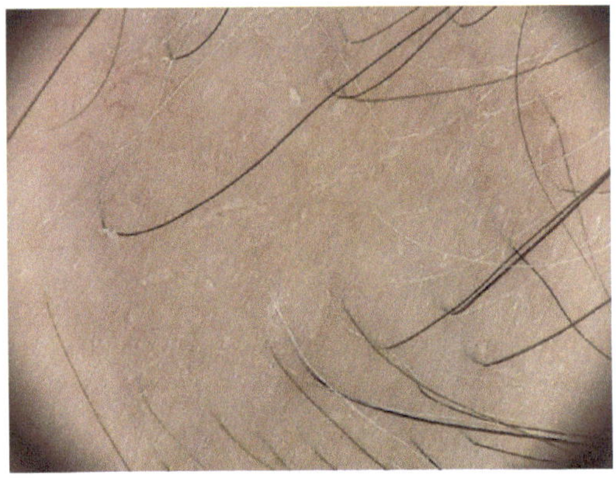

FIGURE 5.9 Frontal fibrosing alopecia. ×20 Loss of vellus hairs, transparent emergences of the proximal hair shafts in the occipital FFA.

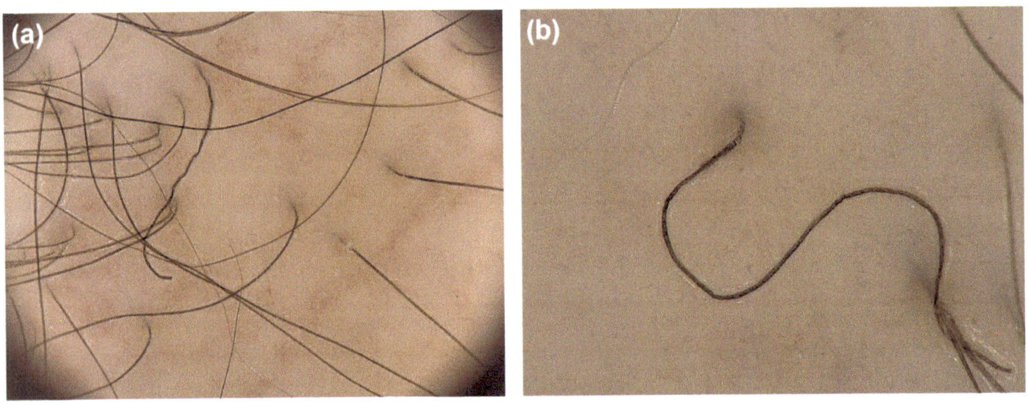

FIGURE 5.10 Frontal fibrosing alopecia. Pili torti seen at ×20 (a) and ×50 (b) magnifications.

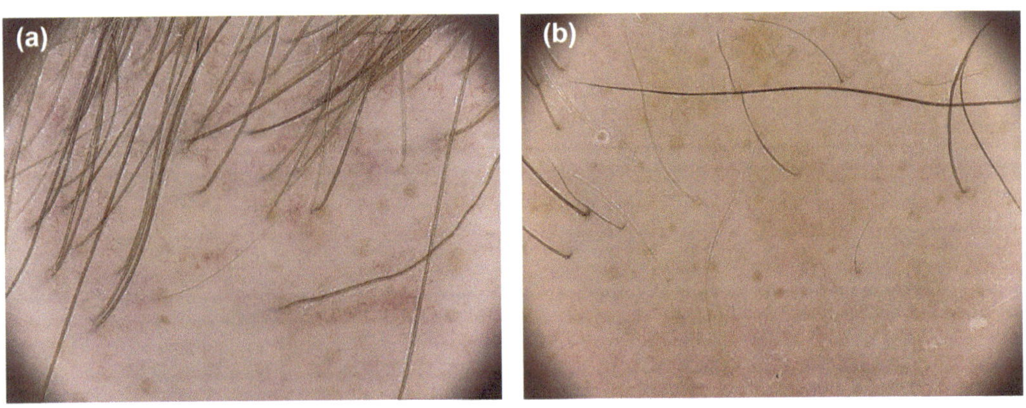

FIGURE 5.11 Yellow dots in FFA. ×20 Absence of vellus hairs and yellow dots at the hairline (a); ×50 absence of vellus hair, yellow dots, short regrowing hairs, and peripilar cast (b).

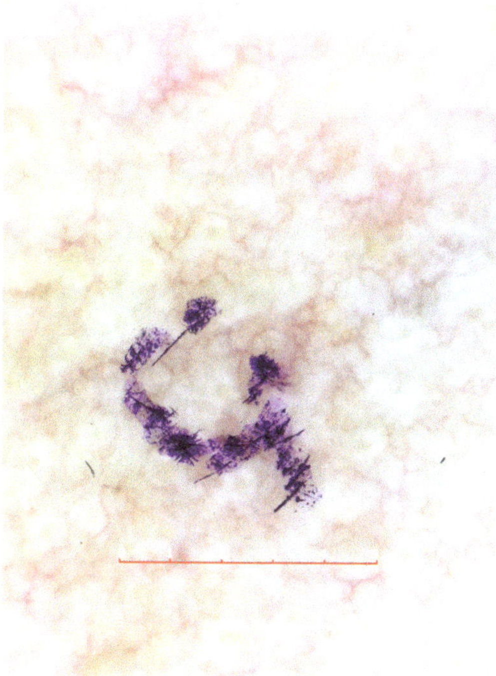

FIGURE 5.12 Facial papules in FFA. ×20 Well-defined homogeneous whitish structures devoid of follicular openings.

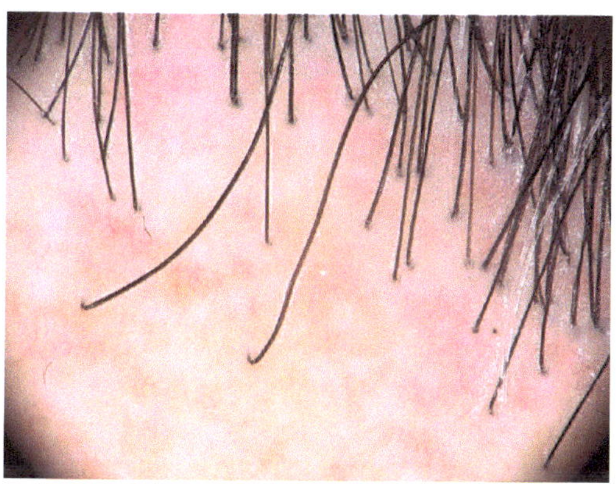

FIGURE 5.15 FFA. ×50 White hypopigmented patches along the hairline.

FIGURE 5.13 Lichen planus pigmentosus in a patient with FFA. ×20 regularly arranged brownish globule.

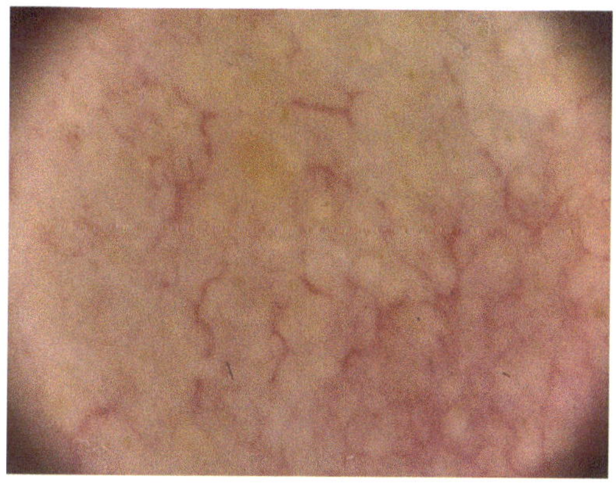

FIGURE 5.14 ×20 Facial papules and rosacea-like lesions in a fair skin phototype patient.

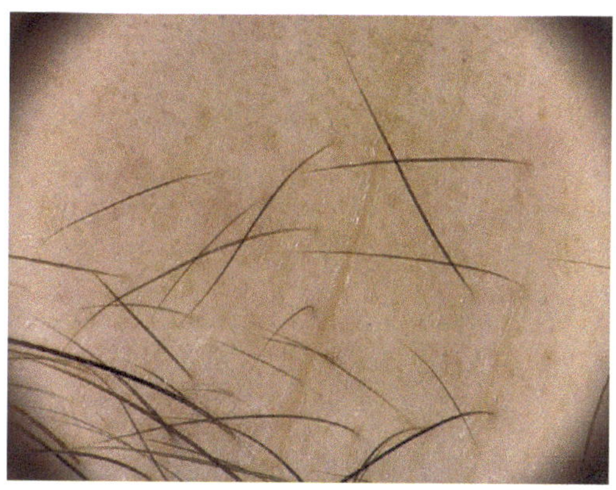

FIGURE 5.16 FFA. 50x Eyebrows growing in different directions.

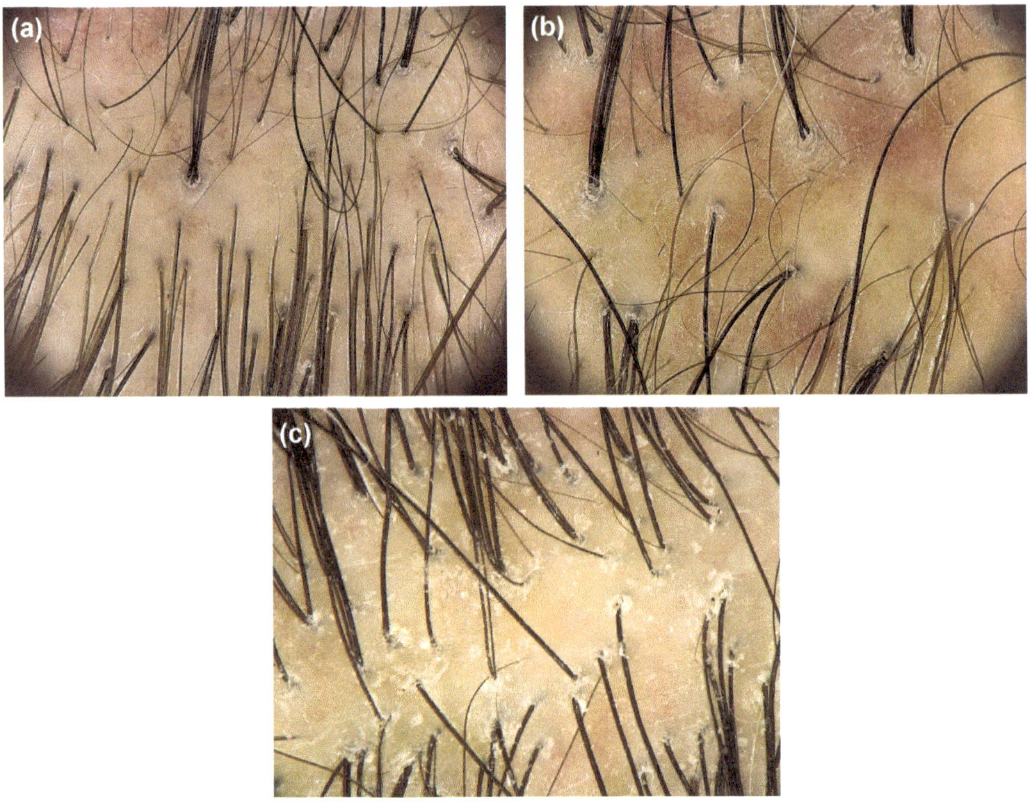

FIGURE 5.17 FADP. ×20 Peripilar casts, hair tufting, and hair shaft variability (a); ×50 higher magnification showing the V-sign, consisting of a peripilar cast encircling two hair shafts (b); ×50 diffuse interfollicular scaling can be present (c).

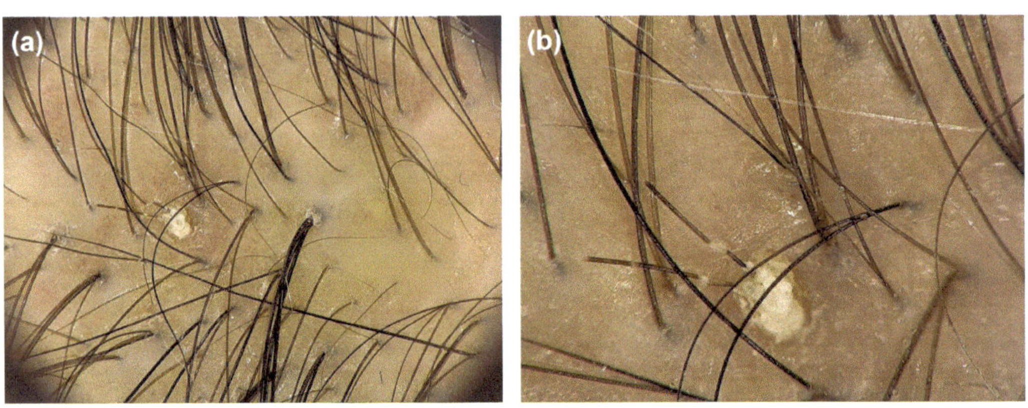

FIGURE 5.18 FAPD. ×20 Loss of follicular openings, peripilar casts, hair shaft variability, and proximal trichorrhexis nodosa due to scratching (a); ×50 higher magnification of proximal trichorrhexis nodosa affecting a tuft of hair surrounded by a cast (b).

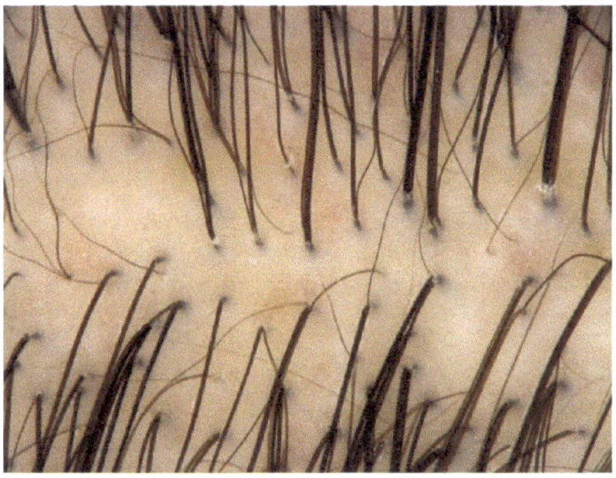

FIGURE 5.19 FAPD early case. ×20 Small white areas of scarring, hair shaft variability, tufting, and peripilar casts.

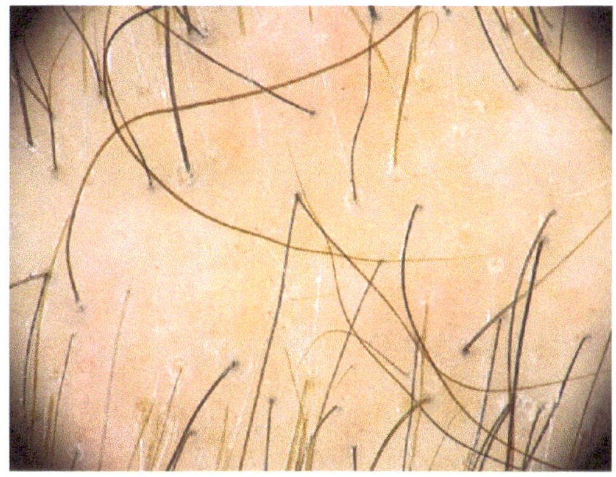

FIGURE 5.20 FAPD advanced case. ×20 Loss of follicular openings, hair shaft variability, and peripilar casts.

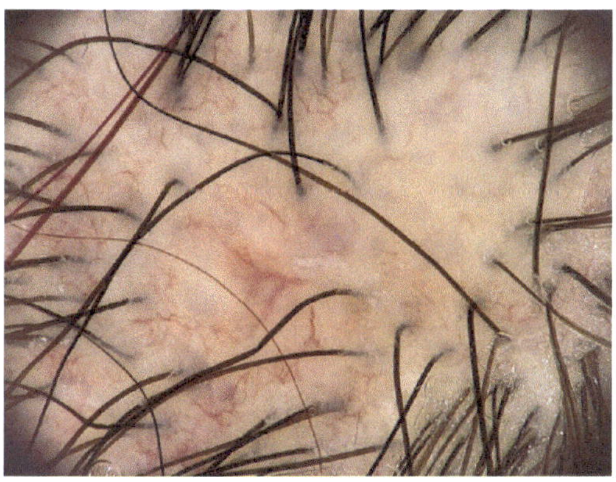

FIGURE 5.21 ×20 Enlarged tortuous vessels of DLE.

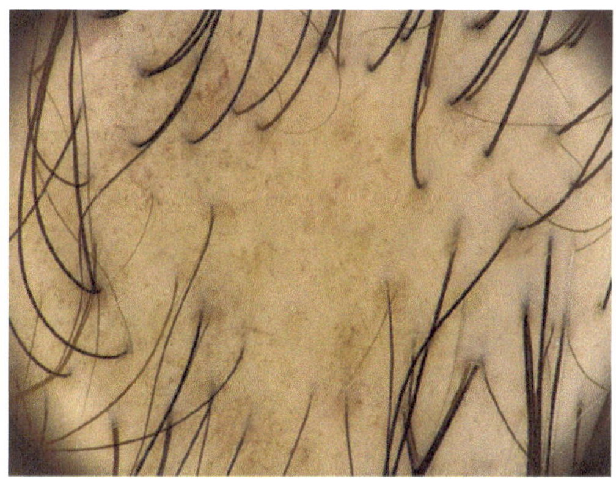

FIGURE 5.22 DLE. ×20 Speckled brown dots in the interfollicular scalp of non-pigmented scalp.

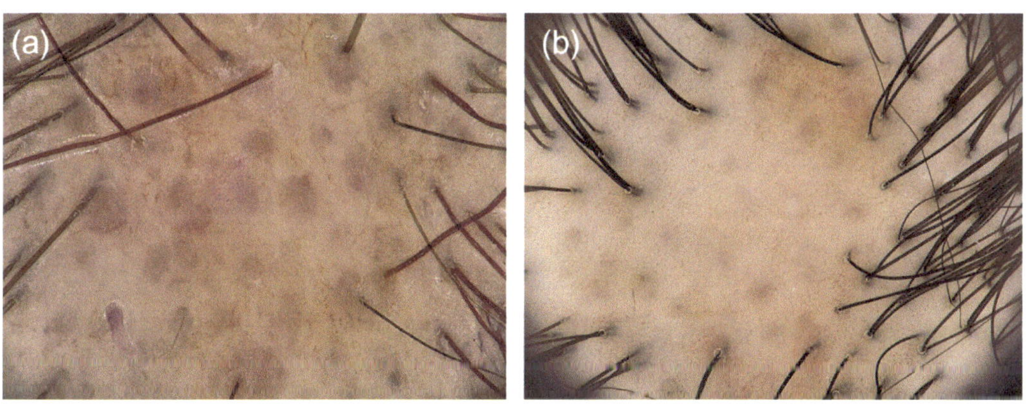

FIGURE 5.23 DLE. ×40 Follicular red dots.

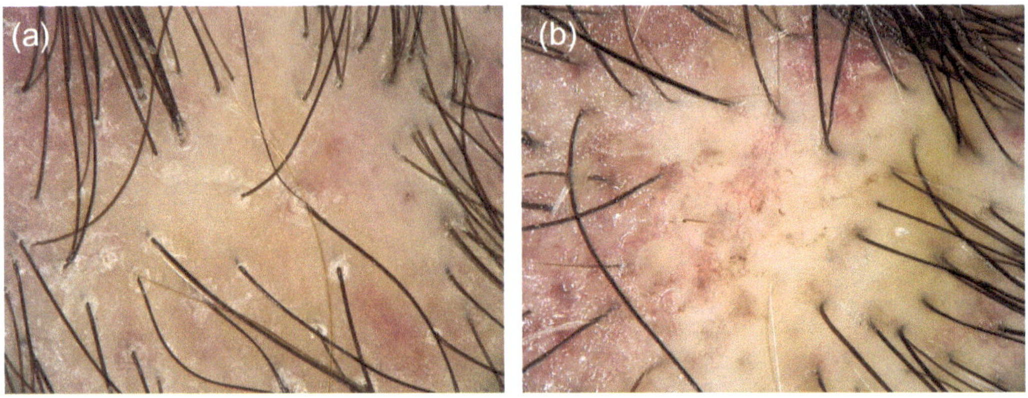

FIGURE 5.24 DLE. ×50 Peripilar casts (a) and ×50 tortuous vessels (b); the presence of thick tortuous vessels is a clue to differentiate DLE from LPP.

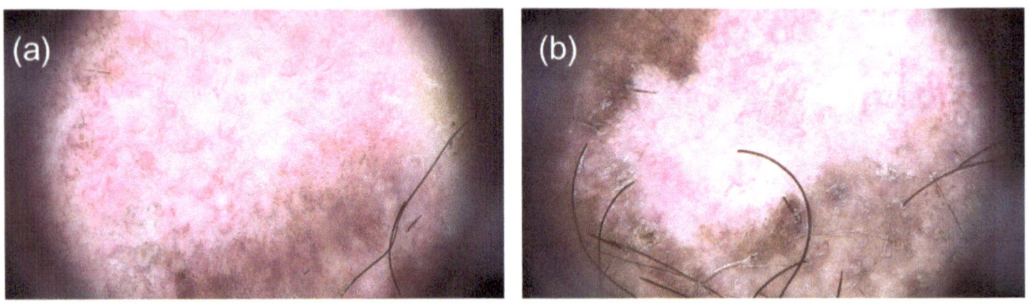

FIGURE 5.25 DLE. ×20 Loss of pigmented network and prominent vessels in the black scalp (a); ×20 also note the presence of keratotic plugs, speckled brown dots in the interfollicular scalp, and brown heterogeneous patches at the periphery of the patch (b).

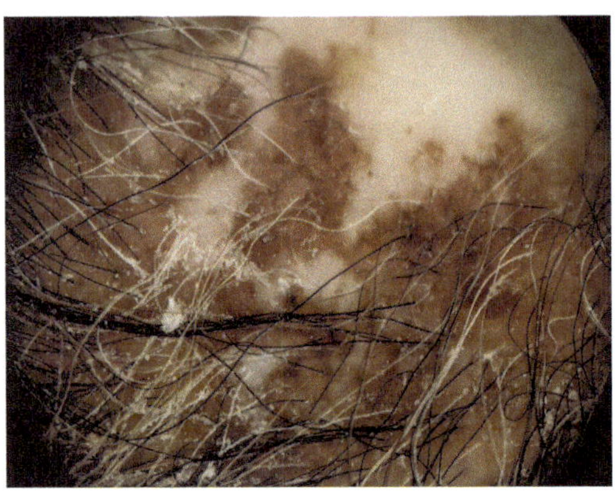

FIGURE 5.26 DLE. ×20 Loss of pigmented network also affects the scalp surrounding the patch that shows heterogeneous brown black patches, without the reticular pattern.

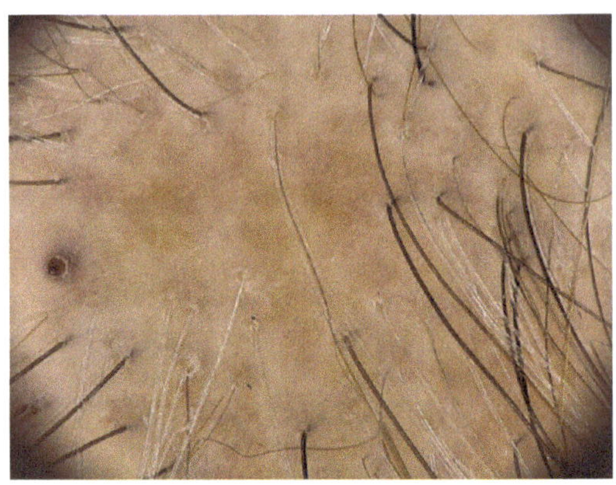

FIGURE 5.27 DLE. ×20 Keratotic plug associated with loss of follicular openings.

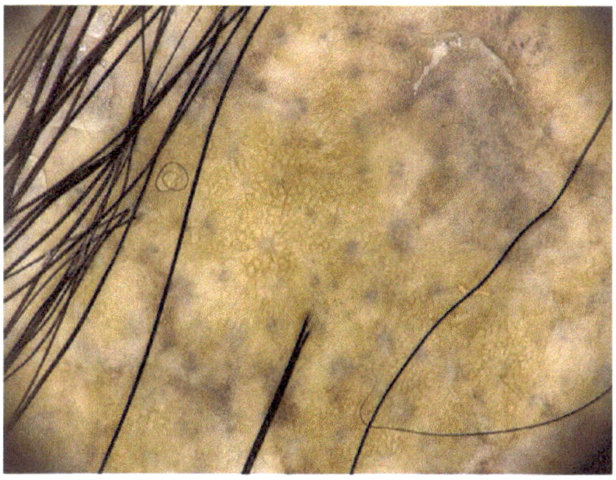

FIGURE 5.28 DLE. ×20 Speckled peri- and interfollicular blue-gray dots in the pigmented scalp.

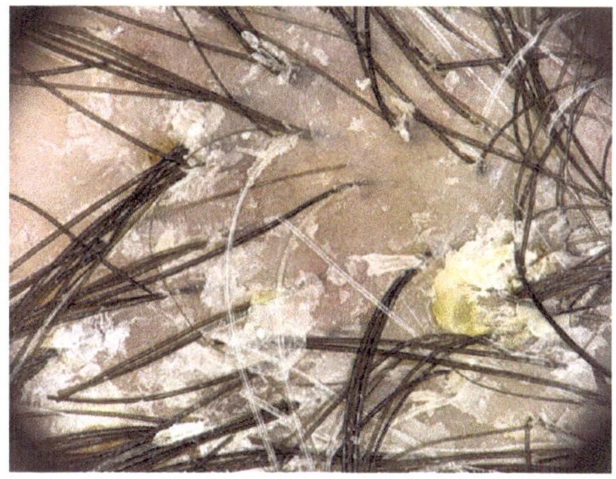

FIGURE 5.29 FD. ×50 Scaling and exudative yellowish crusting in folliculitis decalvans.

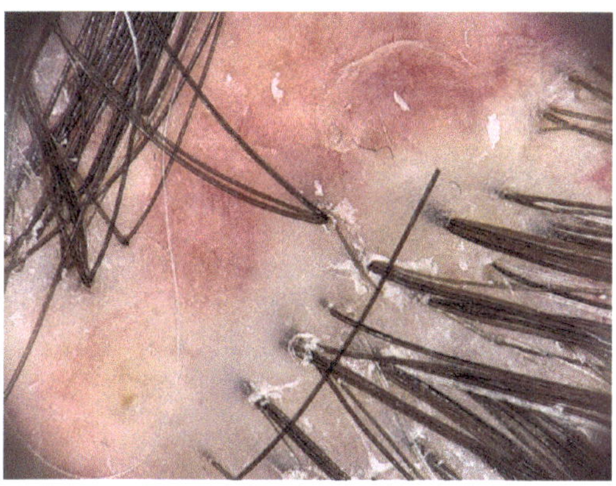

FIGURE 5.30 FD. ×50 Hair tufting surrounded by peripilar casts and white and milky-red areas.

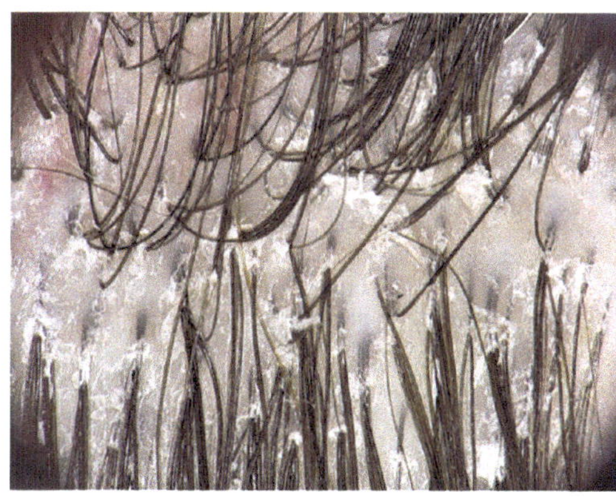

FIGURE 5.31 FD. ×20 Hair tufting with inter- and perifollicular scaling in an apparently normal-appearing scalp.

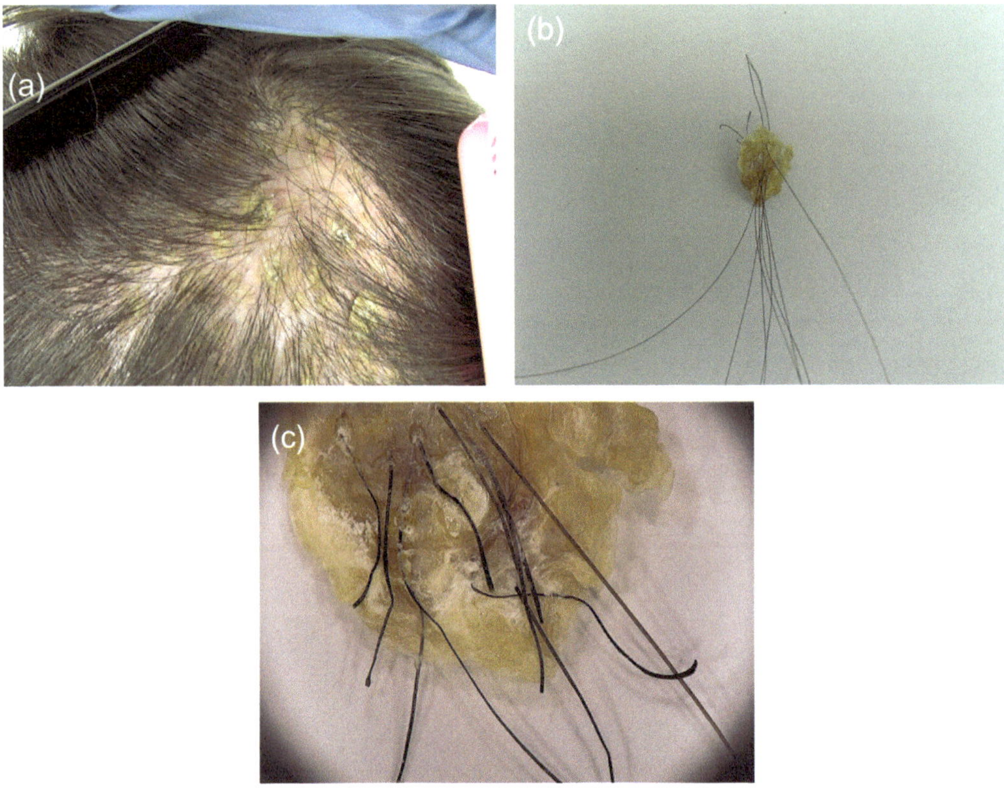

FIGURE 5.32 Folliculitis decalvans with severe scalp inflammation and scaling (a); ×20 the yellowish scales entrap multiple hair shafts (b); ×40 higher magnification shows dystrophic and anagen roots (c).

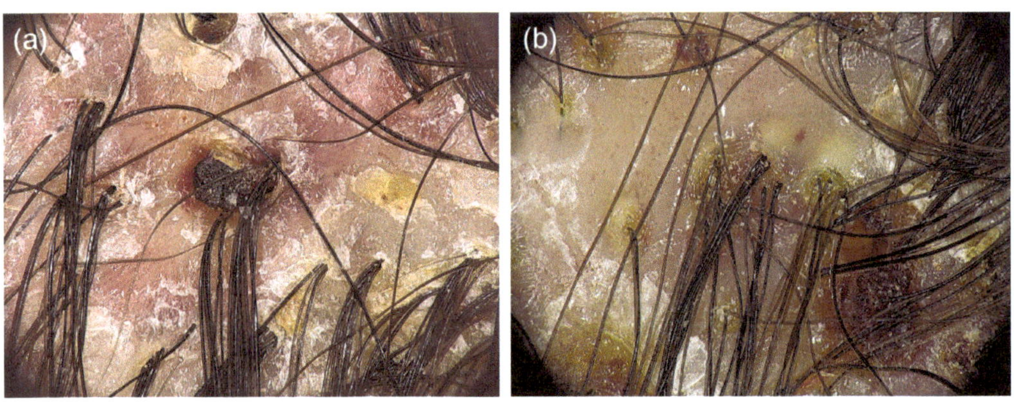

FIGURE 5.33 Folliculitis decalvans. ×50 Acute case with hemorrhagic crusts and purulent yellowish interfollicular and perifollicular scales (a); ×20 follicular pustules, tufting, and hemorrhagic crusting (b).

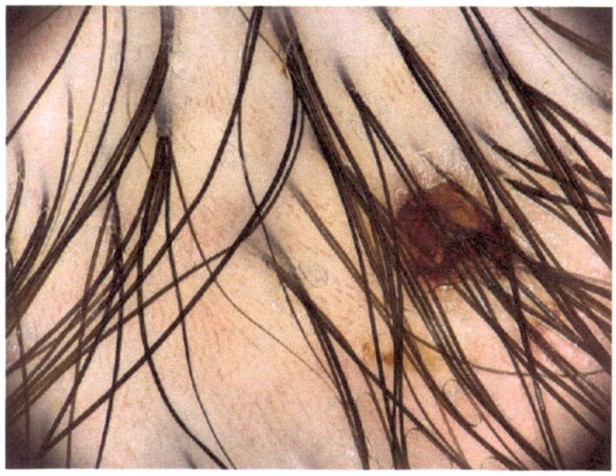

FIGURE 5.34 FD. ×40 Linear radial-arranged vessels similar to twisted vessels of psoriasis.

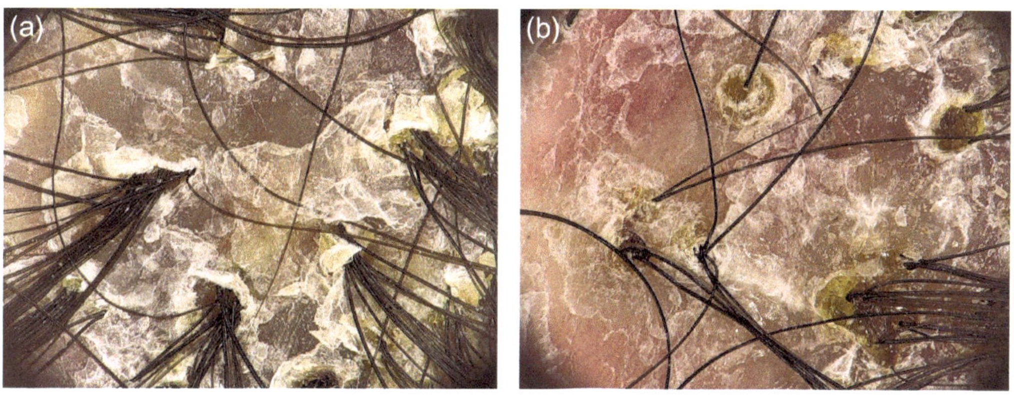

FIGURE 5.35 FD. ×50 Hair tufting and scaling with fibrous remodeling causing a volcano-like appearance (a); ×50 yellowish crusts can be associated (b).

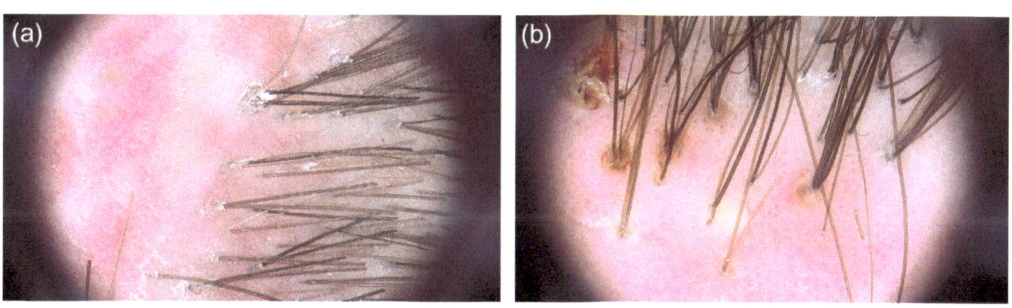

FIGURE 5.36 Acne keloidalis. ×20 Periphery of the lesions shows peripilar casts, follicular pustules/hemorrhagic crusts, and coiled vessels (a,b).

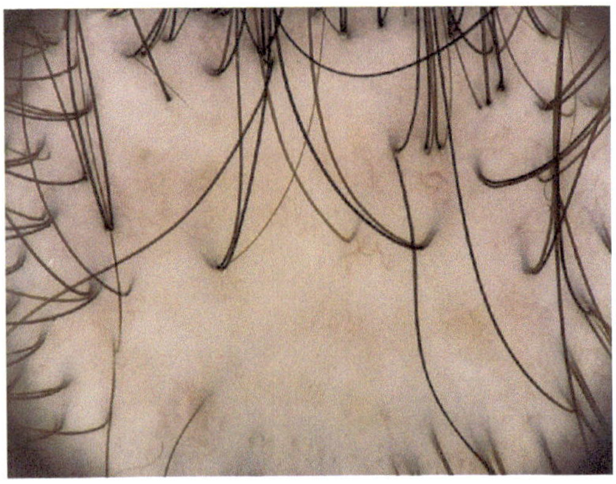

FIGURE 5.37 Biopsy scars. ×20 Loss of follicular openings.

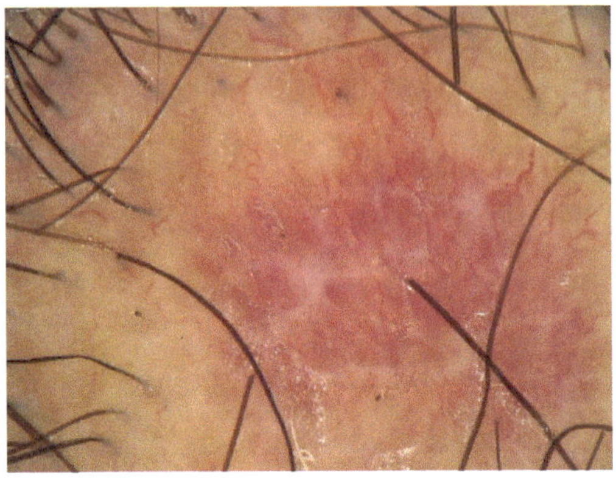

FIGURE 5.38 ×20 Scar after a thick bite. Note broken hairs at the periphery, erythema, white patches, and arborizing vessels in the center of the patch.

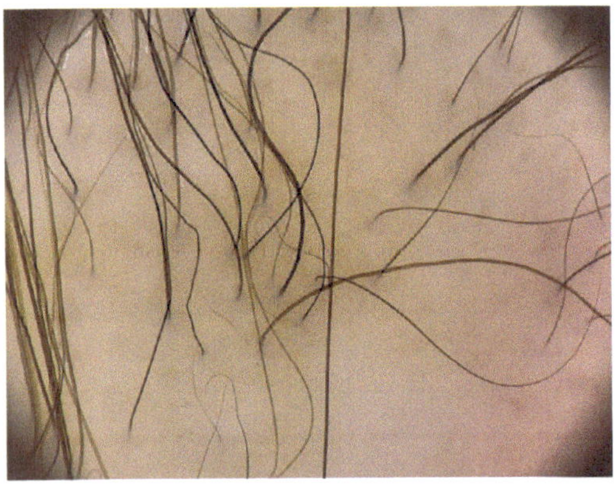

FIGURE 5.39 ×20 Morphea with loss of follicular openings and pili torti.

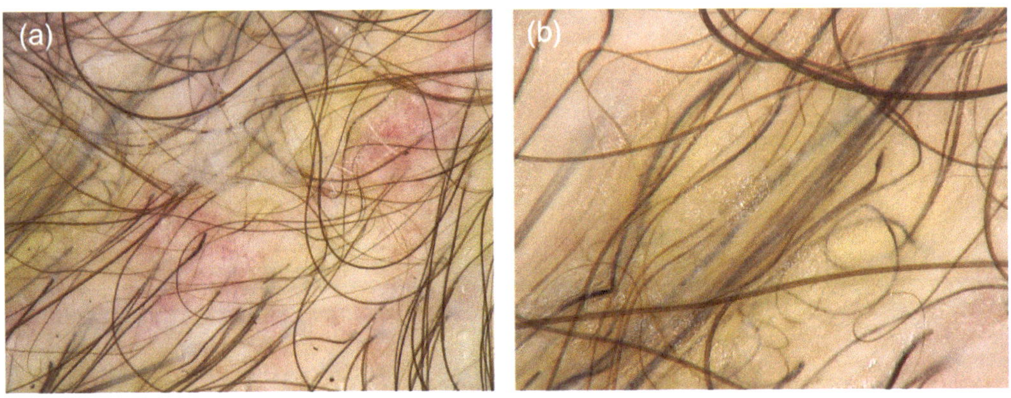

FIGURE 5.40 Erosive pustular dermatosis. ×20 Yellowish exudate and hair roots through the scalp (a); ×50 high magnification (b).

SUGGESTED READING

Duque-Estrada B, Tamler C, Sodré CT et al . Dermoscopy patterns of cicatricial alopecia resulting from discoid lupus erythematosus and lichen planopilaris. *An Bras Dermatol.* 2010;85(2):179–83. Erratum in: *An Bras Dermatol.* 2010;85(4):578.

Lacarrubba F, Micali G, Tosti A. Absence of vellus hair in the hairline: a videodermatoscopic feature of frontal fibrosing alopecia. *Br J Dermatol.* 2013;169(2):473–4.

Lanuti E, Miteva M, Romanelli P, Tosti A. Trichoscopy and histopathology of follicular keratotic plugs in scalp discoid lupus erythematosus. *Int J Trichology.* 2012;4(1):36–8.

Martínez-Velasco MA, Vázquez-Herrera NE, Misciali C, Vincenzi C, Maddy AJ, Asz-Sigall D, Tosti A. Frontal fibrosing alopecia severity index: a trichoscopic visual scale that correlates thickness of peripilar casts with severity of inflammatory changes at pathology. *Skin Appendage Disord.* 2018;4(4):277–80.

Martinez-Velasco MA, Burroway B, Thompson C, Silyuk T, Tosti A. Occipital fibrosing alopecia. *Int J Dermatol.* 2021;60(2):e44–e45.

Miteva M, Tosti A. Dermoscopy guided scalp biopsy in cicatricial alopecia. *J Eur Acad Dermatol Venereol.* 2013;27(10):1299–303.

Ocampo-Garza J, Tosti A. Trichoscopy of dark scalp. *Skin Appendage Disord.* 2018;5(1):1–8.

Pirmez R, Donati A, Valente NS, Sodré CT, Tosti A. Glabellar red dots in frontal fibrosing alopecia: a further clinical sign of vellus follicle involvement. *Br J Dermatol.* 2014;170(3):745–6.

Pirmez R, Duque-Estrada B, Donati A, Campos-do-Carmo G, Valente NS, Romiti R, Sodré CT, Tosti A. Clinical and dermoscopic features of lichen planus pigmentosus in 37 patients with frontal fibrosing alopecia. *Br J Dermatol.* 2016;175(6):1387–90.

Ross EK, Vincenzi C, Tosti A. Videodermoscopy in the evaluation of hair and scalp disorders. *J Am Acad Dermatol.* 2006;55(5):799–806.

Saceda-Corralo D, Tosti A. Trichoscopic features of linear morphea on the scalp. *Skin Appendage Disord.* 2018;4(1):31–33.

Starace M, Loi C, Bruni F, Alessandrini A, Misciali C, Patrizi A, Piraccini BM. Erosive pustular dermatosis of the scalp: clinical, trichoscopic, and histopathologic features of 20 cases. *J Am Acad Dermatol.* 2017;76(6):1109–1114.e2.

Thompson CT, Martínez-Velasco MA, Tosti A. Yellow dots in frontal fibrosing alopecia. *J Eur Acad Dermatol Venereol.* 2021;35(1):e75–e76.

Thompson CT, Martinez Velasco MA, Tosti A. Three-dimensional imaging of a peripilar cast and compound follicle in frontal fibrosing alopecia. *JAAD Case Rep.* 2022;23:46–48.

Tosti A, Miteva M, Torres F, Vincenzi C, Romanelli P. Hair casts are a dermoscopic clue for the diagnosis of traction alopecia. *Br J Dermatol.* 2010;163(6):1353–5.

Tosti A, Torres F, Misciali C, Vincenzi C, Starace M, Miteva M, Romanelli P. Follicular red dots: a novel dermoscopic pattern observed in scalp discoid lupus erythematosus. *Arch Dermatol.* 2009;145(12):1406–9.

6 Hair Shaft Disorders

- Dermoscopy is effective for diagnosing congenital and acquired hair shaft disorders.
- It allows fast examination of all hairy regions, including eyebrows, eyelashes, and body hairs, and it is also very useful in the case of short or brittle hairs.
- In children it has the advantage of being painless and non-invasive avoiding the necessity of plucking or cutting.

CONGENITAL DISORDERS ASSOCIATED WITH HAIR FRAGILITY

- Monilethrix
- Trichorrhexis invaginata
- Trichothiodystrophy
- Pili torti
- Pili annulati

CONGENITAL DISORDERS WITHOUT HAIR FRAGILITY

- Pili trianguli and canaliculi

ACQUIRED DISORDERS WITH HAIR FRAGILITY

- Trichorrhexis nodosa

CONGENITAL DISORDERS ASSOCIATED WITH HAIR FRAGILITY

Monilethrix (Figure 6.1, 6.2, 6.3)

Monilethrix is an autosomal dominant or rarely X-linked hair disorder characterized by a beaded or moniliform appearance of the hair shaft.

Disease severity ranges from very mild cases with only a few hair shafts affected and few broken hairs, to severe cases with involvement of terminal and vellus hairs as well as body hairs.

- The hair shaft has regular intermittent constriction characterized by elliptical nodes separated by internodes. The thickness of swellings and constrictions and their spacing vary among patients.
- Regularly bended ribbon sign: Bending of the hair in different directions with breakage occurring at internode level.
- Black dots and broken hairs.
- The typical monilethrix hairs can sometimes be difficult to detect in the scalp and can only be found in eyebrows and eyelashes.

Trichorrhexis Invaginata (Bamboo Hair) (Figure 6.4)

Trichorrhexis invaginata, commonly referred to as "bamboo hair," is a rare hair shaft abnormality primarily observed in individuals with Netherton syndrome, an autosomal recessive genetic condition. The name "bamboo hair" describes the unique structural change of the hair shaft where one segment telescopes into another, closely resembling the nodes of a bamboo stick.

Dermoscopy

- The typical hair shaft abnormality affects only a few hairs and needs to be searched carefully.
- Hair shaft knots at irregular intervals, caused by the "ball-and-cup" hair shaft deformity, where the distal shaft is invaginated into the proximal shaft.
- Hair breakage mostly occurs in correspondence with the knots, and the broken ends have either a concave shape (golf-tea sign) or a round shape (matchstick sign).
- Broken hairs at different lengths, mostly occur in the scalp areas where friction occurs.

DOI: 10.1201/9780429351433-6

Trichothiodystrophy (Figure 6.5)

Trichothiodystrophy (TTD) is a very rare genetic disorder characterized by a "tiger tail" banding pattern consisting of alternating light and dark bands when the hair is examined under polarized light microscopy.

- Skin findings: Ichthyosis and photosensitivity.

Dermoscopy

- Dermoscopy helps to identify the hair shafts with abnormalities to be collected for polarized light microscopy analysis.
- Polarizing transilluminating dermoscopy could be an alternative to polarized light microscopy for diagnosis: It requires a dermoscope, a glass slide, and either a light source (such as the LED of a mobile phone) or a mirror.
- When using polarizing transilluminating dermoscopy, the characteristic feature of TTD, known as the "tiger tail" banding pattern, becomes visible.
- Procedure:

Method 1: A LED from a cellular phone is projected into a polarizing dermoscope to generate polarized light. The intensity of the light is adjusted using tissue paper. The hair sample with surface irregularities is clipped and placed on a glass slide. A second polarizing dermatoscope is used to view the hair sample under transillumination.

Method 2: The hair specimen is placed on a mirror. When a polarizing dermatoscope is used to view the specimen, polarized light reflects off the mirror, allowing transillumination of the target hairs.

Pili Torti (Figure 6.6)

Pili torti are characterized by the hair shaft being flattened at irregular intervals and twisted 180° along its long axis.

- Inherited pili torti are very rare and only seen in association with genetic syndromes, such as Menkes disease (ATP7A gene), Björnstad syndrome (BCS1L gene), and Bazex-Dupré-Christol syndrome (ACTRT1 gene). Clinical features depend on the associated syndrome.
- Pili torti are often seen as an associated finding in patients affected by other hair shaft abnormalities and even in the normal scalp.
- Acquired pili torti are common in scarring alopecia.

Dermoscopy

- The hair shaft is flat and twisted at various angles and at irregular intervals.
- Broken hairs at different lengths.

Pili Annulati (Figures 6.7, 6.8)

Pili annulati, also known as "ringed hair," is a hair shaft disorder which is rarely associated with fragility. The hair shaft is characterized by the presence of alternating light and dark bands, corresponding to air-filled cavities within the hair shafts, which cause an increased light reflex.

Dermoscopy

- The hair shaft presents multiple irregularly spaced fusiform well-defined whitish areas of different size within its length.
- These whitish alternating bands should be distinguished from the "intermittent medulla."

CONGENITAL HAIR SHAFT ABNORMALITIES WITHOUT HAIR FRAGILITY

Pili Trianguli and Canaliculi (Figure 6.9)

Pili trianguli and canaliculi, commonly known as uncombable hair syndrome or "spun glass hair syndrome," is a rare congenital hair shaft disorder. This condition is characterized by hair that is dry and unruly.

Dermoscopy

- Should be performed at high magnification after sectioning the hair shaft.

ACQUIRED WITH HAIR FRAGILITY

Trichorrhexis Nodosa (Figures 6.10–6.12)

Trichorrhexis nodosa (TN) is a common hair disorder characterized by the presence of nodes or weak points along the hair shaft where the hair tends to fracture.

Distal TN is related to weathering, and proximal TN is related to friction (see Chapter 1).

Very rarely, TN can be a consequence of very severe malnutrition.

Dermoscopy

- Multiple transparent white transversal areas within the hair shaft.
- At high magnification fraying of the inner hair shaft (cortex) is evident.
- Brush-like hair fracturing can be seen before complete breakage.
- The broken end of the shaft presents a frayed tip.
- Fragments obtained with the tug test show frayed tips.

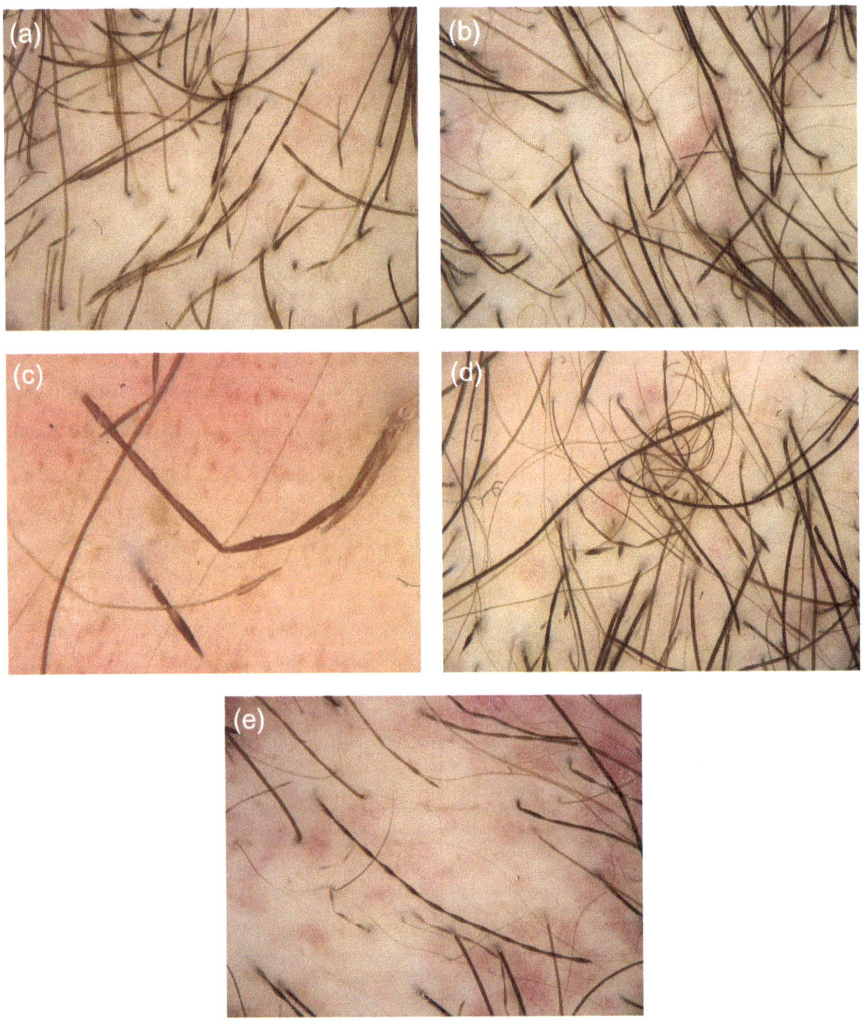

FIGURE 6.1 Monilethrix. ×20 The length and thickness of constrictions vary in the different shafts; note that breakage occurs at constriction level (a). ×20 The abnormality can affect a few hairs (b). ×50 Note the presence of the medulla at node level (c). ×20 Presence of small ovaloid hair fragments is common (d). ×20 Vellus hairs can also be affected (e).

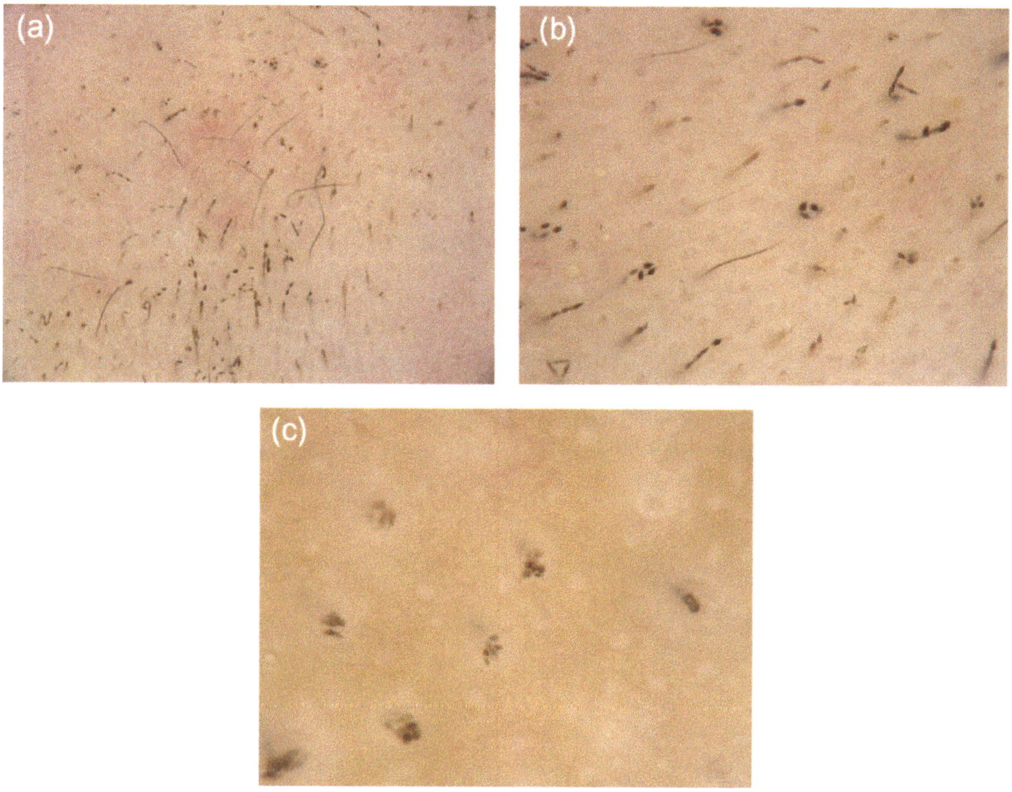

FIGURE 6.2 Monilethrix. ×20 Severe case with involvement of eyebrows (a). ×40–×70 At higher magnification the nodes may take the shape of flower petals (b,c).

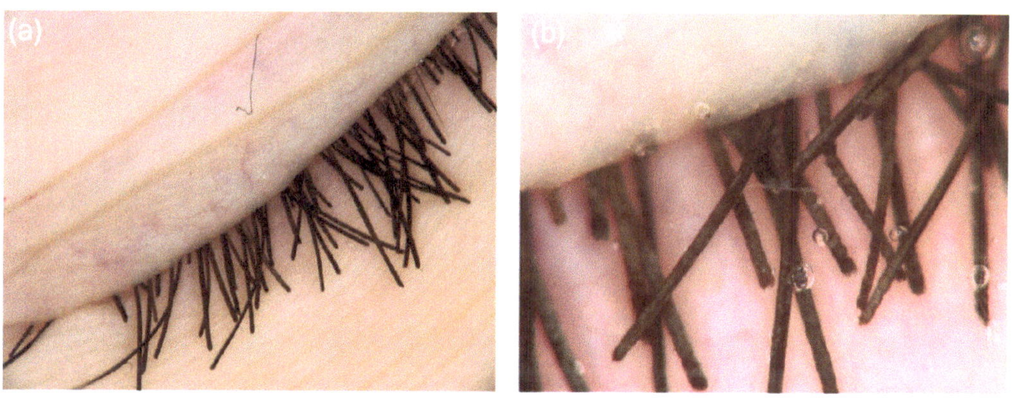

FIGURE 6.3 Monilethrix of the eyelashes. ×20 The lashes have a short length and broken tips (a). ×50 At higher magnification the abnormality is visible, but the constrictions are less evident since internodes have a reduced length (b).

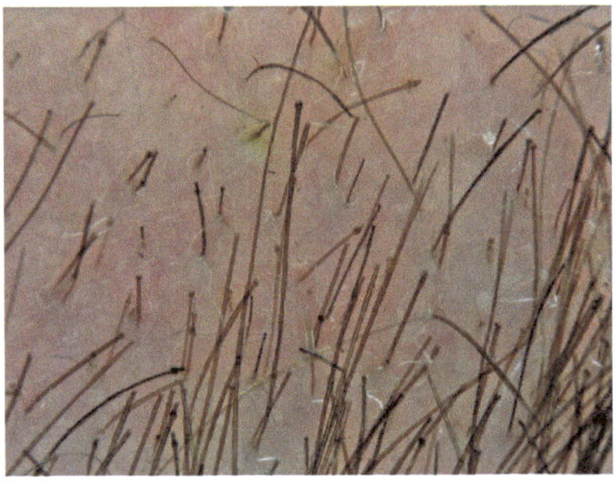

FIGURE 6.4 x20 Hairs presenting matchstick sign and golf-tea sign in trichorrhexis invaginata.

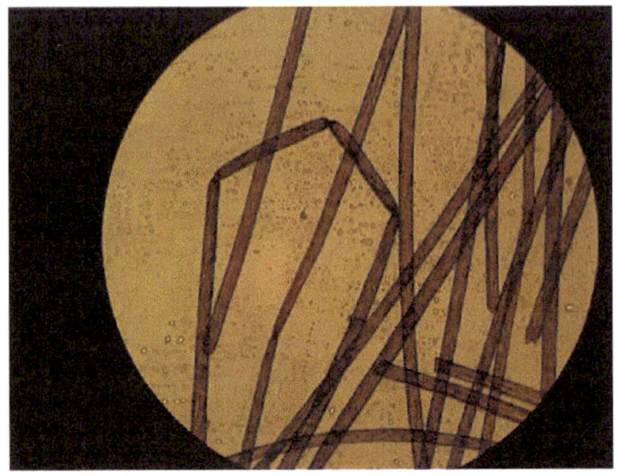

FIGURE 6.5 Trichothiodystrophy. ×40 Abnormal hair shaft that should be selected for polarized microscopic examination. (Courtesy of Dr. Mario Cutrone.)

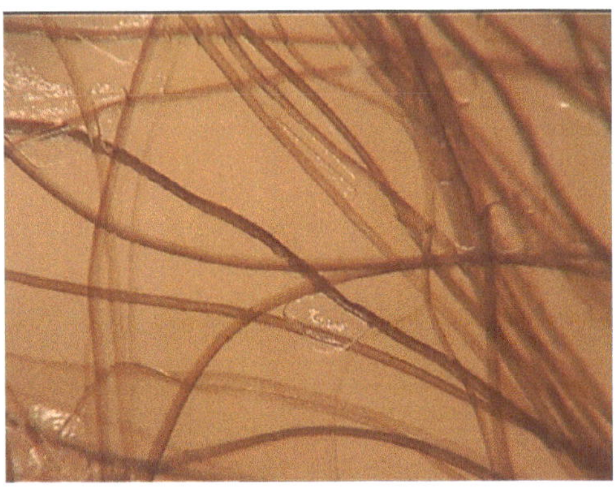

FIGURE 6.6 ×20 Pili torti in Bazex-Dupré-Christol syndrome.

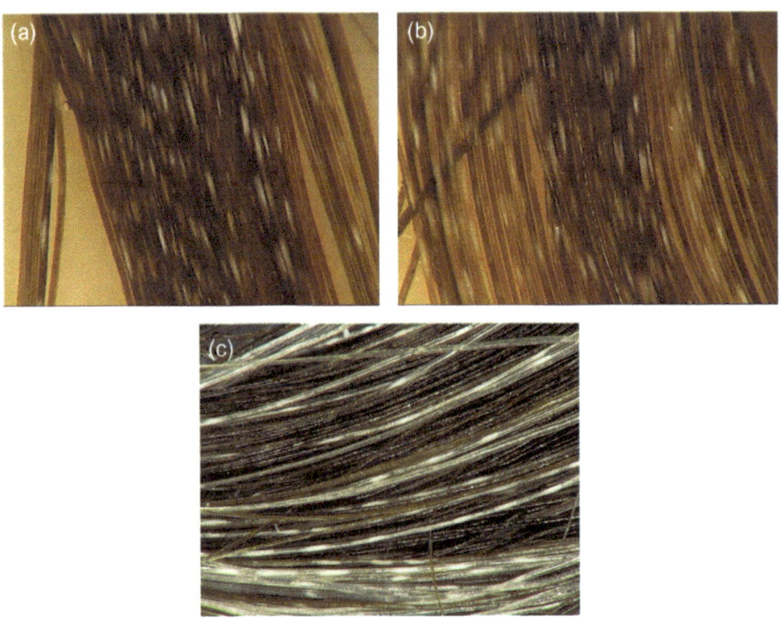

FIGURE 6.7 ×70 Fusiform whitish alternating bands typical of pili annulati (a); ×70 note the difference between the white bands of pili annulati and the hair shaft medulla (b); ×70 the abnormality is more evident in white hairs (c).

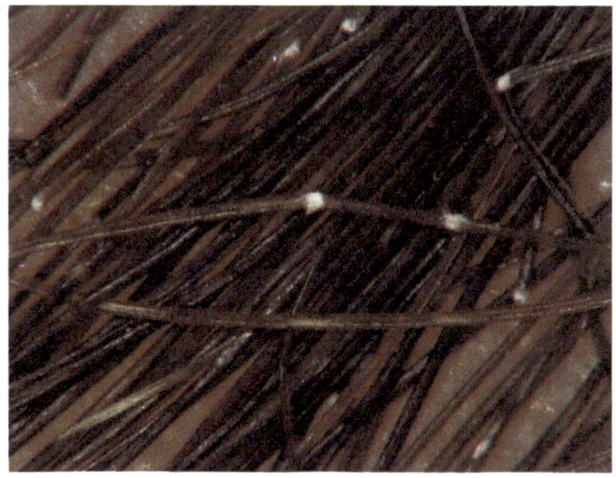

FIGURE 6.8 ×50 Pili annulati with trichorrhexis nodosa.

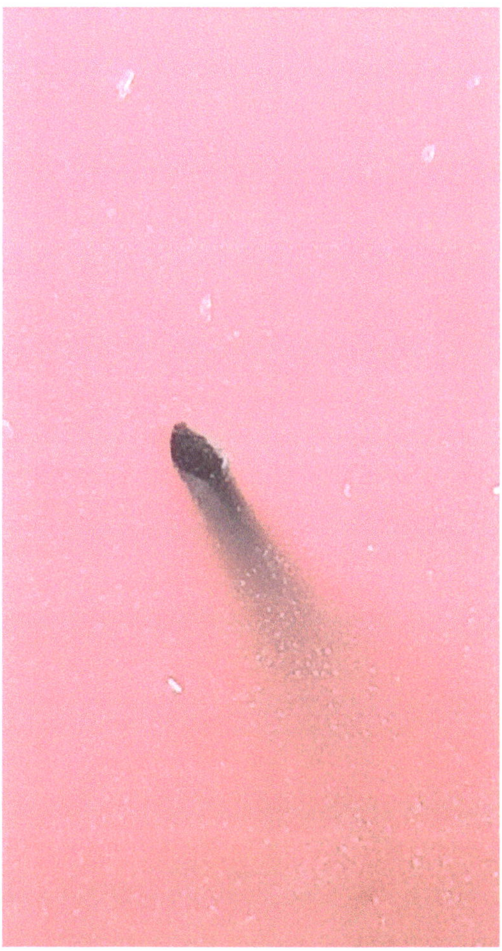

FIGURE 6.9 Pili trianguli and canaliculi. ×70 Note triangular shape of the hair shaft section. (Adapted from Sechi et al. Videodermoscopy as a diagnostic tool for pili trianguli and canaliculi syndrome. *Pediatr Dermatol*. 2024. doi: 10.1111/pde.15846, with permission.)

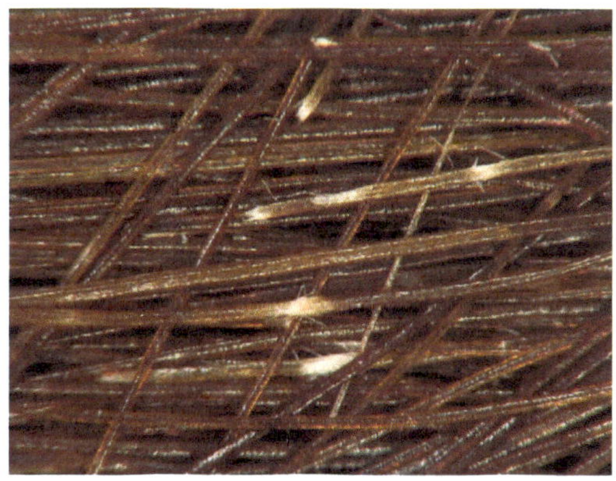

FIGURE 6.10 Trichorrexis nodosa. ×70 Multiple white areas of exposed frayed cortex along the shaft.

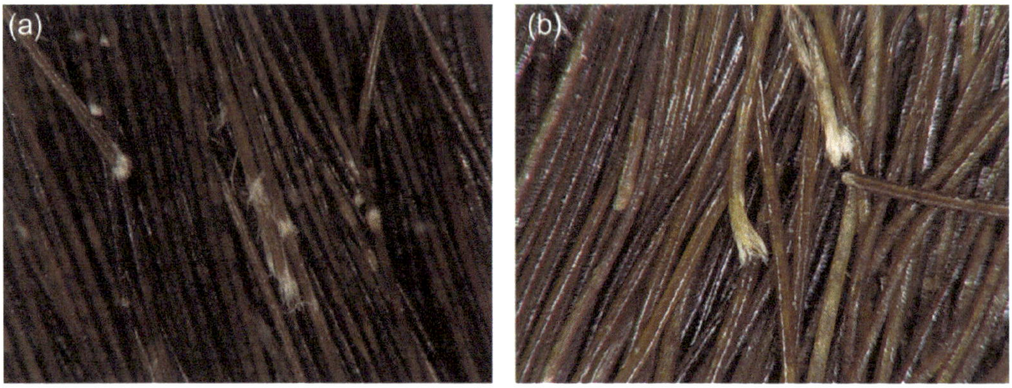

FIGURE 6.11 Trichorrhexis nodosa. ×40 Brush-like frayed tips (a); ×70 affected hairs are lighter in color (b).

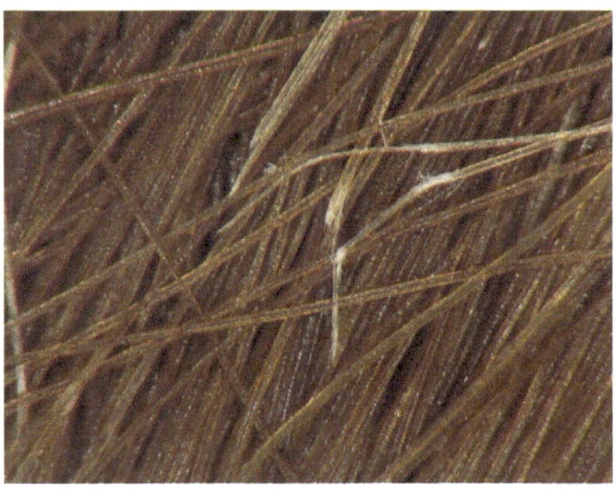

FIGURE 6.12 ×70 Trichorrhexis nodosa associated with distal disruption of the hair shaft and trichoptilosis.

SUGGESTED READING

Ahmed A, Almohanna H, Griggs J, Tosti A. Genetic hair disorders: a review. *Dermatol Ther.* 2019;9(3):421–48.

Burk C, Hu S, Lee C, Connelly EA. Netherton syndrome and trichorrhexis invaginata–a novel diagnostic approach. *Pediatr Dermatol.* 2008;25(2):287–8.

Gonzalez AM, Borda LJ, Tosti A. Pili Annulati with severe trichorrhexis nodosa: a case report and review of the literature. *Skin Appendage Disord.* 2019;5(2):114–16.

Lacarrubba F, Tosti A. Polarized transilluminating dermoscopy. *Pediatr Dermatol.* 2018;35(1):150–51.

Lencastre A, Tosti A. Monilethrix. *J Pediatr.* 2012;161(6):1176.

Lencastre A, Tosti A. Role of trichoscopy in children's scalp and hair disorders. *Pediatr Dermatol.* 2013;30(6):674–82.

Miteva M, Tosti A. Dermatoscopy of hair shaft disorders. *J Am Acad Dermatol.* 2013;68(3):473–81.

Rakowska A, Kowalska-Oledzka E, Slowinska M, Rosinska D, Rudnicka L. Hair shaft videodermoscopy in Netherton syndrome. *Pediatr Dermatol.* 2009;26(3):320–2.

Rakowska A, Slowinska M, Kowalska-Oledzka E, Rudnicka L. Trichoscopy in genetic hair shaft abnormalities. *J Dermatol Case Rep.* 2008;2(2):14–20.

Rudnicka L, Rakowska A, Kerzeja M, Olszewska M. Hair shafts in trichoscopy: clues for diagnosis of hair and scalp diseases. *Dermatol Clin.* 2013;31(4):695–708.

Silverberg NB, Silverberg JI, Wong ML. Trichoscopy using a handheld dermoscope: an in-office technique to diagnose genetic disease of the hair. *Arch Dermatol.* 2009;145(5):600–1.

Yang YW, Yarbrough K, Mitkov M, Russi D, Price HN, Swanson DL. Polarized transilluminating dermoscopy: bedside trichoscopic diagnosis of trichothiodystrophy. *Pediatr Dermatol.* 2018;35(1):147–49.

7 Pediatric Hair Disorders

APLASIA CUTIS CONGENITA (FIGURE 7.1)

Aplasia cutis congenita is a rare congenital condition characterized by the absence of a portion of skin at birth. This defect can vary in size, shape, and most commonly occurs on the scalp.

Dermoscopy

- Loss of follicular openings.
- Skin atrophy with a translucent appearance.
- Hair bulbs visible through the thin epidermis.
- In a typical case, these are arranged in a starburst pattern or as a golf club set.
- Telangiectatic vessels.
- In dark-skinned individuals, there is a disruption of the honeycomb pattern and loss of pinpoint white dots.

SEBACEOUS NEVUS (FIGURES 7.2–7.4)

Sebaceous nevus (SN) most commonly manifests on the scalp, particularly near the vertex or occipital regions.

- Infancy stage: In neonates and infants, SN typically presents as a smooth, hairless plaque.
- At puberty SN lesions can thicken and develop nodular or verrucous changes.
- Risk of various appendageal tumors (e.g., trichoblastoma, syringocystadenoma papilliferum, basal cell carcinoma) increases with age.

Dermoscopy

- Loss of follicular openings.
- Infant stage: Non-follicular bright yellow dots: Associated with sebaceous glands but do not correlate with follicular openings.
- Adult lesions: Cobblestone pattern with yellowish/orange globules due to sebaceous hyperplasia, or cerebriform pattern due to the epithelial hyperplasia and papillomatosis.
- Multiple brown globules can be seen in the cerebriform pattern in the pigmented scalp.
- In adults dermoscopy is useful to identify the development of possible neoplastic lesions.
- Linear, dotted vessels are frequently associated with SN; arborizing vessels should raise the concern for the growth of basal cell carcinoma within the SN, especially when associated with blue-gray globules.

CONGENITAL TRIANGULAR ALOPECIA (FIGURE 7.5)

Congenital triangular alopecia is a non-scarring hair loss condition that primarily affects the temporal region of the scalp.

Dermoscopy

- The patch is not bald but contains numerous vellus hairs (carpet of vellus hairs).
- Vellus hairs may vary in length and may have a white color.

DOI: 10.1201/9780429351433-7

- Dermoscopy helps to easily differentiate it from alopecia areata due to the lack of black dots, exclamation mark hairs, or broken hairs.

LOOSE ANAGEN HAIR SYNDROME (FIGURES 7.6–7.8)

Loose anagen hair syndrome is a hair disorder characterized by the premature shedding of hair in the anagen phase due to a defective attachment of the hair shaft to the follicle.

Dermoscopy

- Rectangular granular structures: Pigmented structures with a rectangular shape in the interfollicular scalp. Usually not numerous, need to be searched for.
- Broken hairs with a pigmented tip.
- Anagen roots: Can occasionally be seen on the scalp surface.
- Dermoscopy can be utilized to confirm diagnosis on plucked hairs, showing anagen roots without sheaths with a raffled cuticle (see Chapter 15).

SHORT ANAGEN SYNDROME

Short anagen syndrome is characterized by a shortening of the anagen phase of the hair cycle, leading to the inability of the hair to reach a normal length.

Dermoscopy

- Dermoscopy can be utilized to confirm diagnosis on hairs extracted with the pull test to show that the short hairs have not been cut (see Chapter 15).

KERATOSIS FOLLICULARIS SPINULOSA DECALVANS (FIGURE 7.9)

Keratosis follicularis spinulosa decalvans is a rare, X-linked or autosomal dominant disorder characterized by keratosis pilaris and progressive scarring alopecia primarily affecting the scalp, eyebrows, and eyelashes.

Dermoscopy

- Overall features might resemble lichen planopilaris/folliculitis decalvans.
- Loss of follicular openings.
- Peripilar casts surrounding the emergences of the hair shafts, often associated with hair tufting.
- Follicular papules and pustules with crusting and exudation.
- Encircling tubular scales around the hair shaft of terminal hairs.
- Diffuse interfollicular erythema and scaling.
- Elongated linear or twisted vessels.
- Broken hairs and black dots.

PERIPILAR KERATIN CASTS (FIGURE 7.10)

A rare condition reported in children, mostly girls. Multiple elongated whitish structures surround the hair shafts at multiple levels from scalp to tips.

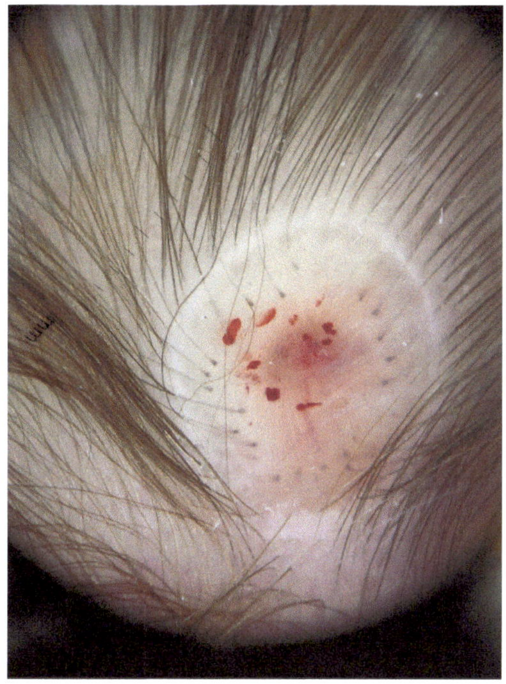

FIGURE 7.1 ×10 Anagen roots arranged in a starburst pattern and loss of follicular openings in aplasia cutis. (Courtesy of Dr. Mario Cutrone.)

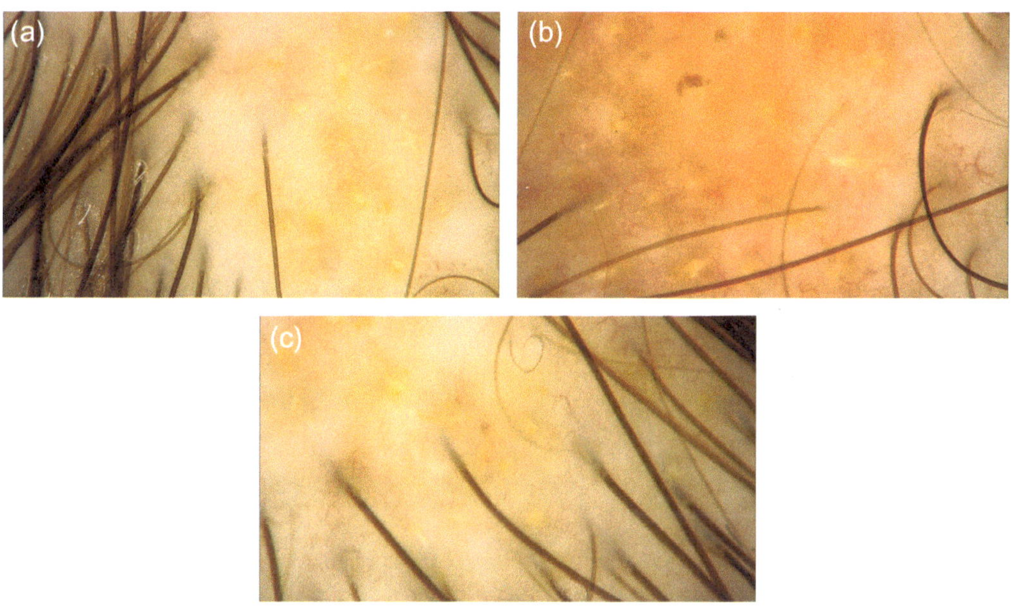

FIGURE 7.2 Sebaceous nevus in children. ×40 Bright yellow dots not corresponding with follicular opening (a); ×70 note irregular shape and size (b,c).

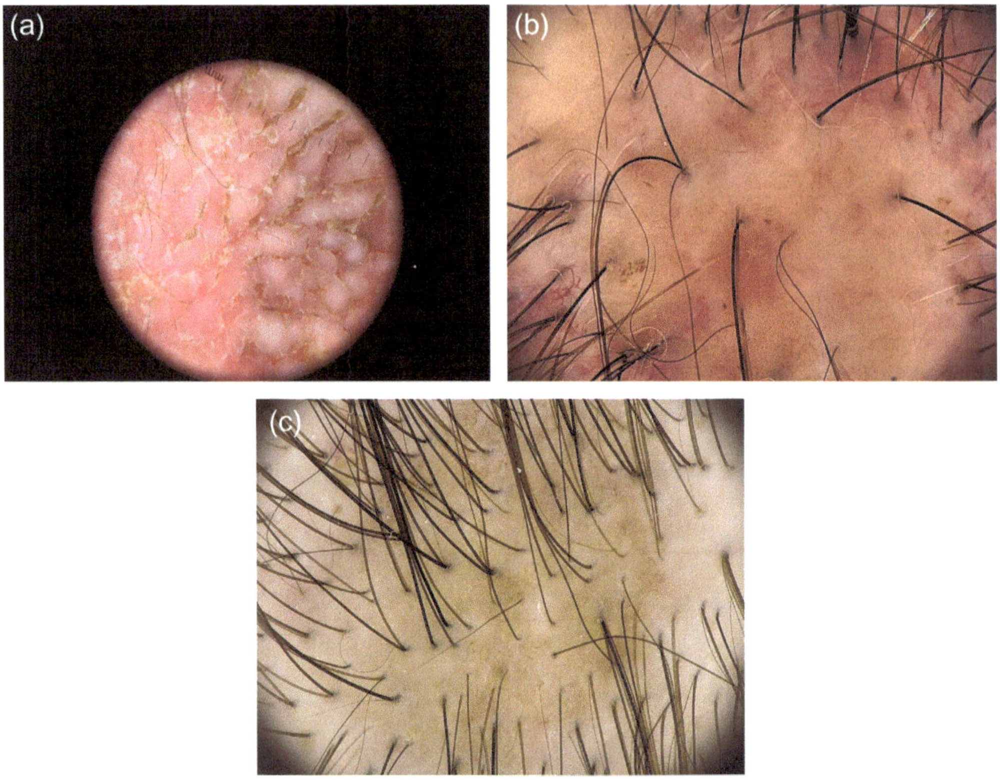

FIGURE 7.3 Sebaceous nevus in adults. ×10 Cerebriform pattern (a) (Courtesy of Dr. Mario Cutrone); ×20 cobblestone pattern (b,c).

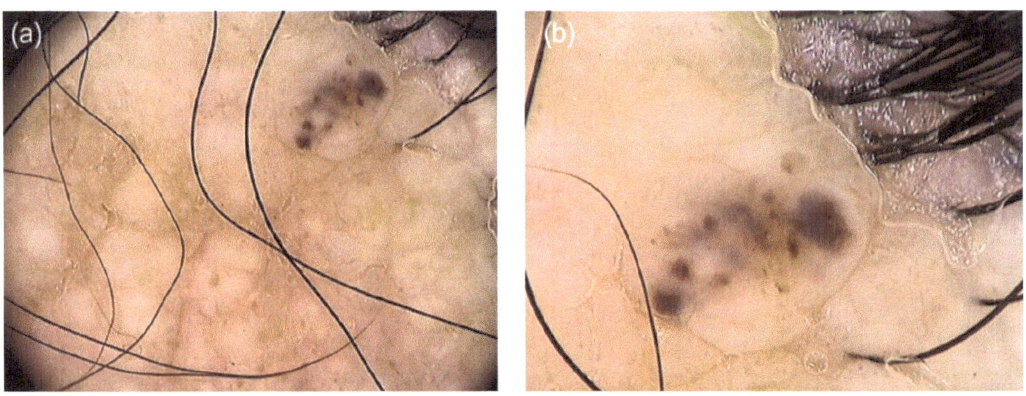

FIGURE 7.4 Basal cell carcinoma on a sebaceous nevus. ×20 (a); ×50 (b).

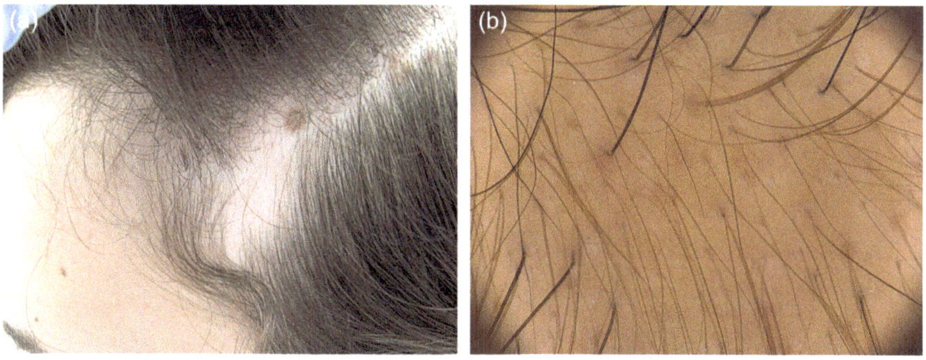

FIGURE 7.5 Triangular alopecia (a); ×20 carpet of vellus hairs of different length (b).

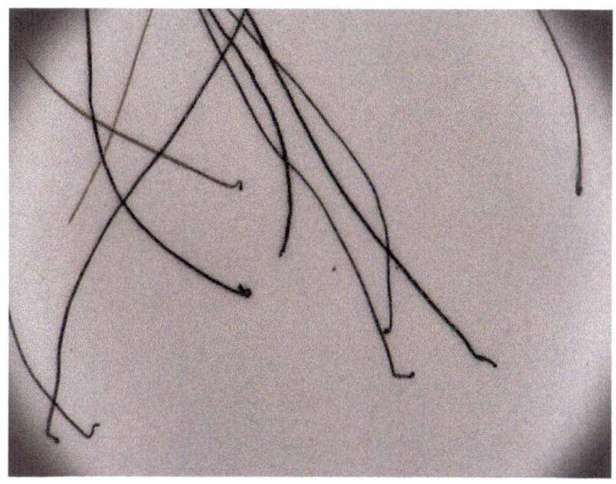

FIGURE 7.6 Loose anagen hair syndrome. ×20 Trichogram showing anagen hairs with absence of sheaths and misshaped anagen bulbs.

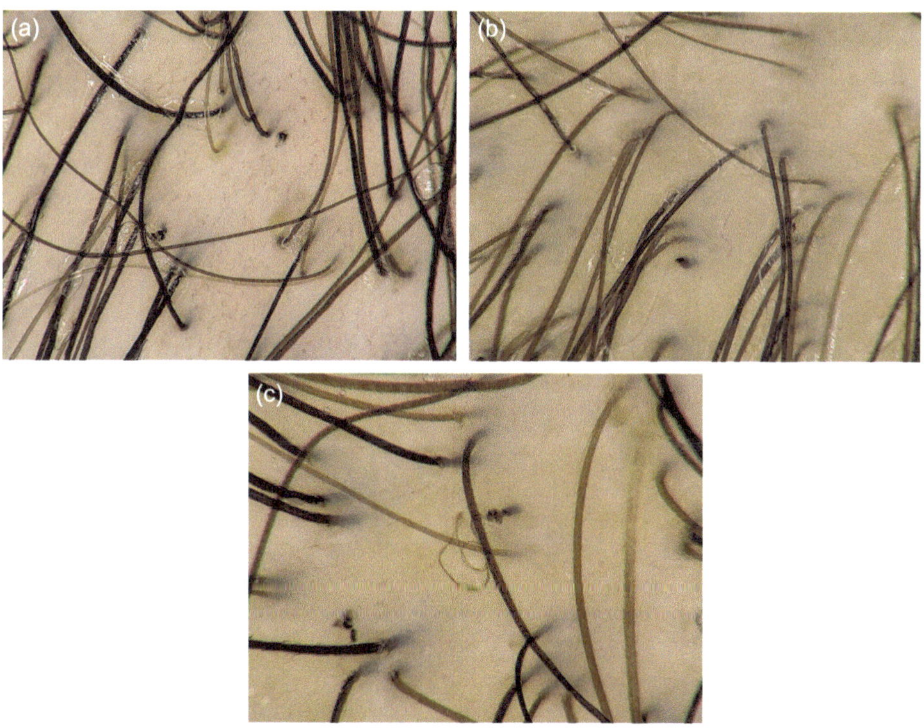

FIGURE 7.7 Loose anagen hair syndrome x20 (a,b). ×50 Rectangular structures found in the interfollicular scalp (a,b,c).

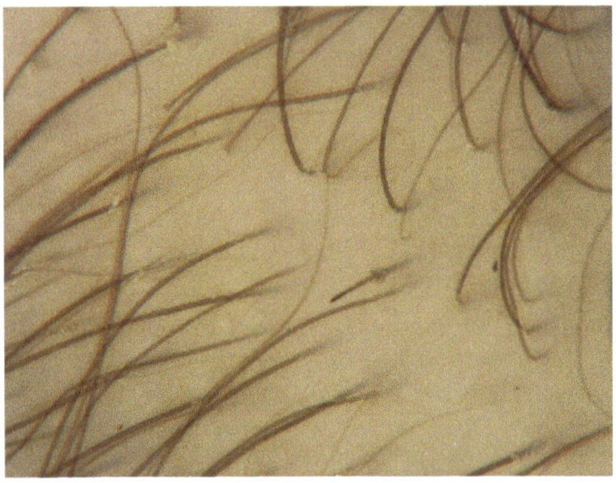

FIGURE 7.8 Loose anagen hair syndrome. ×20 Broken hair and rectangular structure.

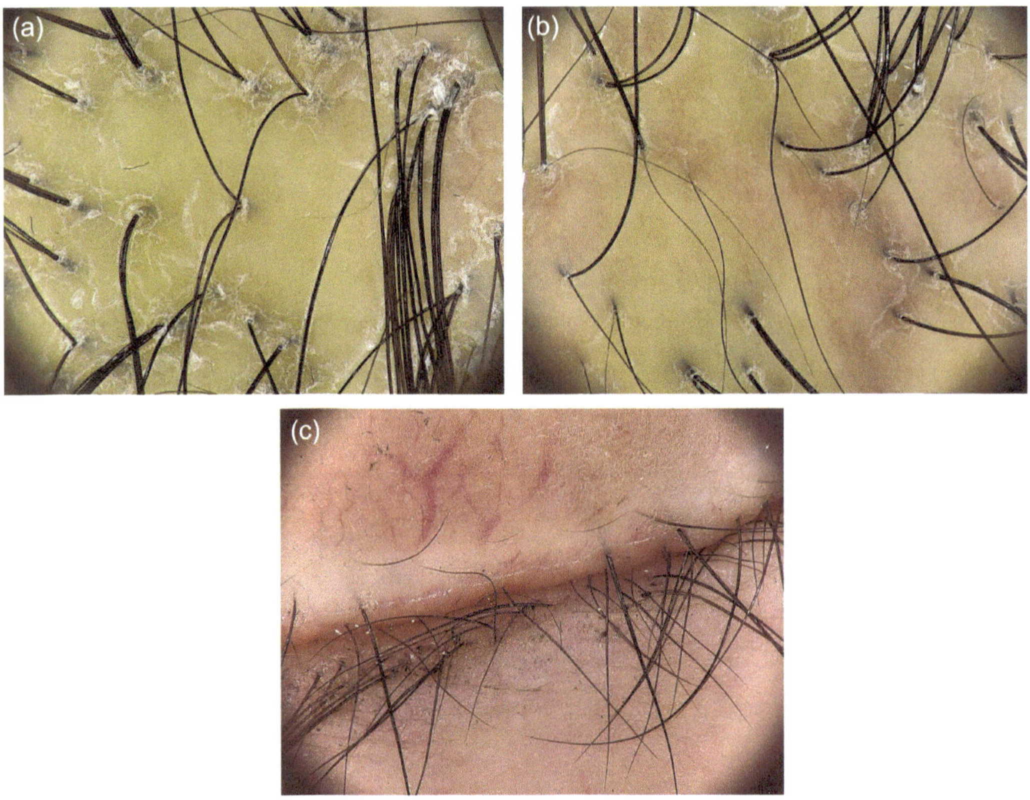

FIGURE 7.9 KFSD. ×20 Loss of follicular openings, peripilar cast, and hair tufting (a); ×20 also note diffuse erythema and elongated and twisted vessels (b); ×50 involvement of eyelashes with peripilar casts and atrichia with loss of follicular openings (c).

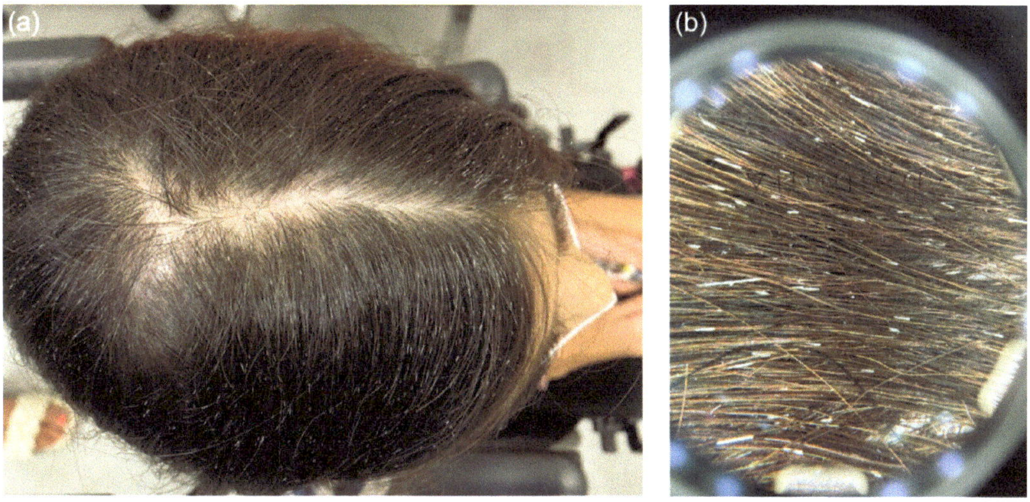

FIGURE 7.10 Peripilar keratin casts (a); ×10 encircling tubular casts of different length irregularly distributed along each shaft (b).

SUGGESTED READING

Alessandrini A, Brattoli G, Piraccini BM, Di Altobrando A, Starace M. The role of trichoscopy in keratosis follicularis spinulosa decalvans: case report and review of the literature. *Skin Appendage Disord.* 2021;7:29–35.

Iorizzo M, Pazzaglia M, Starace M, Militello G, Tosti A. Videodermoscopy: a useful tool for diagnosing congenital triangular alopecia. *Pediatr Dermatol.* 2008;25(6):652–4.

Lacarrubba F, Micali G. Congenital triangular alopecia. *BMJ Case Rep.* 2014:bcr2013202918.

Lencastre A, Tosti A. Role of trichoscopy in children's scalp and hair disorders. Pediatr Dermatol. 2013;30(6):674–82.

Neri I, Savoia F, Giacomini F, Raone B, Aprile S, Patrizi A. Usefulness of dermatoscopy for the early diagnosis of sebaceous naevus and differentiation from aplasia cutis congenita. *Clin Exp Dermatol.* 2009;34(5):e50–2.

Oberlin KE, Maddy AJ, Martínez-Velasco MA, Vázquez-Herrera NE, Schachner LA, Tosti A. Short anagen syndrome: case series and literature review. *Pediatr Dermatol.* 2018;35(3):388–91.

Rakowska A, Zadurska M, Czuwara J, Warszawik-Hendzel O, Kurzeja M, Maj M, Olszewska M, Rudnicka L. Trichoscopy findings in loose anagen hair syndrome: rectangular granular structures and solitary yellow dots. *J Dermatol Case Rep.* 2015;9(1):1–5.

Verzì AE, Lacarrubba F, Micali G. Starburst hair follicles: a dermoscopic clue for aplasia cutis congenita. *J Am Acad Dermatol.* 2016;75(4):e141–e142.

8 Dermoscopy of the Black Scalp

- Trichoscopic examination of dark-skinned scalps reveals a variation in the scalp skin tone, ranging from light brown to dark black, which may not necessarily correlate with the individual's skin tone in exposed skin areas.
- Hair density in the African scalp is lower as compared to Caucasians and Asians, the hair shaft diameter is larger, and the shaft is flat in shape. Hairs usually emerge in groups of two from the scalp.
- The African scalp often presents scales and residues of styling products.
- A characteristic pigmented network known as honeycomb pattern consists of pigmented lines (rete ridge melanocytes) surrounding hypochromic areas (suprapapillary epidermis containing fewer melanocytes).
- Accentuation of the pigmented network is common around the follicular openings. The presence of a fingertip pattern with hypopigmented asterisk-like macules can be observed in the sun-exposed scalp.
- A distinctive feature of the pigmented scalp is the presence of pinpoint white dots.
- Pinpoint white dots are small (0.2- to 0.3-mm) white dots that are regularly distributed between hair emergences and correspond to sweat glands and follicular openings.
- The number of pinpoint white dots increases both in non-scarring and primary scarring alopecias (except for discoid lupus erythematosus), and the scalp has a starry-sky appearance.
- Absence of follicular openings is not evident in the pigmented scalp, because of the presence of pinpoint white dots. This makes the differentiation between scarring and non-scarring alopecia difficult.
- In non-scarring alopecias, pinpoint white dots are regularly distributed, and often contain miniaturized or broken hair shafts.
- In scarring alopecias pinpoint white dots have an irregular distribution and are often interspersed with irregular white patches (follicular scars).
- Co-occurrence of multiple hair disorders in a single patient is common in patients of African descent, and dermoscopy plays a crucial role in aiding clinicians by revealing distinct characteristics of each condition.

DERMOSCOPY

Non-Scarring: Regular Pinpoint White Dots Often Containing Miniaturized or Broken Hair Shafts (Figure 8.1)

- Androgenetic alopecia (male and female pattern hair loss)
- Alopecia areata
- Trichotillomania
- Traction alopecia (non-scarring phase)
- Dissecting cellulitis (non-scarring phase)

Scarring: Irregular Pinpoint White Dots and Irregular White Patches (Follicular Scars)

- Traction alopecia (scarring phase)
- Dissecting cellulitis (scarring phase)
- Central centrifugal cicatricial alopecia
- Lichen planopilaris
- Frontal fibrosing alopecia
- Folliculitis decalvans
- Acne keloidalis nuchae

DOI: 10.1201/9780429351433-8

Scarring: Loss of Pigmented Network and Loss of Pinpoint White Dots

- Discoid lupus erythematosus

Hair Shaft

- Hair breakage common in patients of African descent

NON-SCARRING ALOPECIAS

Androgenetic Alopecia (AGA) (Figure 8.2)

- Differential diagnosis with early central centrifugal cicatricial alopecia may be difficult.

Dermoscopy

- Hair shaft variability: More than 20% hair shaft variability is diagnostic.
- Presence of short, thin (0.03 mm in diameter) regrowing hairs in the frontal scalp.
- Yellow dots and empty follicles might not be visible.
- Preservation of honeycomb pattern.
- Regularly distributed pinpoint white dots.
- Peripilar sign: The peripilar sign has often a brown hue.

Alopecia Areata (Figures 8.3, 8.4)

Dermoscopy

- Preservation of the honeycomb-like pigment network.
- Regularly distributed pinpoint white dots.
- Exclamation mark hairs, broken hairs, and black dots are usually found within pinpoint white dots.
- Numerous circle hairs are a common finding.
- Yellow dots are barely detected.

Trichotillomania

Dermoscopy (See Chapter 4)

- Question mark hairs (coiled hair)
- Broken hairs of varying lengths
- Short split hairs (hamburger sign)
- Black dots
- Flame hairs, which have a frayed end resembling a flame
- Preserved honeycomb-like pigmented network
- Regularly arranged pinpoint white dots
- Detection of hair powder, which are fine particles of broken hair shafts

Traction Alopecia (TA) (Figure 8.5)

A biphasic form of hair loss that is directly related to the mechanical stress on hair follicles.

Dermoscopy

- Preservation of the honeycomb pattern and pinpoint white dots.
- Perifollicular papules and pustules.
- Perifollicular and interfollicular erythema.
- Broken hairs: Are generally few and should be searched.
- Black dots: Correspond to hair breakage at the scalp level.
- Persistence of miniaturized and vellus hairs: Their presence is more noticeable if the terminal hairs are lost due to traction.
- Linear orientation of hair emergences with whitish linear halo (Flambeau's sign).
- Tubular casts: A very important clue to detect ongoing traction is the presence of tubular structures encircling the hair shafts in the scalp surrounding the area of traction. They are freely mobile, nonadherent, and can be seen along the length of the hairs. Their number is related to the severity of traction.

SCARRING ALOPECIAS

Traction Alopecia—Scarring Phase (Figure 8.6)

Interfollicular Patterns

- Preservation of the pigmented network

- Irregular pinpoint white dots
- Scalp erythema
- Reduced hair density with persistence of vellus hairs

Dissecting Cellulitis of the Scalp—Scarring Phase

Dermoscopy

- Polytrichia: Multiple hairs emerging from a single follicle
- White patches/structureless white areas: Inter/perifollicular scalp fibrosis
- Hair tufts emerging from skin clefts
- Pili torti, irregularly shaped and twisted hair shafts

In dissecting cellulitis, trichoscopic features of advanced keloidal phase can often coexist with active phase trichoscopic findings.

Central Centrifugal Cicatricial Alopecia (CCCA) (Figures 8.7–8.9)

Central centrifugal cicatricial alopecia is a lymphocytic primary scarring alopecia that affects the central scalp and extends centrifugally

A genetic linkage with PADI3 mutations, which is also seen for pili trianguli and canaliculi, has been reported.

Dermoscopy

- Irregularly distributed pinpoint white dots and white patches.
- Peripilar white-gray halos: The follicular ostia are encircled by round white-gray halo surrounding either a single hair or a group of two–three hairs.
- Broken hairs and black dots are rarely found in active disease, mainly at the border of the alopecic patches.
- Hair shaft diameter variability.
- Patchy interfollicular erythema.

Early CCCA may be difficult to distinguish from androgenetic alopecia on clinical and dermoscopic grounds.

CCCA and TA are commonly associated.

CCCA can be distinguished from lichen planopilaris (or fibrosing alopecia in a pattern distribution) due to the lack of peripilar casts and tufting.

Lichen Planopilaris (Figure 8.10)

Dermoscopy

- Preservation of the honeycomb pattern.
- Irregular distributed pinpoint white dots and white patches; in frontal fibrosing alopecia (FFA) the pinpoint white dots can be regularly distributed and scarring not be so evident.
- Peripilar cast, usually surrounding a tuft of two terminal hairs emerging together.
- Hair tufting.
- Encircling tubular structures.
- Broken hairs and black dots (few).
- Pili torti (few).
- Blue-gray dots with an annular or "target" pattern, located on the area where previous viable follicles have been destroyed by the disease; correspond to melanin particles within melanophages or free on the papillary dermis.
- Scalp erythema can be subtle.
- Interfollicular scales are common.

Frontal Fibrosing Alopecia (Figures 8.11–8.13)

- FFA is often associated with lichen planus pigmentosus in patients of color.
- FFA is often found concurrently with traction alopecia in women of African descent.

Dermoscopy

- Absence of vellus hairs in the receding hairline is a very important clue to distinguish FFA from traction.
- Peripilar casts, which range from subtle to very prominent.
- Transparent emergences of the proximal hair shafts in the temporal/occipital scalp.
- Black dots (sparse).
- Broken hairs (sparse).
- Pili torti (sparse).

- Pinpoint white dots might not look irregularly distributed and white patches might or might not be present.

Lichen Pigmentosus

- Pseudo-reticular pigmentary network, dotted pattern, speckled blue-gray dots, and blue-gray dots arranged in circles.

Folliculitis Decalvans (see Chapter 5)

Acne Keloidalis Nuchae (AKN) (Figure 8.14)

AKN is a mixed lymphocytic and neutrophilic primary scarring alopecia that affects the occipital scalp and posterior neck of young men of African or Hispanic descent. Shaving is considered a main factor for the development of the disease.

Dermoscopy

- Perifollicular erythema, perifollicular scaling, follicular papules/pustules with embedded hairs
- White halos surrounding the emergence of hair shafts due to fibrosis
- Hair tufting with peripilar casts
- Keloidal scars with loss of pigmented network and irregular pinpoint white dots with white patches

Discoid Lupus Erythematosus (DLE) (Figures 8.15, 8.16)

- Discoid lupus erythematosus is more prevalent in patients of African descent.
- Both hypo- and hyperpigmentation are pronounced.

Dermoscopy

- Disruption of the pigmented network and disappearance of the pinpoint white dots are a unique feature of DLE.
- Loss of honeycomb pattern in the affected scalp.
- Almost complete disappearance of pinpoint white dots in affected scalp.
- Patches of melanic heterogeneous staining in the scalp surrounding and within the hypopigmented patches.
- Enlarged tortuous vessels that are thicker than the hair shafts are typical.
- Peri- and interfollicular erythema and scaling can be a prominent feature.
- Keratotic follicular plugs.
- Follicular red dots.
- Peripilar casts.
- Peri- and interfollicular speckled blue-gray dots: Resulting from pigment incontinence involving both the hair follicle and interfollicular epidermis due to basal layer damage.

HAIR BREAKAGE (FIGURE 8.17)

- Hair breakage is particularly common in individuals of African descent due to the natural fragility of African hair.
- The tug test is positive and dermoscopy is useful to evaluate the hair fragments.

Dermoscopy of hair fragments extracted with the tug test shows:

- Trichorrhexis nodosa with brush-like ends
- Longitudinal splitting within the hair length
- Hair knots
- Split ends (trichoptilosis)

Dermoscopy of the hair shaft tips shows:

- Trichorrhexis nodosa and trichoptilosis

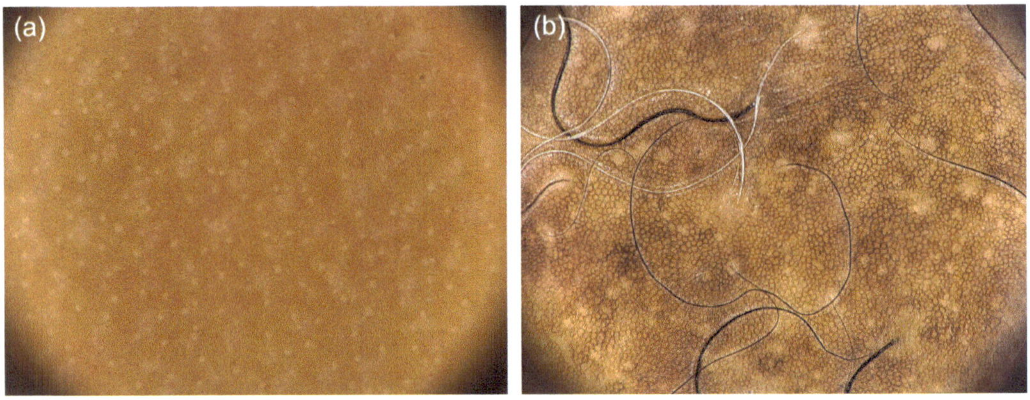

FIGURE 8.1 ×20 Non-scarring alopecia showing regularly distributed pinpoint white dots (a); ×20 scarring alopecia showing irregularly distributed pinpoint white dots and white patches (b).

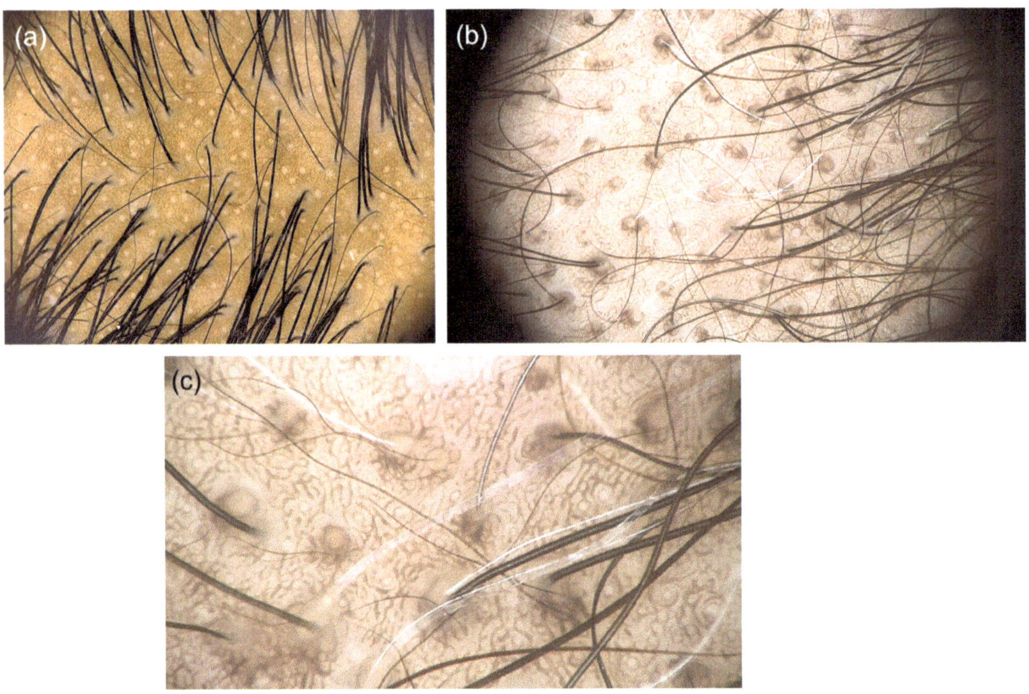

FIGURE 8.2 AGA ×20 Hair shaft variability (a); ×20 note accentuation of the pigmented network around the follicular openings (b); ×50 (c).

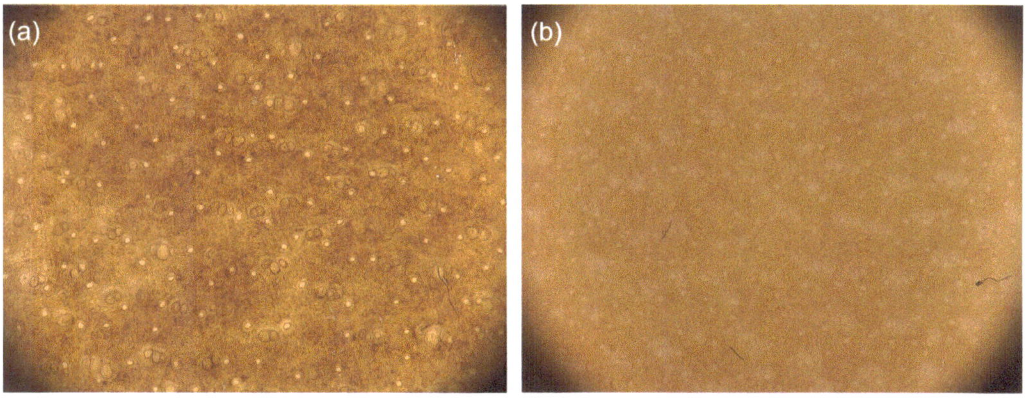

FIGURE 8.3 (a) ×20; (b) ×40: Regularly distributed pinpoint white dots in alopecia totalis.

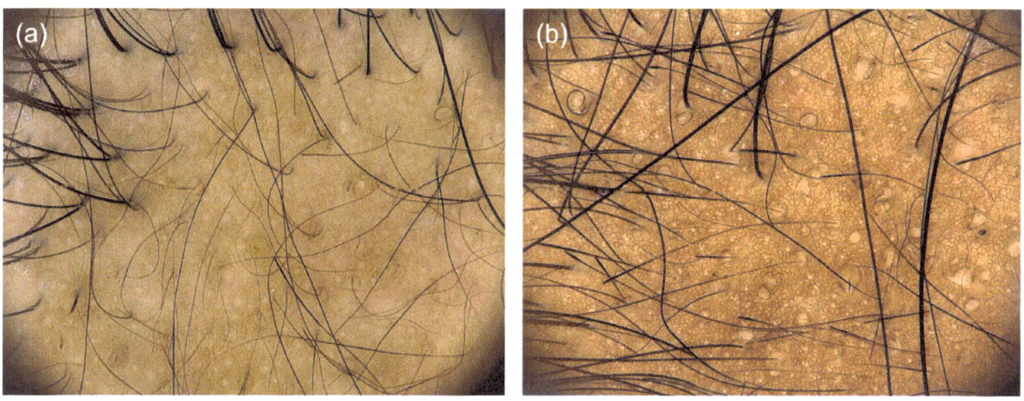

FIGURE 8.4 Alopecia areata. ×20 Broken hairs (a); and pigtail and exclamation mark hairs (b).

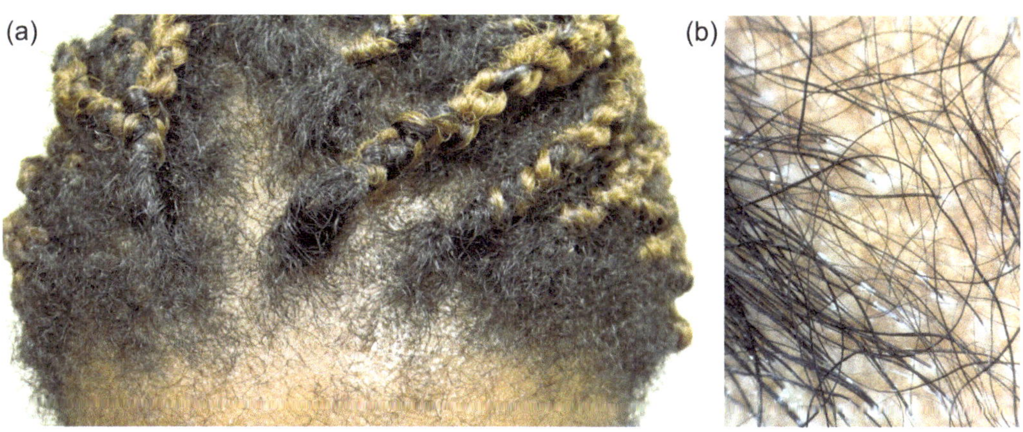

FIGURE 8.5 Marginal traction alopecia (a); ×20 tubular structure encircling the shafts surrounding the patch (b).

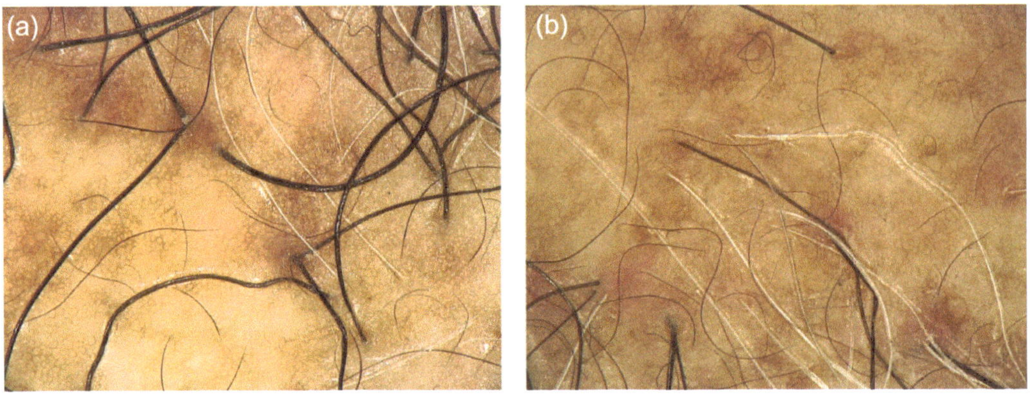

FIGURE 8.6 (a,b) Traction alopecia scarring phase. ×50 Reduced density, increased number of vellus hairs, and scalp erythema.

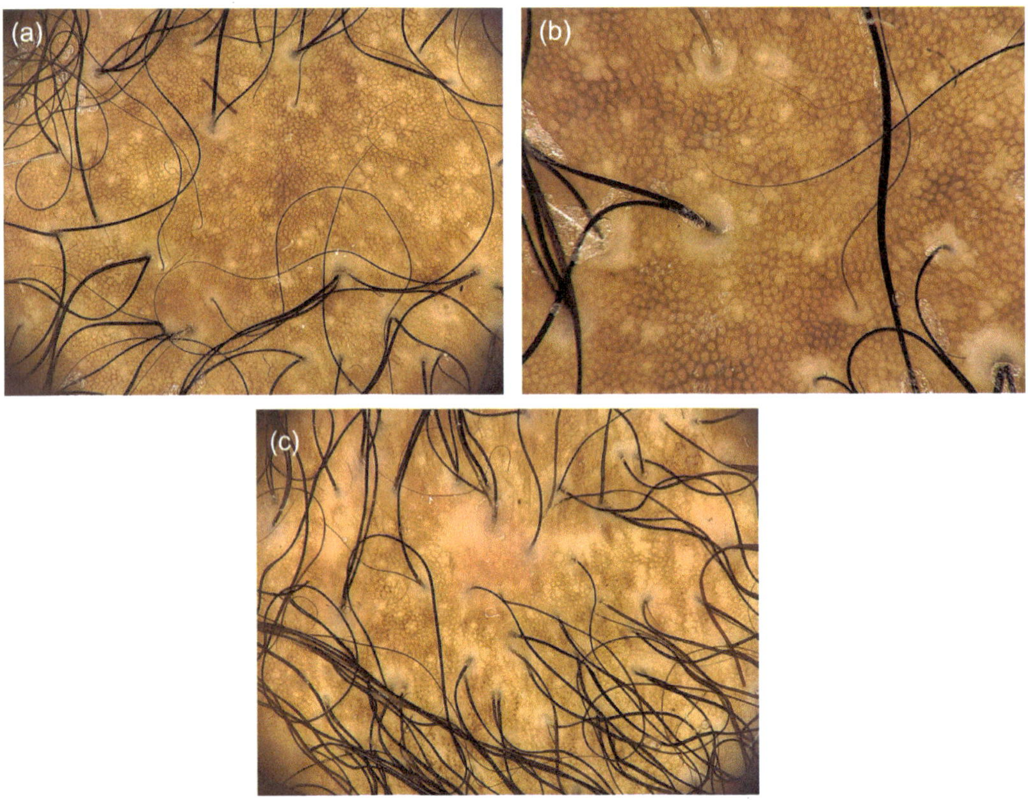

FIGURE 8.7 CCCA. ×20 Alopecic patch with irregular distributed pinpoint white dots, and peripilar gray-white halos (a); ×50 peripilar gray-white halos surrounding the follicular openings, that are often composed of two hairs (b); ×40 also note erythema and whitish patches (c).

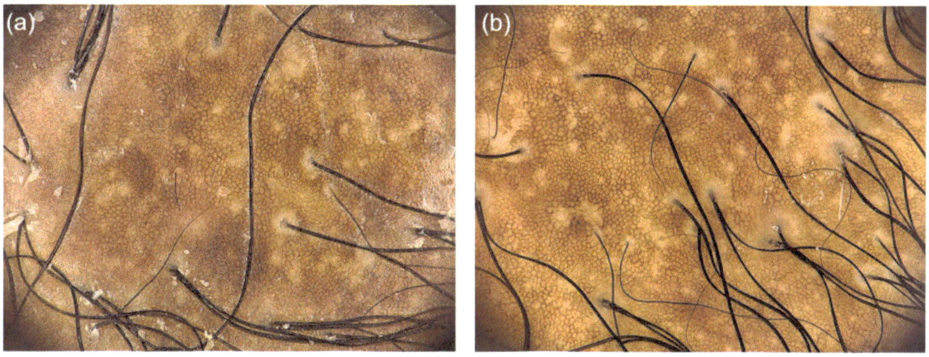

FIGURE 8.8 CCCA. ×20 Preservation of the honeycomb pattern, irregularly distributed pinpoint white dots, and gray-white halos (a); ×50 higher magnification of the gray-white halo (b).

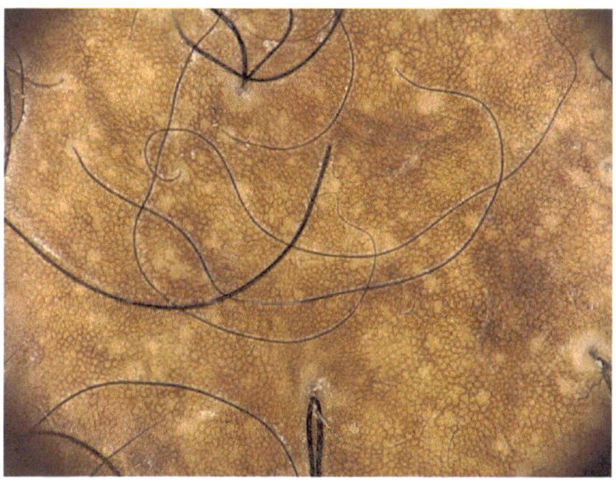

FIGURE 8.9 CCCA. ×20 Gray-white halos and asterisk-like hypopigmented macules.

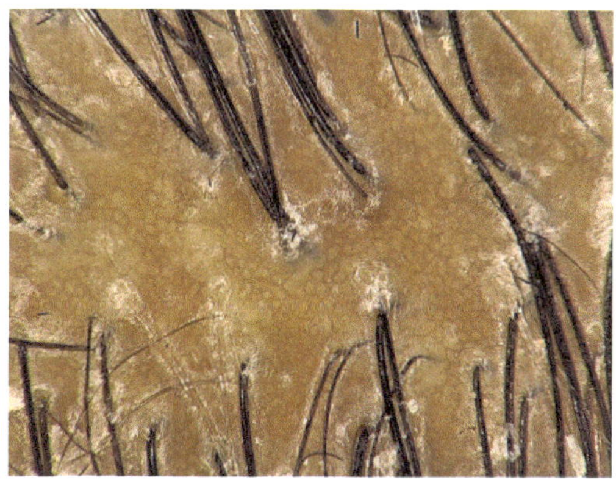

FIGURE 8.10 ×50 Peripilar casts and hair tufting in lichen planopilaris/fibrosing alopecia in a pattern distribution.

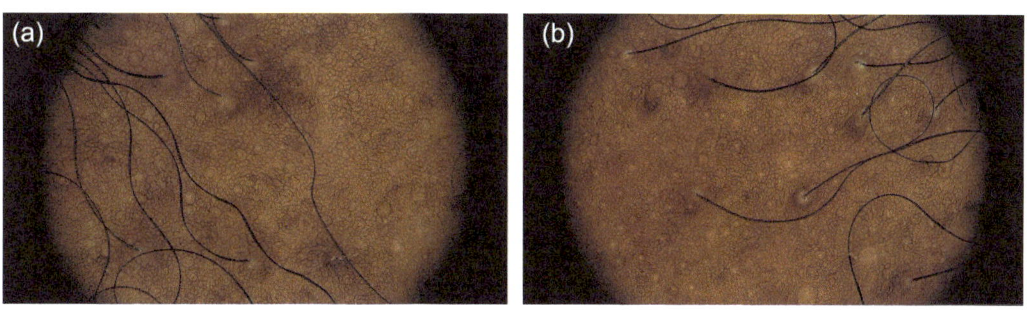

FIGURE 8.11 ×50 Frontal fibrosing alopecia on the hairline, showing loss of vellus hairs and peripilar casts (a,b). Note that pinpoint white dots are regularly distributed and there are not white patches.

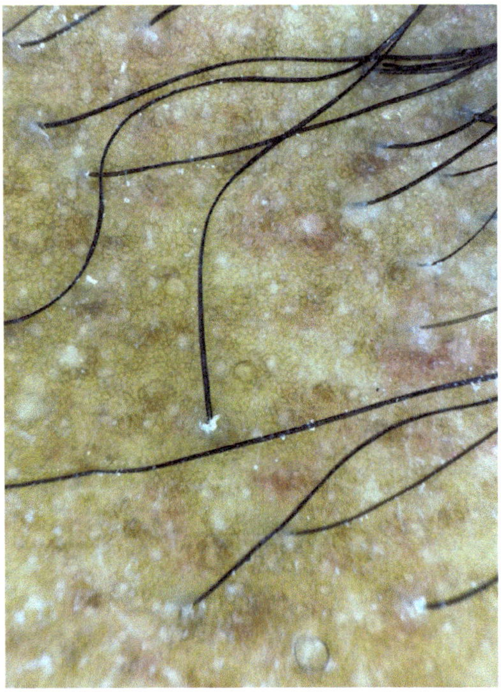

FIGURE 8.12 FFA. ×20 loss of vellus hair, irregularly distributed pinpoint white dots, erythema, and peripilar casts.

FIGURE 8.13 ×20 Lichen planus pigmentosus: Pseudo-reticular pigmentary network.

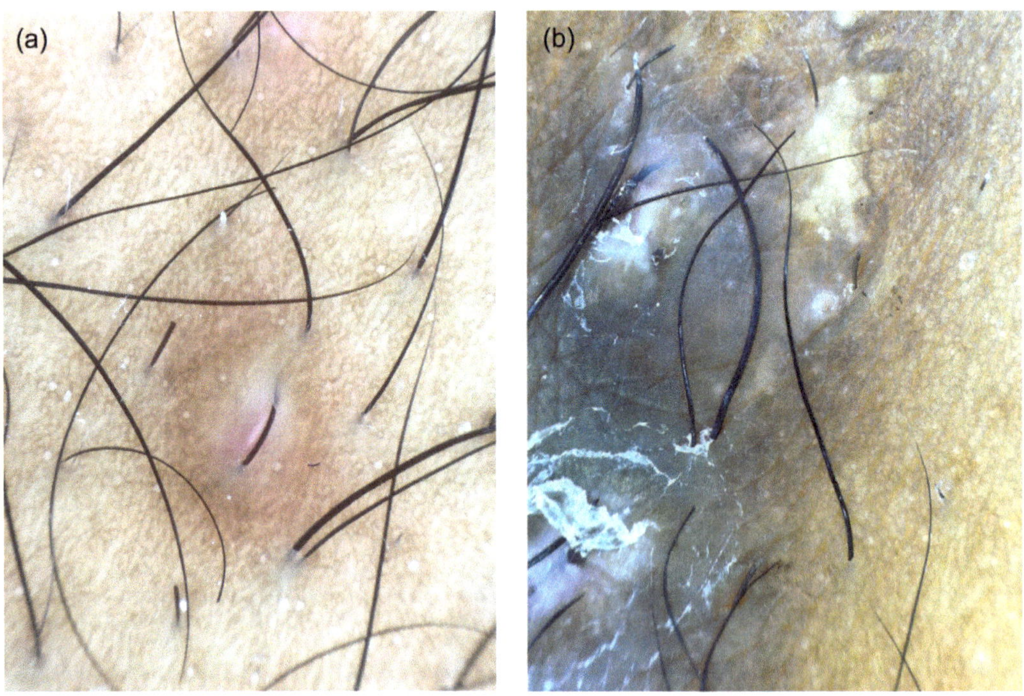

FIGURE 8.14 Acne keloidalis nuchae. ×20 Pseudo folliculitis with extra follicular penetration and erythema in early disease (a); ×20 extra follicular penetration and white patch due to scarring in late disease (b).

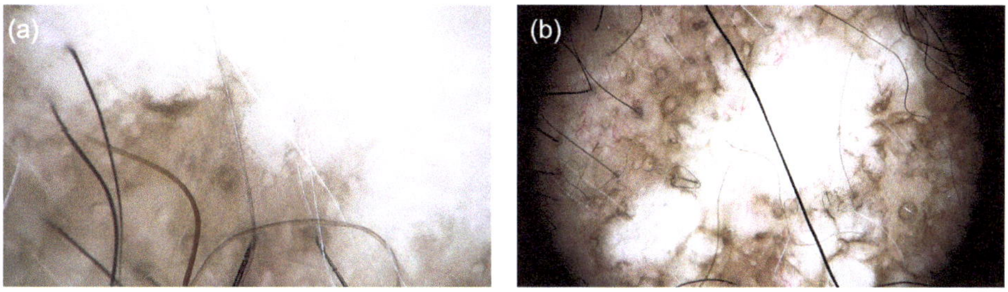

FIGURE 8.15 DLE: ×50 Loss of pigmented network and brownish dots due to incontinentia pigmenti at the periphery of the hypopigmented area (a); ×20 hypopigmented patch with loss of the honeycomb pattern and the pinpoint white dots. Note tortuous vessels within the patch and in the surrounding area (b).

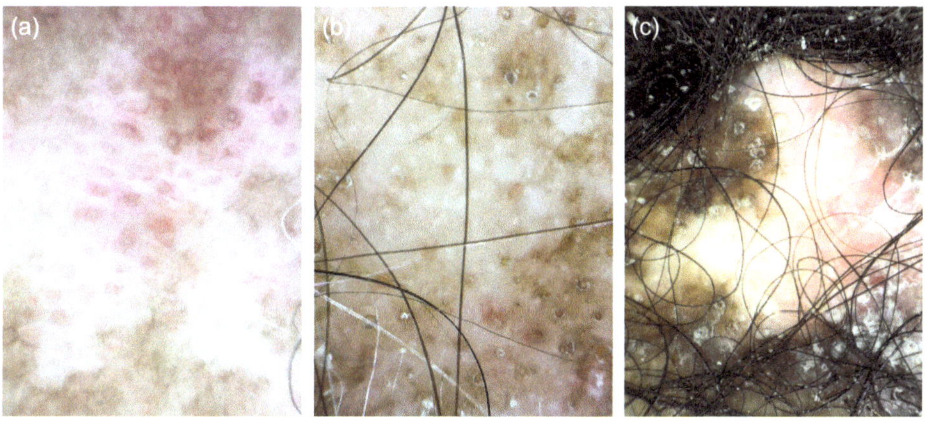

FIGURE 8.16 DLE. ×20 Loss of pigmented network and red dots (a); ×20 loss of pigmented network and keratotic plugs (b); ×20 loss of pigmented network, keratotic plugs, and patches of melanic heterogeneous staining (c).

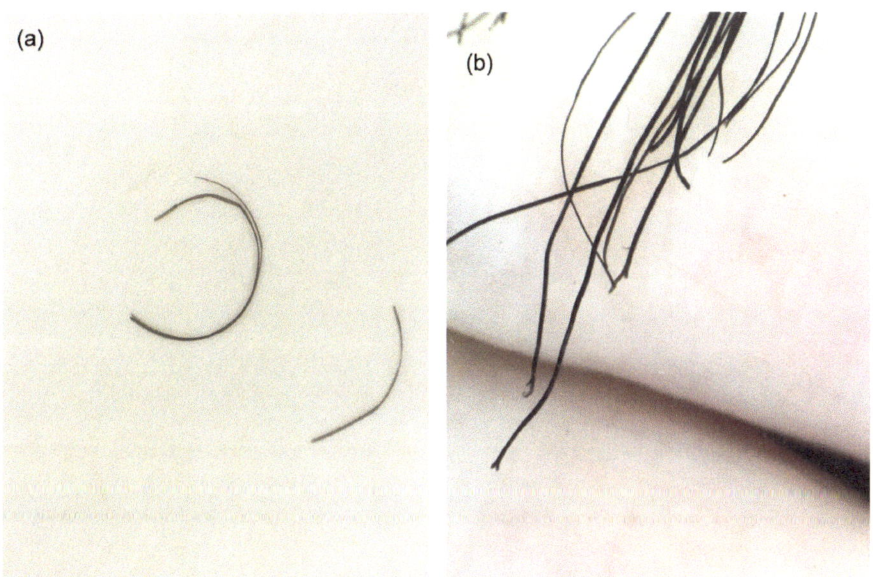

FIGURE 8.17 Dermoscopy of the hair shafts extracted with the tug test and of the distal tips: ×20 longitudinal splitting (a); ×40 trichorrhexis nodosa and trichoptilosis (b).

SUGGESTED READING

Abraham LS, Piñeiro-Maceira J, Duque-Estrada B, Barcaui CB, Sodré CT. Pinpoint white dots in the scalp: dermoscopic and histopathologic correlation. *J Am Acad Dermatol.* 2010;63(4):721–2.

Duque-Estrada B, Tamler C, Sodré CT, Barcaui CB, Pereira FB. Dermoscopy patterns of cicatricial alopecia resulting from discoid lupus erythematosus and lichen planopilaris. *An Bras Dermatol.* 2010;85(2):179–83. Erratum in: *An Bras Dermatol.* 2010;85(4):578.

Miteva M, Tosti A. Dermatoscopic features of central centrifugal cicatricial alopecia. *J Am Acad Dermatol.* 2014;71(3):443–9.

Ocampo-Garza J, Tosti A. Trichoscopy of dark scalp. *Skin Appendage Disord.* 2018;5(1):1–8.

Pirmez R, Duque-Estrada B, Donati A, Campos-do-Carmo G, Valente NS, Romiti R, Sodré CT, Tosti A. Clinical and dermoscopic features of lichen planus pigmentosus in 37 patients with frontal fibrosing alopecia. *Br J Dermatol.* 2016;175(6):1387–90.

Quaresma MV, Martinez Velasco MA, Tosti A. Hair breakage in patients of African descent: role of dermoscopy. *Skin Appendage Disord.* 2015;1(2):99–104.

Tosti A, Miteva M, Torres F, Vincenzi C, Romanelli P. Hair casts are a dermoscopic clue for the diagnosis of traction alopecia. *Br J Dermatol.* 2010;163(6):1353–5.

Tosti A, Torres F, Miteva M. Dermoscopy of early dissecting cellulitis of the scalp simulates alopecia areata. *Actas Dermosifiliogr.* 2013;104(1):92–3.

Vander Does A, Larrondo J, McMichael A. Flambeau sign: a trichoscopic finding of traction alopecia in Black patients. *J Am Acad Dermatol.* 2024;91(4):e93–e94.

Yin NC, Tosti A. A systematic approach to Afro-textured hair disorders: dermatoscopy and when to biopsy. *Dermatol Clin.* 2014;32(2):145–51.

9 Hair Weathering

- Hair weathering refers to the progressive degeneration of the hair shaft from the root to the tip.
- Dermoscopy is very useful to detect weathering in patients complaining of slow hair growth with short hair length or shedding of short hairs.
- Dermoscopic signs of weathering include: Trichorrhexis nodosa, trichoclasis, trichoschisis, trichoptilosis, and bubble hair.
- Dermoscopy examination should be performed on the hairs that appear lighter and shorter, using the finger as a support
- Interface solution is not necessary.

TRICHORRHEXIS NODOSA (FIGURE 9.1)

Dermoscopy

- White transversal transparent areas within the hair shaft
- More frequent in hair that has lighter coloration from sun exposure or chemical bleaching
- Fraying of the cortex
- Brush-like terminal endings
- Frayed tips

TRICHOPTILOSIS

Commonly known as "split ends," affecting the distal hair shaft.

Dermoscopy

- Split ends appear as longitudinal fissures of different length.
- Multiple splits from a single shaft create a "tree-branch" or "feather-like" pattern.
- In African hairs, hair splitting is common in the middle of the shaft.

BUBBLE HAIRS (FIGURES 9.2, 9.3)

Occur when wet hair is exposed to very high temperatures from electric straighteners, curlers, or blow dryers.

Dermoscopy

- Should be performed at high magnification (×70).
- "Swiss cheese" or "honeycomb-like" pattern: Aligned bubbles of various sizes are visible within the hair shaft, and increase its thickness.

TRICHONODOSIS

- Characterized by the formation of knots within the shaft (also known as "hair knotting").
- Dermoscopy shows trichorrhexis nodosa and raised cuticles.

DOI: 10.1201/9780429351433-9

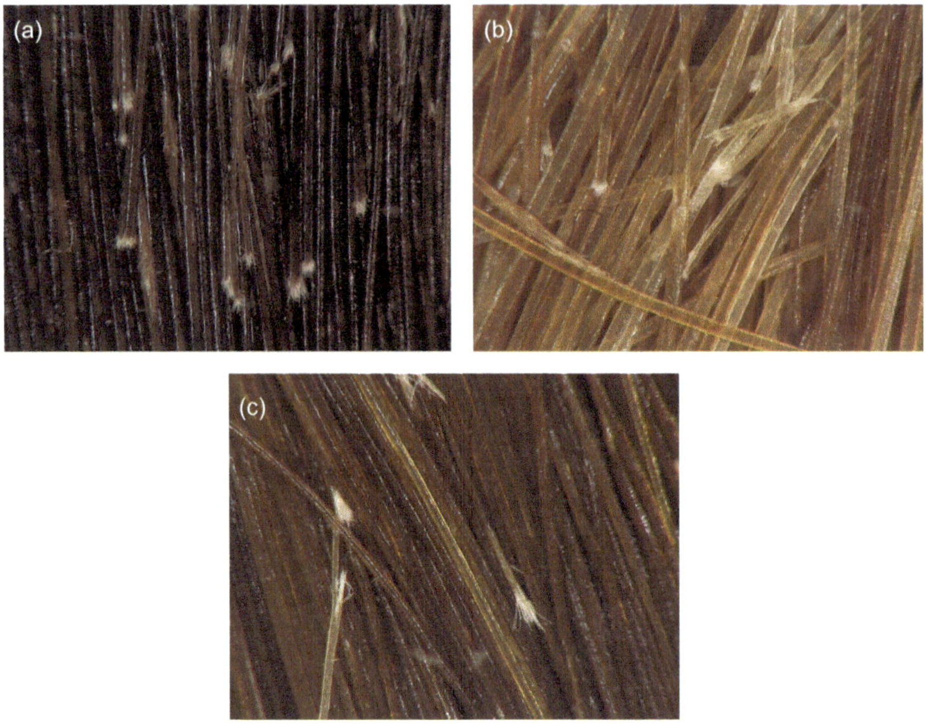

FIGURE 9.1 ×40 Multiple whitish area of breakage with brush-like terminal endings (a); ×70 higher magnification (b); ×70 brush-like tips (c).

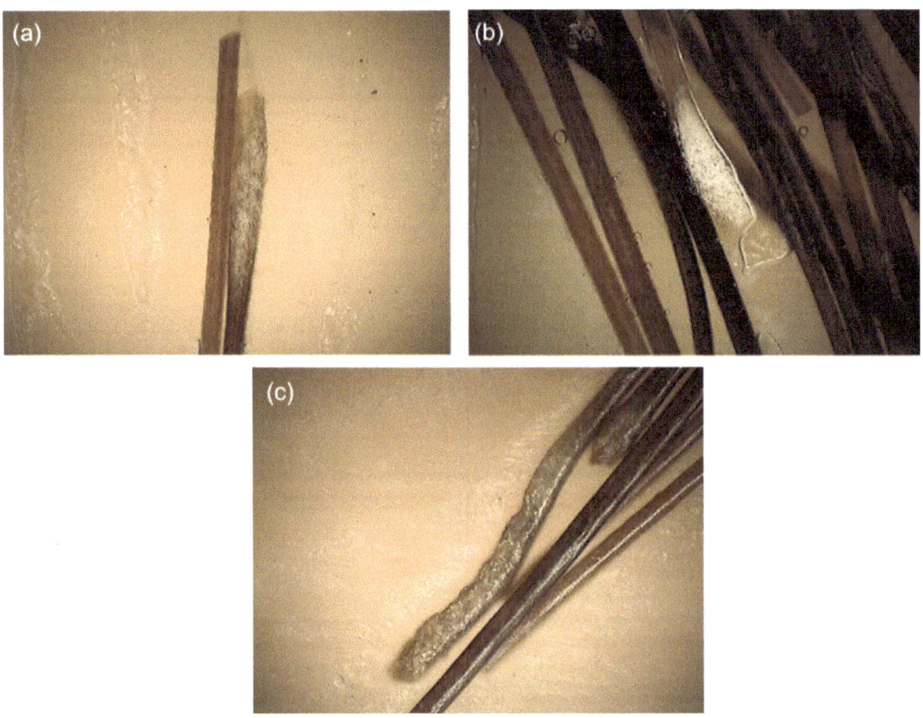

FIGURE 9.2 Bubble hair. ×50 The hair shaft is swollen and shows whitish granular areas (a); at higher magnification (×70) has a bubble appearance (b); ×50 bubble hair compared with the normal hair shaft (c).

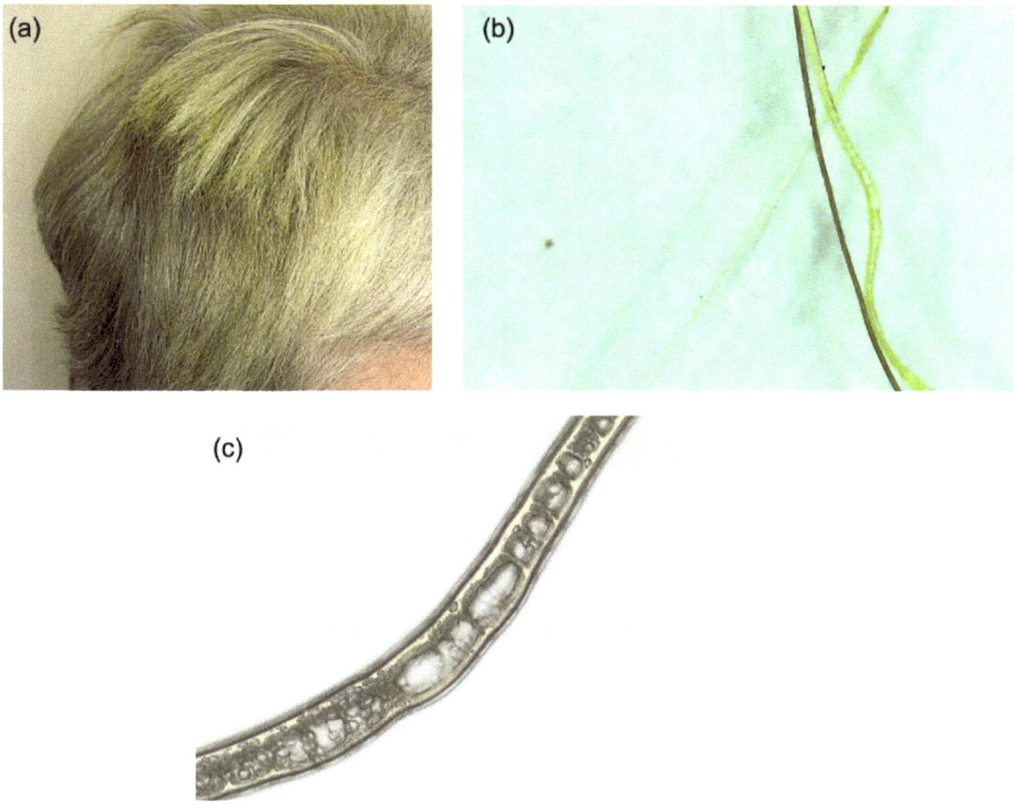

FIGURE 9.3 Bubble hair. Presenting as yellowish frizzy hair (a); ×20 note swelling and cavities within the shaft in comparison with the normal hair (b); cavities are very evident under the microscope (c).

SUGGESTED READING

Li YM, Diaz-Perez JA, Obayomi A, Galimberti F, Romanelli P, Tosti A. A review of bubble hair deformity. *Int J Dermatol.* 2023;62(3):428–31.

Osorio F, Tosti A Hair weathering part 2: clinical features, diagnosis, prevention, and treatment. *Cosm Dermatol.* 2011,24:255–59.

10 Systemic Diseases

SYSTEMIC LUPUS ERYTHEMATOSUS (SLE) (FIGURES 10.1–10.4)

In lupus erythematosus (LE), patients frequently experience various patterns of hair loss, including both scarring and non-scarring types.

LE-Specific Alopecia

- DLE causing scarring alopecia in most cases (see Chapter 5)
- Patchy alopecia areata-like of LE (see Chapter 4): Non-scarring but may be associated with DLE
- Linear and annular lupus panniculitis of the scalp: Non-scarring but may be associated with DLE
- Diffuse alopecia of systemic LE

Trichoscopy

- Thick tortuous convoluted vessels
- Preservation (SLE)/disruption (DLE) of the pigmented network and pinpoint white dots in the dark scalp
- Follicular red dots/diffuse erythema
- Keratotic plugs
- Peripilar casts
- Speckled blue-gray dots

DERMATOMYOSITIS (FIGURES 10.5–10.7)

Dermoscopy

- Enlarged thick tortuous vessels: Thicker than the hair shaft of terminal hairs
- Bushy capillaries: Are similar to those observed in the proximal nail fold
- Blotchy lake-like structures: Correspond to ectatic vascular structures and resemble red ink spots caused by a leaking pen
- Peripilar casts with occasional tufting
- Interfollicular scaling and perifollicular pigmentation

SARCOIDOSIS (FIGURE 10.8)

Dermoscopy

- Loss of follicular openings
- Diffuse or spotted yellowish to pale-orange discoloration of the interfollicular and perifollicular skin
- Orange spots, which do not match with follicular openings and are related to well-formed granulomas in the superficial dermis
- Peri- and interfollicular scaling
- Black dots/broken hairs (few)
- Dilated follicular ostia, mostly located at the borders of the patch
- Disruption of pigmented network in black scalp

T-CELL LYMPHOMAS (FIGURES 10.9, 10.10)

Non-Folliculotropic Mycosis Fungoides

Alopecia is typically non-scarring, can involve the whole scalp as well as other hairy areas, and closely resembles alopecia areata.

Dermoscopy

- Yellow dots
- Follicular spicules emerging from the follicular ostia
- Broken hairs and black dots
- Serpentine-like vessels

Folliculotropic Mycosis Fungoides

The hair loss is scarring and may present as:

DOI: 10.1201/9780429351433-10

- Patchy alopecia resembling alopecia areata
- Erythematous plaques of scarring alopecia
- Alopecia affecting eyelashes, eyebrows, and body hairs

Trichoscopy

- Absence of follicular ostia.
- Yellow dots and red dots can be seen in some areas.
- Linear and arborizing vessels.
- Background erythema.

ALOPECIA NEOPLASTICA (FIGURES 10.11, 10.12)

- Scalp metastases, particularly those presenting as scarring alopecic patches, are a relatively uncommon but clinically significant manifestation of advanced cancer, notably breast cancer.

Dermoscopy

- Loss of follicular openings
- Abnormal vascular pattern: Thick telangiectatic, arborizing, serpiginous vessels
- Diffuse pink-whitish erythema

NECROBIOSIS LIPOIDICA

Necrobiosis lipoidica primarily occurs on the lower extremities but can very rarely appear on the face and scalp causing scarring alopecia.

Dermoscopy

- Loss of follicular openings
- Prominent long telangiectatic vessels
- Yellowish-orange background

BULLOUS AUTOIMMUNE DISEASES

Pemphigus (Figure 10.13)

Scalp involvement in pemphigus affects up to 60% of patients during the disease course.

Dermoscopy

- Diffuse yellowish or whitish scaling: Caused by superficial epidermal disruption
- Pronounced vascular network
- Red hemorrhagic areas with sharply demarcated polygonal patterns (extravasation): Correspond to a mixture of serum, blood, and inflammatory cells and are a sign of active blistering and erosion
- Tubular encircling structures: Encircle the hair shaft and are produced by the acantholysis occurring within the outer root sheath
- Dermoscopy of the roots of pulled hairs shows anagen bulbs

Systemic Amyloidosis (Figure 10.14)

Scalp amyloidosis represents a rare clinical entity within the spectrum of systemic amyloidosis, typically presenting as a diffuse nonscarring alopecia.

Dermoscopy

- Salmon-colored halos surrounding the follicular ostia, correlating with perifollicular amyloid deposition
- Broken hairs and black dots

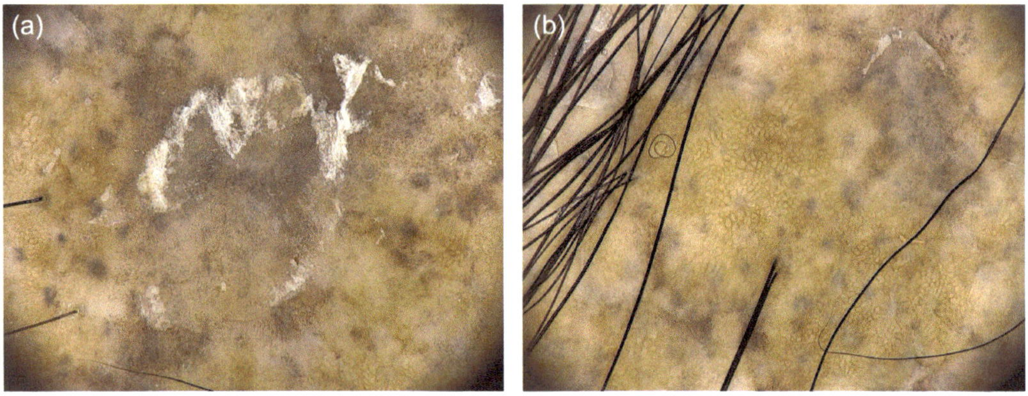

FIGURE 10.1 (a,b) DLE. ×50 The destruction of the pigmented network induces the development of diffuse tiny gray-brown dots before the development of white patches.

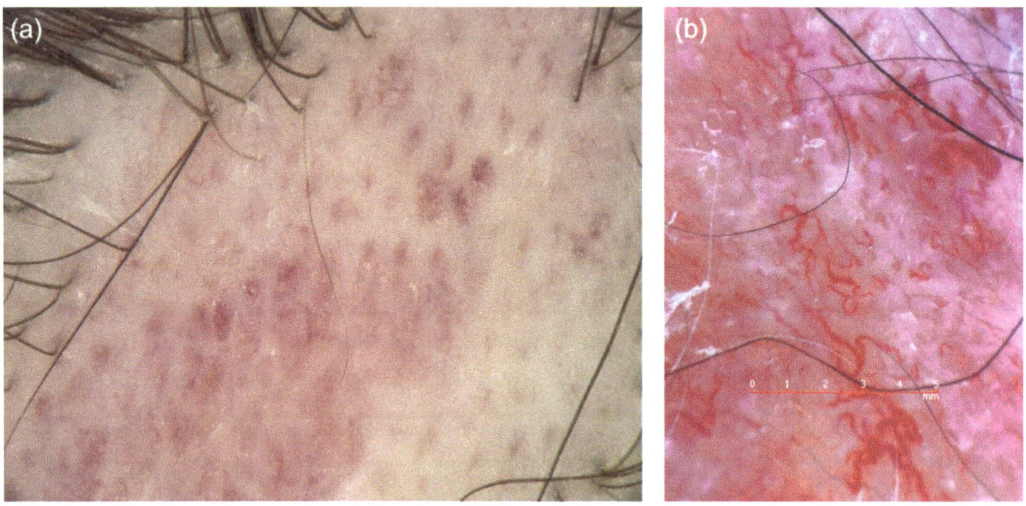

FIGURE 10.2 Systemic lupus with discoid lesions of the scalp. ×20 Multiple red dots (a); ×50 tortuous vessels (b).

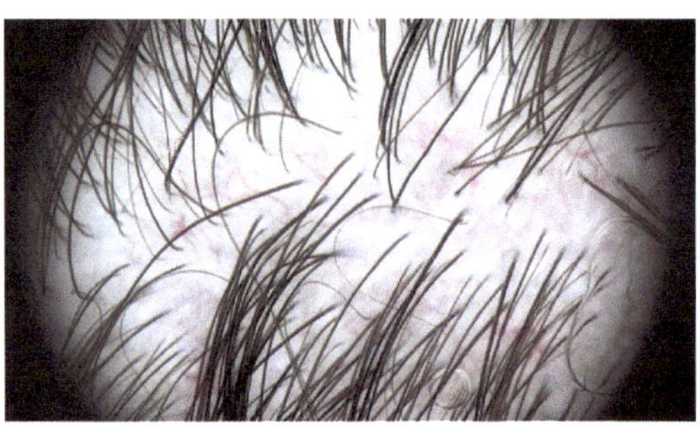

FIGURE 10.3 Systemic lupus with diffuse hair loss. ×20 Enlarged tortuous vessels.

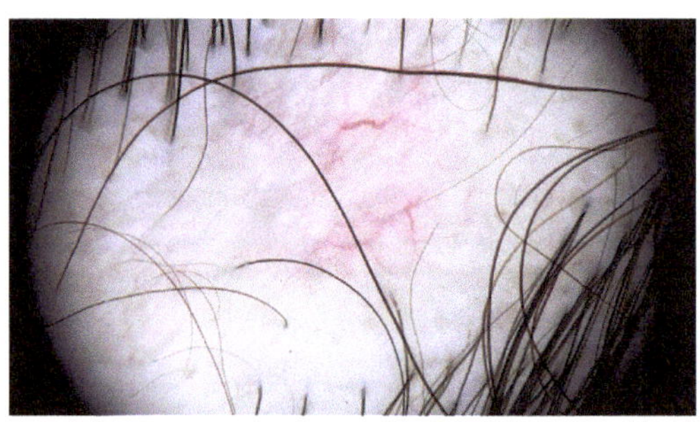

FIGURE 10.4 ×20 Patchy alopecia in lupus panniculitis showing tortuous dilated vessels and some yellow dots.

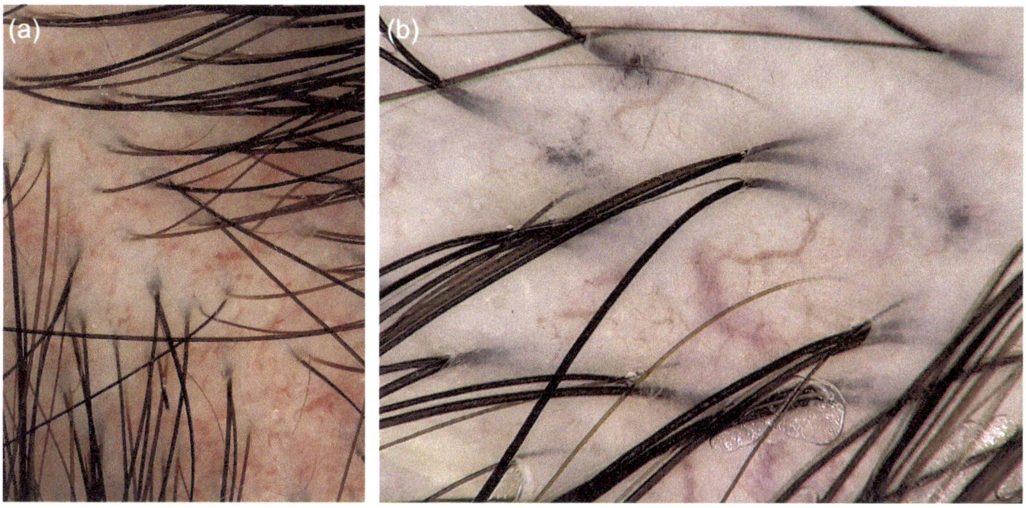

FIGURE 10.5 Dermatomyositis. ×20 Enlarged tortuous vessels and hair breakage due to scratching (a); ×50 the size of the vessels is thicker than that of the hair shaft; black dots are due to micropigmentation (b).

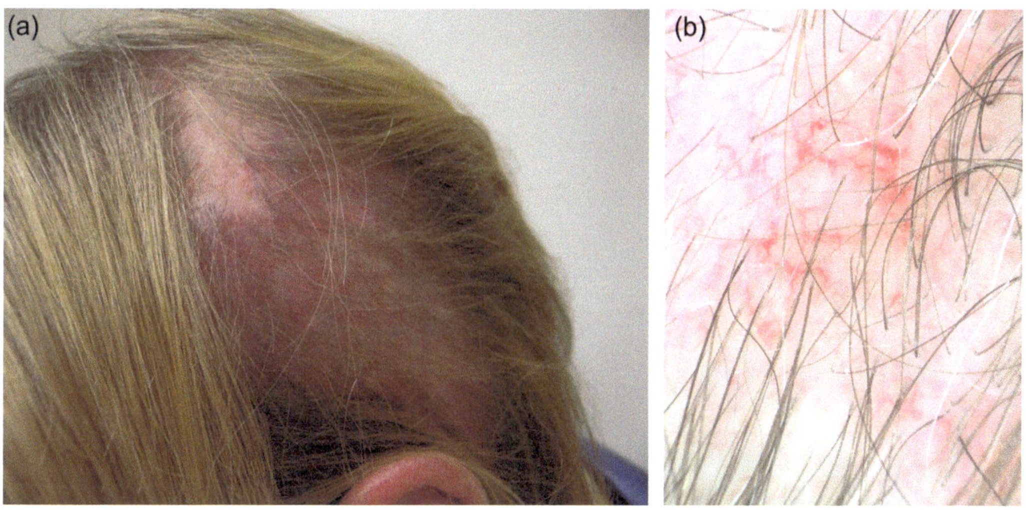

FIGURE 10.6 Scalp erythema and diffuse severe alopecia in dermatomyositis (a); ×20 enlarged tortuous vessels (b).

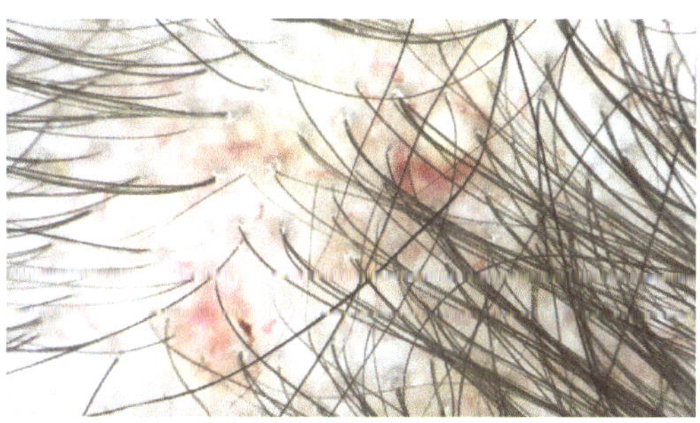

FIGURE 10.7 ×20 Blotchy lake-like structures.

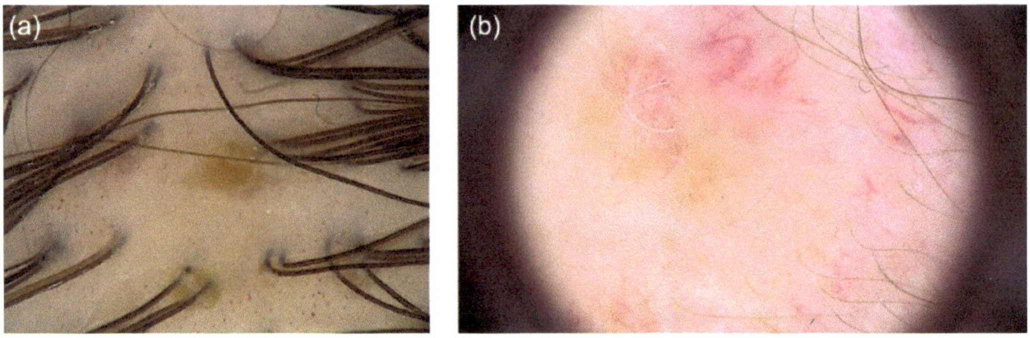

FIGURE 10.8 Sarcoidosis. ×20 Round yellow/orange spots in sarcoidosis presenting with folliculitis (a); ×40 loss of follicular openings, non-follicular orange spots, and tortuous vessels (b).

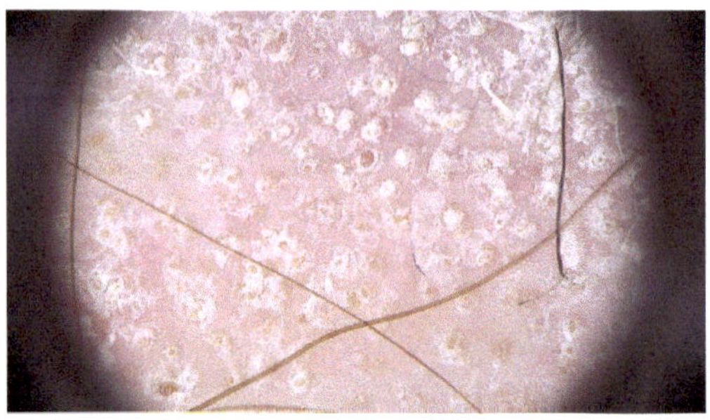

FIGURE 10.9 ×20 Yellow dots and follicular spicules in non-folliculotropic mycosis fungoides.

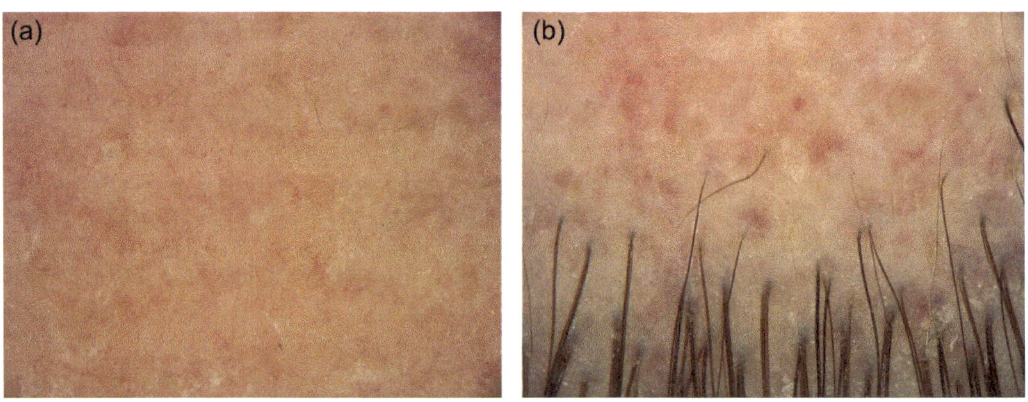

FIGURE 10.10 ×20 Folliculotropic mycosis fungoides showing diffuse erythema, loss of follicular openings and few scales (a); ×20 red dots at the border of the patch (b).

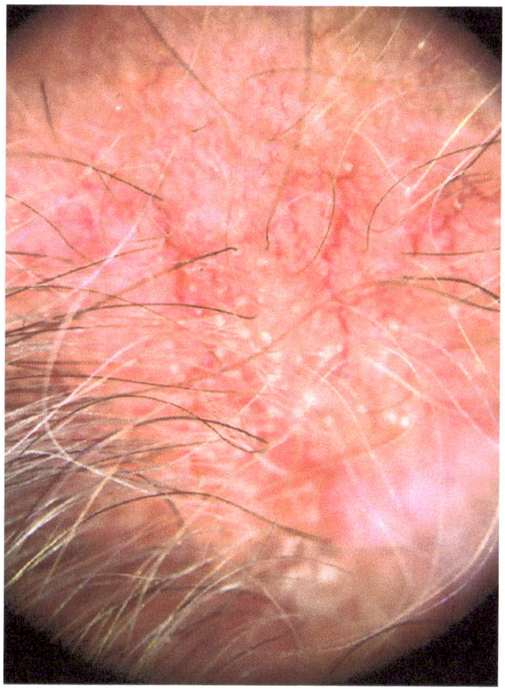

FIGURE 10.11 Scalp metastasis of breast cancer. ×10 Loss of follicular openings and irregular serpiginous vessels. (Courtesy of Dr. Mario Valenti.)

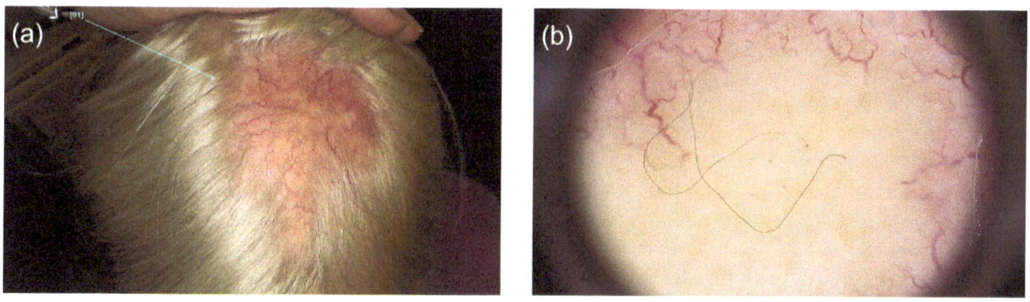

FIGURE 10.12 Scalp metastasis. Large red alopecic patch with evidence of prominent serpiginous vessels (a). ×20 loss of follicular openings with serpiginous enlarged vessels that do not fade with pressure (b). (Courtesy of Dr. Tatiana Siliuk.)

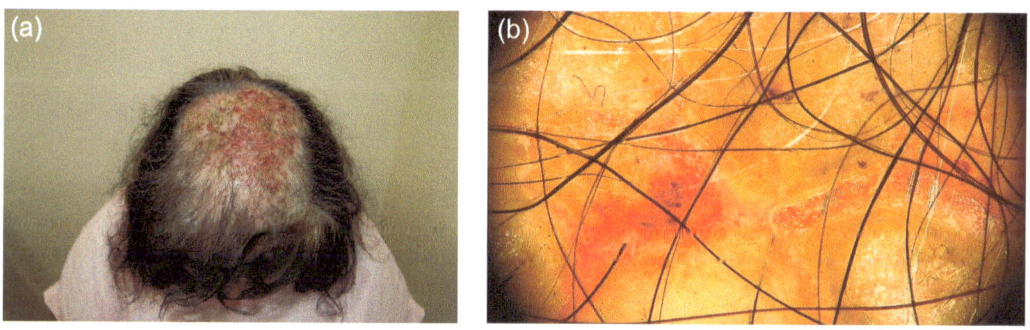

FIGURE 10.13 Pemphigus with severe scalp erosions (a); ×50 red hemorrhagic areas with polygonal patterns (b). (Courtesy of Dr Bianca Maria Piraccini.)

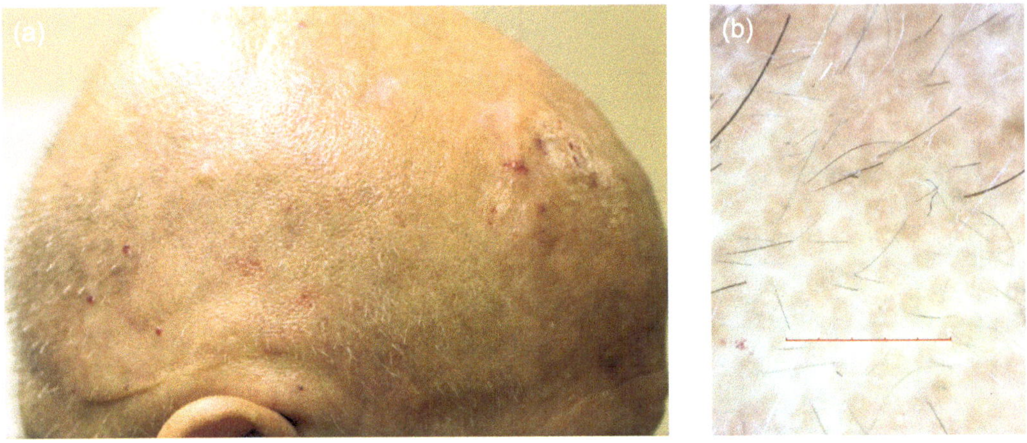

FIGURE 10.14 Systemic amyloidosis. Diffuse alopecia with hemorrhagic lesions in systemic amyloidosis. (a); ×20 follicular openings with salmon-colored halos, black dots, and spotted hemorrhages (b).

SUGGESTED READING

Ardigò M, El Shabrawi-Caelen L, Tosti A. In vivo reflectance confocal microscopy assessment of the therapeutic follow-up of cutaneous T-cell lymphomas causing scalp alopecia. *Dermatol Ther.* 2014;27(4):248–51.

Jasso-Olivares JC, Tosti A, Miteva M, Domínguez-Cherit J, Díaz-González JM. Clinical and dermoscopic features of the scalp in 31 patients with dermatomyositis. *Skin Appendage Disord.* 2017;3(3):119–24.

Miteva M, El Shabrawi-Caelen L, Fink-Puches R, Beham-Schmid C, Romanelli P,Kerdel F, Tosti A. Alopecia universalis associated with cutaneous T cell lymphoma. *Dermatology.* 2014;229(2):65–9.

Miteva M, Wei E, Milikowski C, Tosti A. Alopecia in systemic amyloidosis: trichoscopic-pathologic correlation. *Int J Trichology.* 2015;7(4):176–8.

Pirmez R. Acantholytic hair casts: a dermoscopic sign of pemphigus vulgaris of the scalp. *Int J Trichology.* 2012;4(3):172–73.

Sławińska M, Sokołowska-Wojdyło M, Olszewska B, Nowicki RJ, Sobjanek M, Zalaudek I. Dermoscopic and trichoscopic features of primary cutaneous lymphomas - systematic review. *J Eur Acad Dermatol Venereol.* 2021;35(7):1470–84.

Starace M, Loi C, Cedirian S, Bruni F, Filippi F, La Placa M, Piraccini BM, Bardazzi F. Trichoscopy as a monitoring tool in assessing treatment response in scalp pemphigus. *J Eur Acad Dermatol Venereol.* 2024;38(9):e755–e757.

Torres F, Tosti A, Misciali C, Lorenzi S. Trichoscopy as a clue to the diagnosis of scalp sarcoidosis. *Int J Dermatol.* 2011;50(3):358–61.

Vezzoni R, Toffoli L, Conforti C, Dri A, Retrosi C, di Meo N, Magaton Rizzi G, Signoretto D, Zalaudek I. Breast cancer-related neoplastic alopecia: a case report and review of the literature. *Skin Appendage Disord.* 2021;7(5):339–45.

Yaşar Ş, Kaynak E, Güneş P, Göktay F, Aytekin S. Atypical localization of necrobiosis lipoidica: involvement of the face and scalp. *Skin Appendage Disord.* 2017;3(2):92–94.

Ye Y, Zhao Y, Gong Y, Zhang X, Caulloo S, Zhang B, Cai Z, Yang J, McElwee KJ, Zhang X. Non-scarring patchy alopecia in patients with systemic lupus erythematosus differs from that of alopecia areata. *Lupus.* 2013;22(14):1439–45.

11 Inflammatory Scalp Disorders

SCALP PSORIASIS (FIGURES 11.1–11.5)

Dermoscopy

- The vascular pattern can be detected either in the affected or unaffected scalp and manifests as:
  - Red dots and globules at low magnification (×10–×20).
  - Twisted red loops, glomerular vessels, hairpin vessels at high magnification (×40 and up).
- The vessels are better visualized with the use of interface solution and should be searched in areas without/with few scales.
- They do not or only minimally blanch with pressure.
- Hemorrhagic red spots corresponding to ectatic vessels of papillary dermis can be seen due to scratching.
- Perifollicular and interfollicular silvery-white scales; when very pronounced, like in the psoriatic cap, they can prevent the detection of the vascular pattern.
- Yellowish scales can occasionally be found.
- Pityriasis amiantacea, characterized by thick scales adhering to a tuft of multiple hair shafts, may be followed by scarring alopecia.
- Interfollicular pustules can be seen in pustular psoriasis.
- Hair shaft variability due to androgenetic alopecia can be associated.

SEBORRHEIC DERMATITIS (FIGURES 11.6, 11.7)

Dermoscopy

- Arborizing vessels corresponding to dilation of the subpapillary plexus.
- Since arborizing vessels blanch with pressure, dermoscopy should be performed with minimal pressure.
- Yellowish interfollicular and perifollicular scaling.
- Follicular pustules, crusts, and excoriations.
- "Dandelion" vascular conglomerate consists of a yellow dot surrounded by glomerular and comma vessels, and correlates with a deep *Malassezia* spp. colonization.
- Perifollicular oily material, appearing as a yellowish greasy halo around the emergence of the hair shaft.
- Hair shaft variability due to androgenetic alopecia is commonly associated.

CONTACT DERMATITIS (FIGURES 11.8, 11.9)

Dermoscopy

The dermoscopic features may overlap with scalp psoriasis and seborrheic dermatitis:

- White or yellow interfollicular scales that may adhere to hair shafts.
- Diffuse or patchy erythema.
- In chronic lichenified lesions, dermoscopy shows prominence of follicular openings and proximal trichorrhexis nodosa due to scratching.
- Polymorphic vascular pattern, mainly consisting of arborizing vessels and simple red loops.
- Presence of exudation/crusting or hemorrhagic dots.
- Tiny brown and bluish-gray globules arranged in a reticular pattern, sparing orifices, and eccrine pores are typical signs of post-inflammatory pigmentation.

DOI: 10.1201/9780429351433-11

SCALP ROSACEA (FIGURE 11.10)

Dermoscopy

- Dilated arborizing vessels in the interfollicular skin (caterpillar vessels).
- Perifollicular scales.
- Plugging of follicular ostia in the bald scalp.
- Hair shaft variability can be an associated finding when androgenetic alopecia is present.

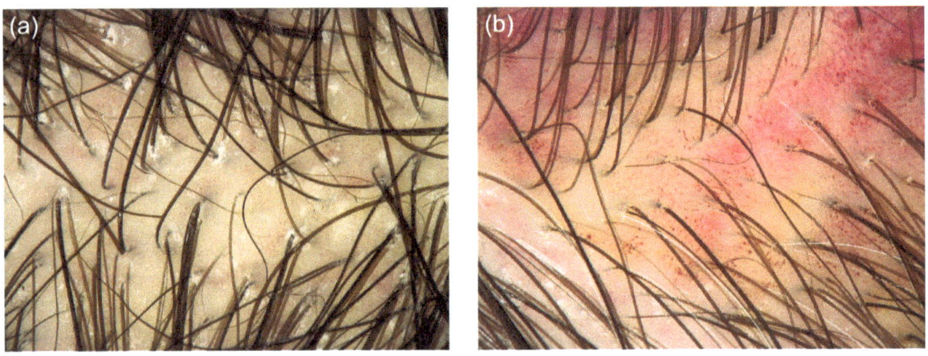

FIGURE 11.1 Scalp psoriasis. ×20 Perifollicular scaling and red dots (a); ×20 twisted capillary loops and hemorrhagic red spots (b).

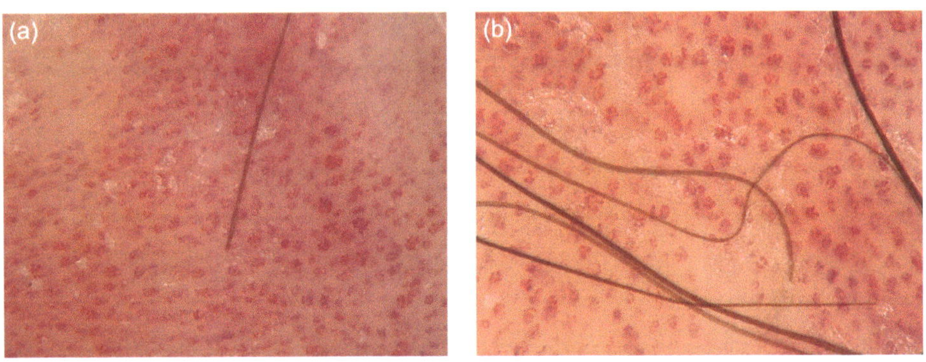

FIGURE 11.2 Scalp psoriasis. Twisted capillary loops seen at ×40 (a) and ×70 (b).

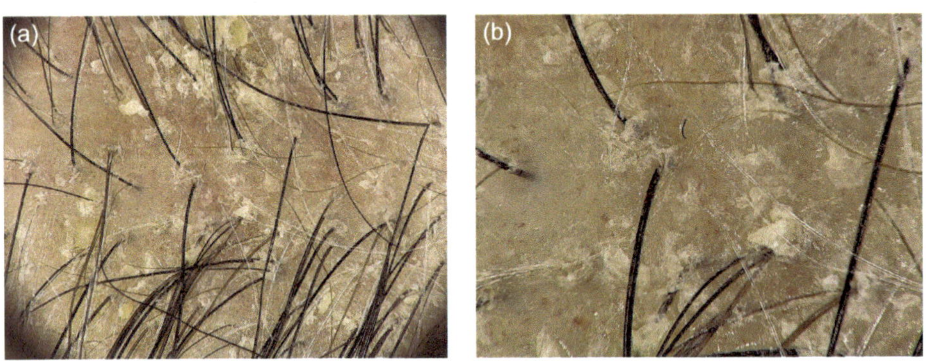

FIGURE 11.3 Scalp psoriasis. ×20 At low magnification the scales are the prominent features (a); ×50 at high magnification twisted capillary loops are evident (b).

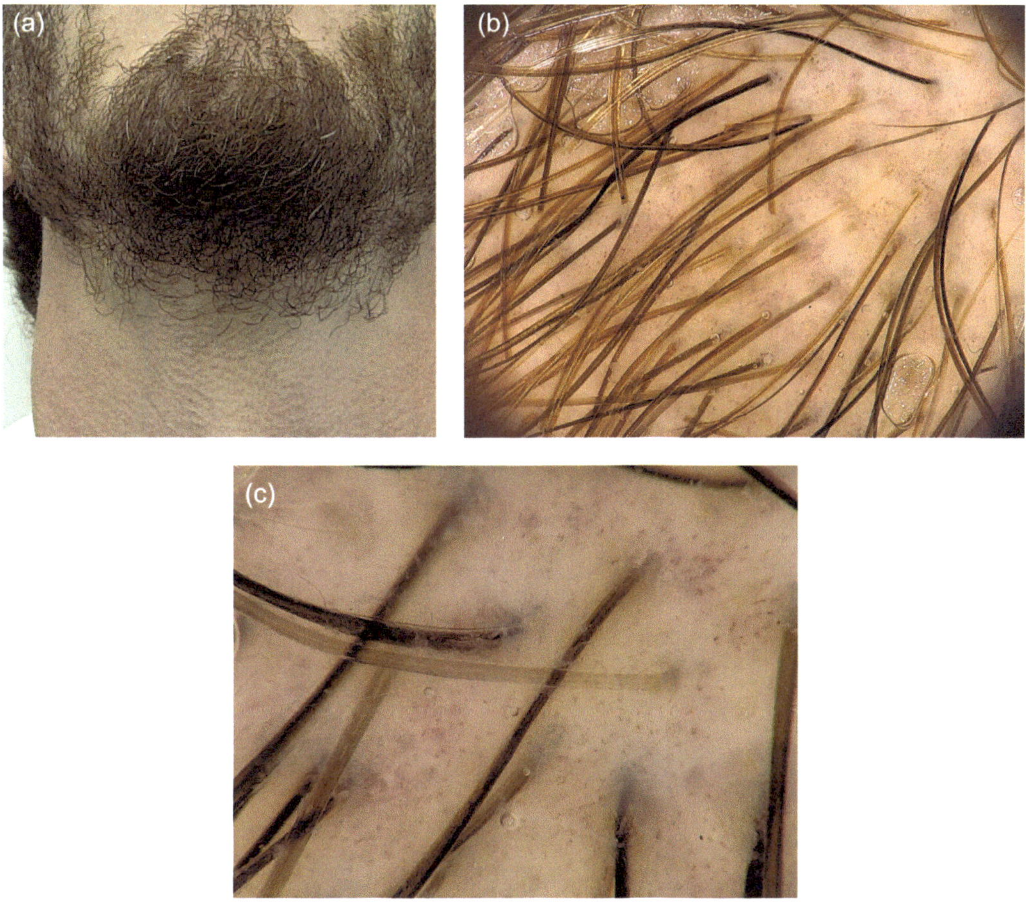

FIGURE 11.4 Psoriasis of the beard. No clinical evidence of scaling (a); ×40 (b) and ×60 (c) twisted capillary loops are seen also in this area.

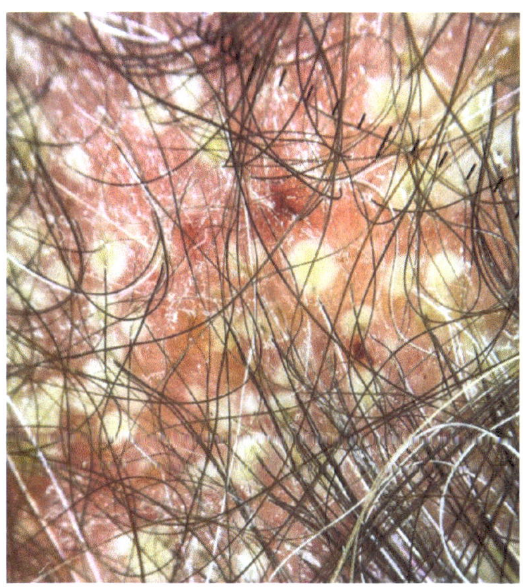

FIGURE 11.5 Pustular psoriasis. ×10 Multiple interfollicular pustules.

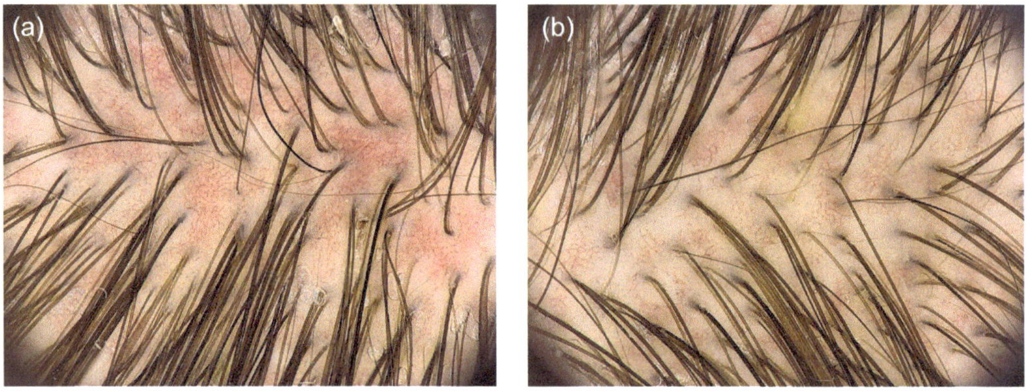

FIGURE 11.6 Seborrheic dermatitis. ×20 Arborizing vessels and yellowish deposits surrounding the hair shafts (a,b).

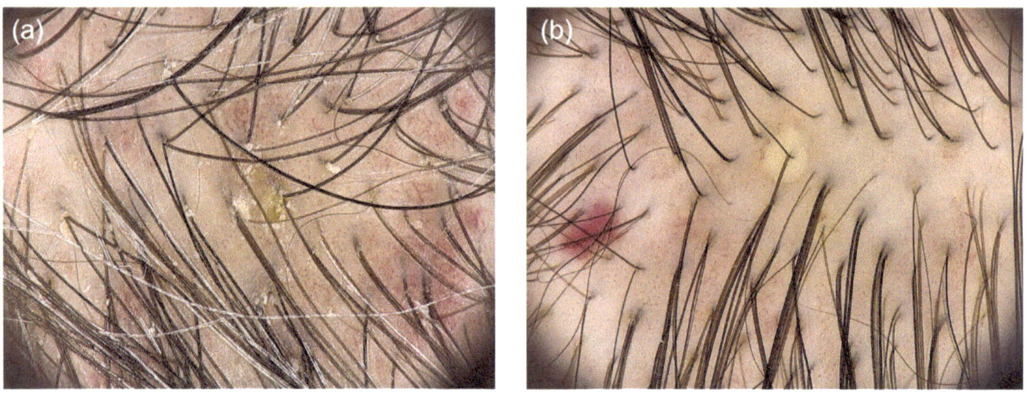

FIGURE 11.7 Seborrheic dermatitis. ×20 Perifollicular yellowish crust (a); follicular pustule associated with arborizing vessels (b).

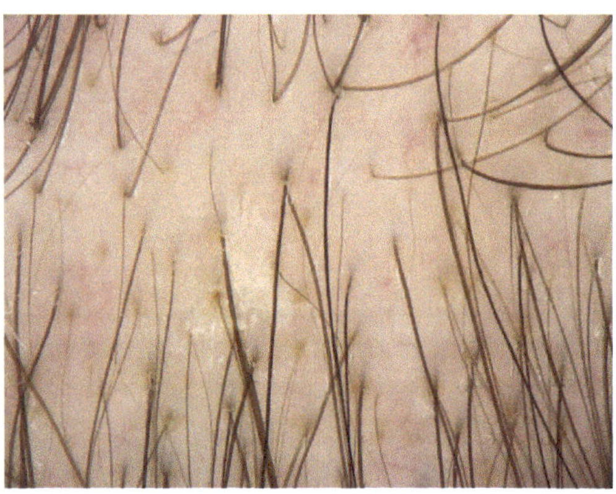

FIGURE 11.8 Scalp contact dermatitis. ×40 White scales and increased number of arborizing vessels.

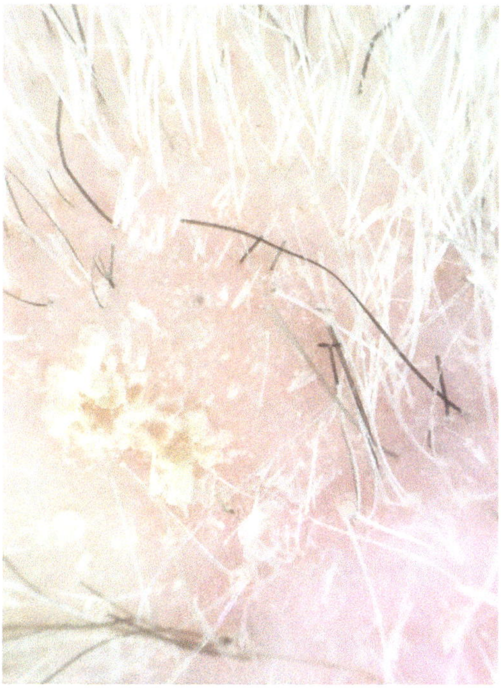

FIGURE 11.9 Chronic scalp contact dermatitis. ×20 Scalp scaling, broom hairs and proximal trichorrhexis nodosa.

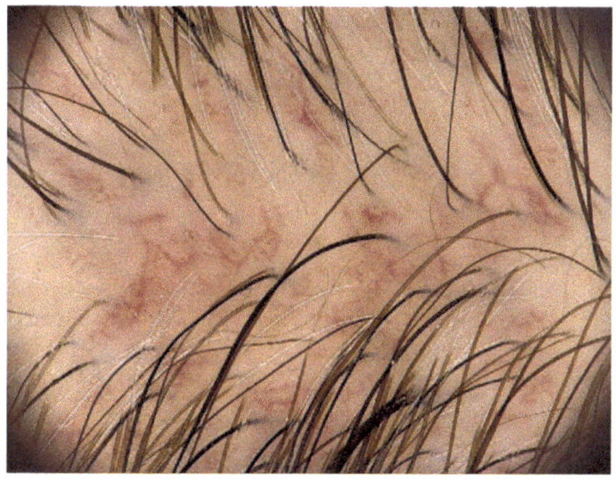

FIGURE 11.10 Scalp rosacea. ×20 Perifollicular scales and dilated arborizing vessels.

SUGGESTED READING

Bruni F, Alessandrini A, Starace M, Orlando G, Piraccini BM, Clinical and trichoscopic features in various forms of scalp psoriasis. *J Eur Acad Dermatol Venereol.* 2021;35: 830–37.

Kim GW, Jung HJ, Ko HC, Kim MB, Lee WJ, Lee SJ, Kim DW, Kim BS. Dermoscopy can be useful in differentiating scalp psoriasis from seborrheic dermatitis. *Br J Dermatol.* 2011;164(3):652–6.

Kłosowicz A, Alsalhi W, Tosti A. How to optimize trichoscopy for evaluation of scalp vessels. *Skin Appendage Disord.* 2020;6(4):216–19.

Ross EK, Vincenzi C, Tosti A. Videodermoscopy in the evaluation of hair and scalp disorders. *J Am Acad Dermatol.* 2006;55(5):799–806.

Tosti A, Donati A, Vincenzi C, Fabbrocini G. Videodermoscopy does not enhance diagnosis of scalp contact dermatitis due to topical minoxidil. *Int J Trichology.* 2009;1(2):134–7.

Vázquez-Herrera NE, Zamora-Benze DM, Garza-Chapa JI, Rodríguez-Baca AB, Tosti A. Scalp rosacea: rethinking peripilar scaling. *Skin Appendage Disord.* 2021;7(5):382–86.

12 Scalp Infections and Infestations

TINEA CAPITIS (FIGURES 12.1–12.7)

Dermoscopy

- Comma hairs: Short broken C shaped hairs, due to bending of the hair shaft filled with fungi
- Corkscrew hairs: Irregularly twisted short hairs
- Morse code-hairs: Broken hairs with multiple transverse translucent white bands corresponding to focal areas of heavy fungal infection. Typical of endothrix infection
- Zig-zag hairs: Broken hairs with multiple bending
- Broken hairs.
- Black dots (in dark hair individuals)
- Perifollicular and interfollicular scales
- Perifollicular crusts and pustules
- Dermoscopy of Kerion is often not diagnostic
- Scutulum (tinea favosa): Yellow concretion on the scalp surface encircling tufts of hairs.

WHITE PIEDRA (FIGURE 12.8)

Epidemiology

- White piedra is a superficial fungal infection of hair shaft primarily caused by *Trichosporon* spp. and is prevalent in South America.
- Presents as soft white non-moveable nodules encasing the hair shafts at irregular intervals.
- Microscopic examination and fungal culture confirm the diagnosis.

Dermoscopy

- Multiple round/fusiform nodules of irregular size encircling completely the hair.
- Differential diagnosis includes nits and cosmetic residues.

BLACK PIEDRA

Epidemiology

- Black piedra is a very rare superficial mycosis of the hair shaft caused by a pigmented fungus named *Piedraia hortae.*
- It usually affects the scalp, but beard and body hair can be involved.
- Affected hairs have small, hard, brown-black nodules that are firmly attached giving the impression of a hair shaft studded with black stones.

Dermoscopy

- Irregularly shaped dark brown or black hard concretions tightly bound to the hair shaft.
- Their shape can range from round to elongated nodules.
- The affected hair shaft presents multiple irregularly spaced nodules.

PEDICULOSIS CAPITIS (FIGURES 12.9, 12.10)

Dermoscopy

- The head louse with one pair of antennae and three pairs of legs can be detected in the interfollicular scalp. It is transparent except for the dark section in the lower abdomen.

DOI: 10.1201/9780429351433-12

- Dark rounded spots that correspond to louse feces can be seen in the interfollicular scalp, along with erosions due to scratching.
- Nits do not encircle entirely the hair shaft but are attached to one side.
- Viable nits: Contain nymphs and appear as ovoid, brown structures with a convex extremity.
- Empty nits: Appear translucent with a flat free ending.
- Vital nits are commonly located near the surface of the scalp.
- Dermoscopy differentiates lice nits from pseudo-nits.

SCALP SCABIES (FIGURE 12.11)

Epidemiology

- Scalp scabies is rare in adult immunocompetent patients but can be seen in children.
- Scalp scabies may persist as a reservoir for mites and can be a source of persistent infestation.

Dermoscopy

Should be performed without interface to enhance the detection of the burrows in the interfollicular scalp, which are identical to those found in other body areas.

- Brownish arrowhead, localized at one extremity of the burrow corresponding to the head of the mite (triangle or delta-wing jet sign).
- Whitish wavy line, corresponding to the mite's burrow (jet contrail sign).
- Interfollicular yellowish/hemorrhagic crusting, due to scratching.

SYPHILIS

Epidemiology

- Non-scarring alopecia can be a manifestation of secondary syphilis.

Dermoscopy

- Empty follicles
- Yellow dots
- Peripheral black dots
- Thin short regrowing hairs
- Broken hairs
- Dilated and tortuous vessels

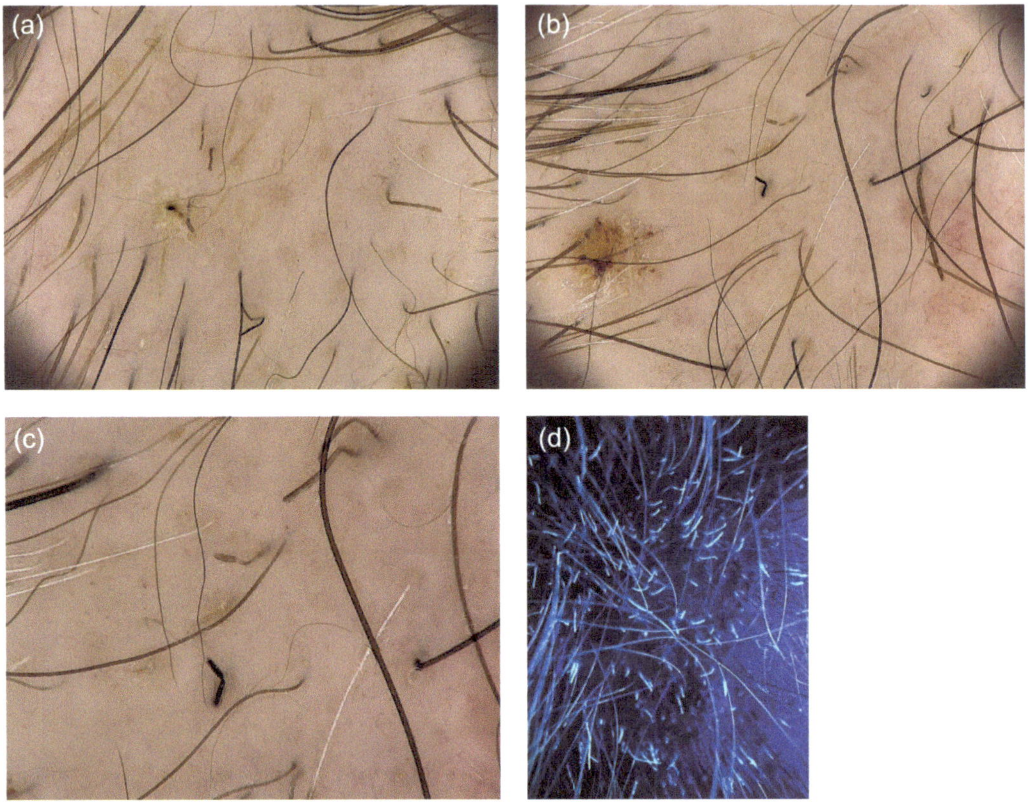

FIGURE 12.1 Tinea capitis. ×20 Broken hairs, comma hairs, and Morse-code hairs (a); also note crusting (b). ×50 Comma hairs at high magnification (c). ×10 Comma hairs can be easily visualized using Wood light in *Microsporum canis* infection (d).

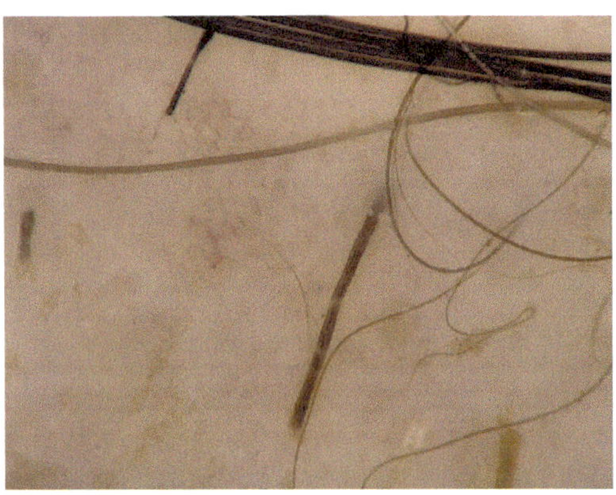

FIGURE 12.2 Tinea capitis. ×50 Morse-code hairs.

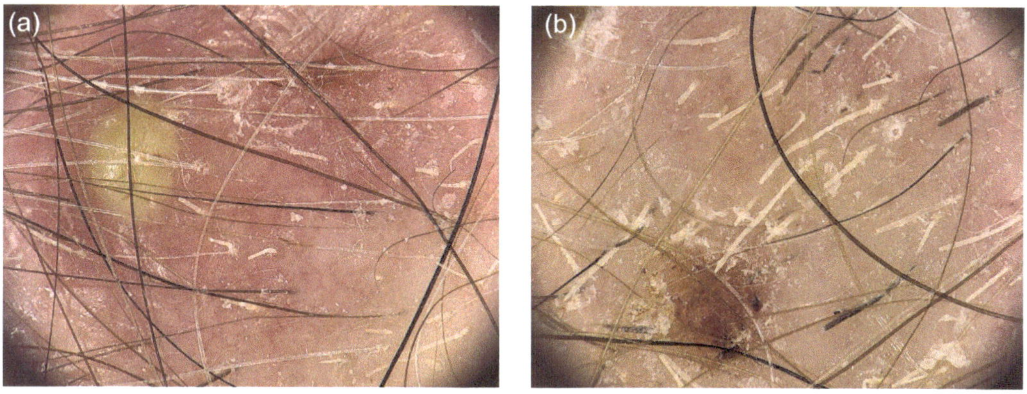

FIGURE 12.3 Tinea capitis in an elderly patient. ×40 Broken hairs, comma hairs, and interfollicular pustule (a) and crusts (b).

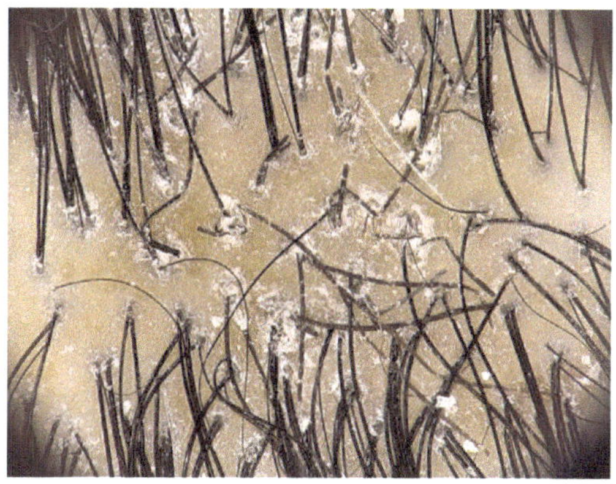

FIGURE 12.4 Tinea capitis. ×20 Diffuse scaling with comma hairs.

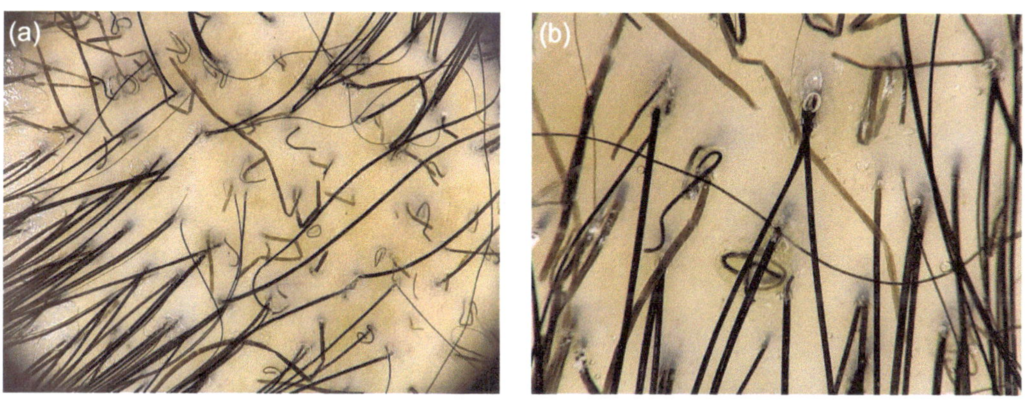

FIGURE 12.5 Tinea capitis. ×20 Corkscrew hairs, comma hairs and zigzag hairs (a), ×50 corkscrew hairs at high magnification (b).

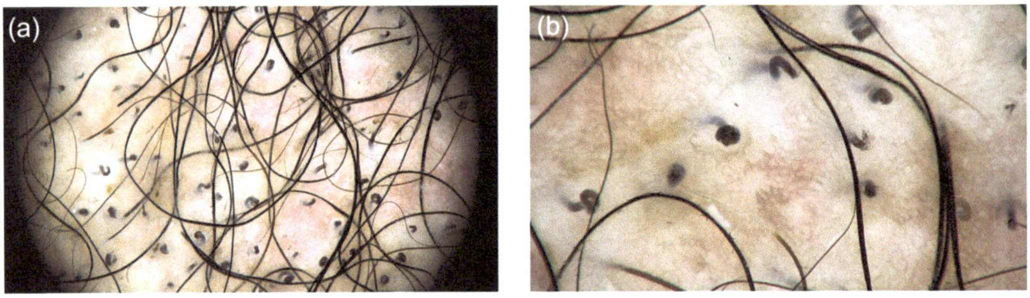

FIGURE 12.6 Tinea capitis in a patient of color. ×40 Corkscrew hairs and comma hairs (a); ×50 corkscrew hair—the hair shaft twisting is very evident (b).

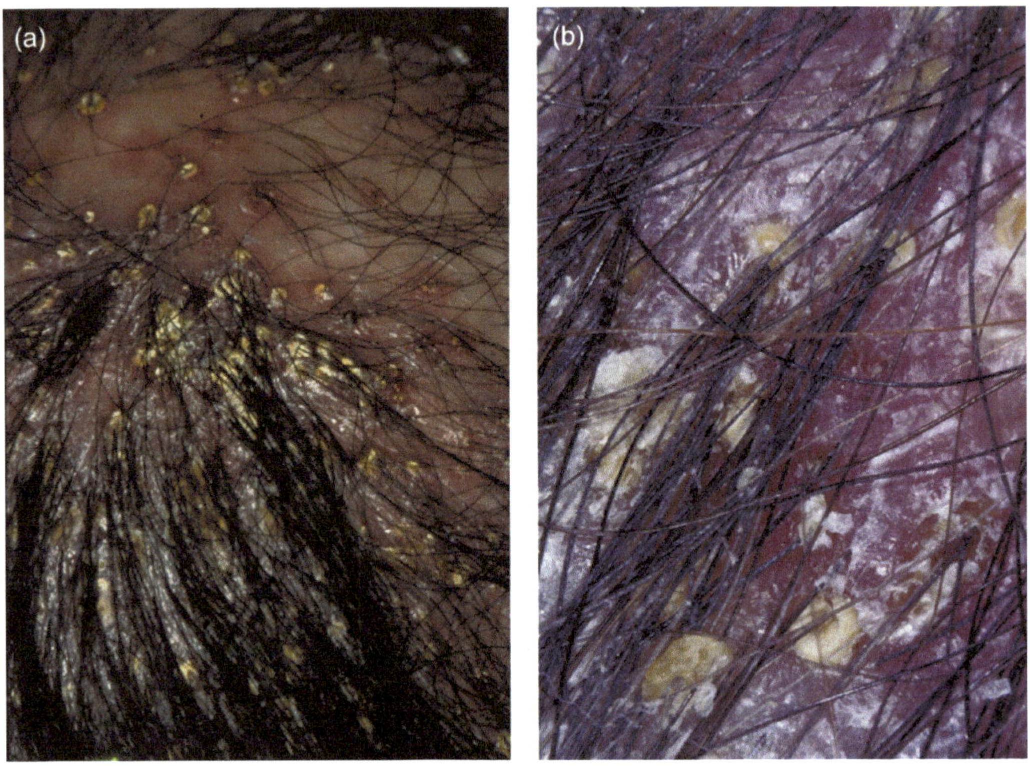

FIGURE 12.7 Tinea favosa. Clinical presentation: ×40 yellow crusts (scutulum) englobing the hair shafts (a). Also note severe erythema and exudation (b).

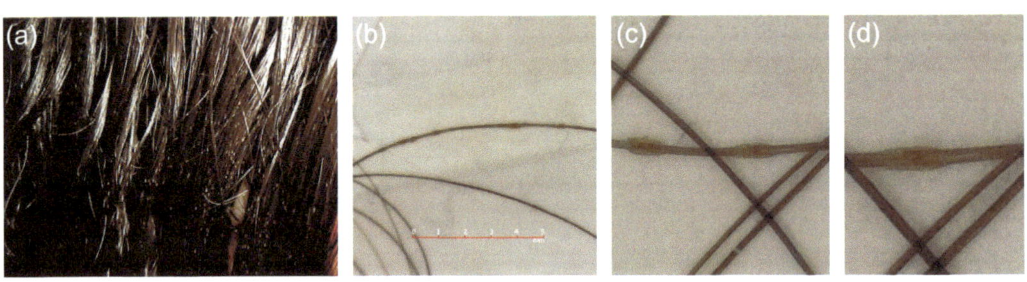

FIGURE 12.8 White piedra. Clinical presentation ×20 regular fusiform nodules along the hair shaft (a) (Courtesy of Dr. Nilton Di Chiacchio); ×50–×70 at high magnifications the hair shaft is visible through the nodules (b,c,d). (Courtesy of Dr Fernanda Torres.)

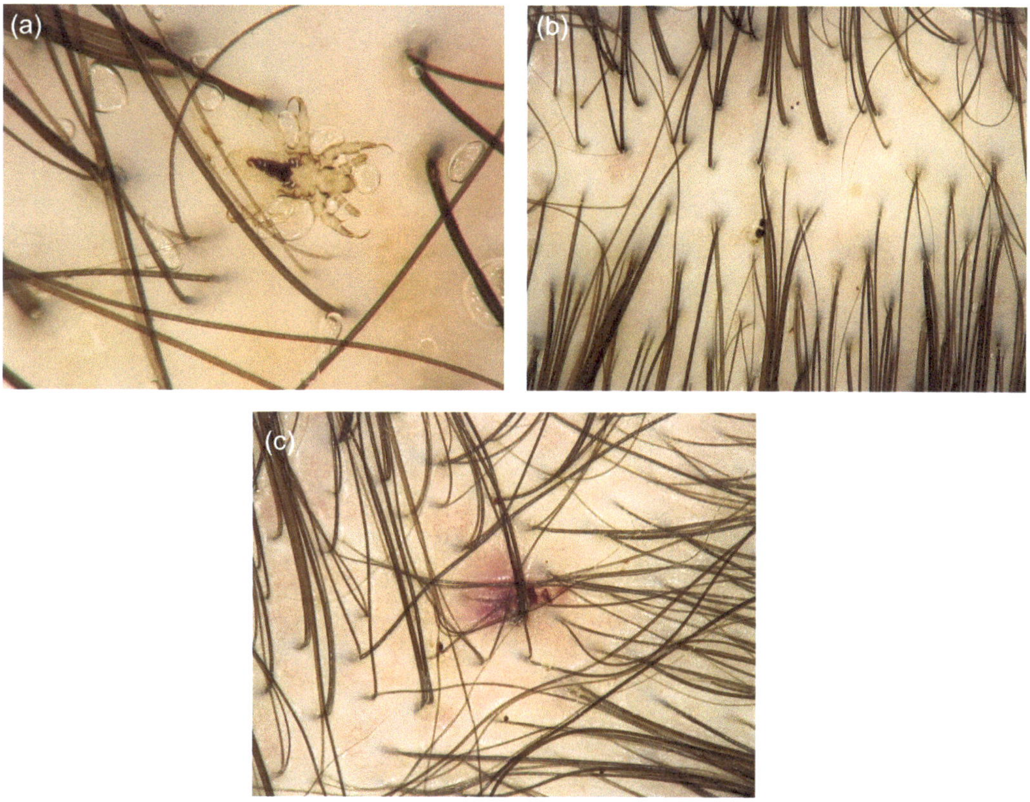

FIGURE 12.9 Pediculosis. ×40 *Pediculus humanus capitis* on the scalp surface (a); ×20 dark rounded spots corresponding to feces (b); ×20 also note hemorrhagic lesions due to bites (c).

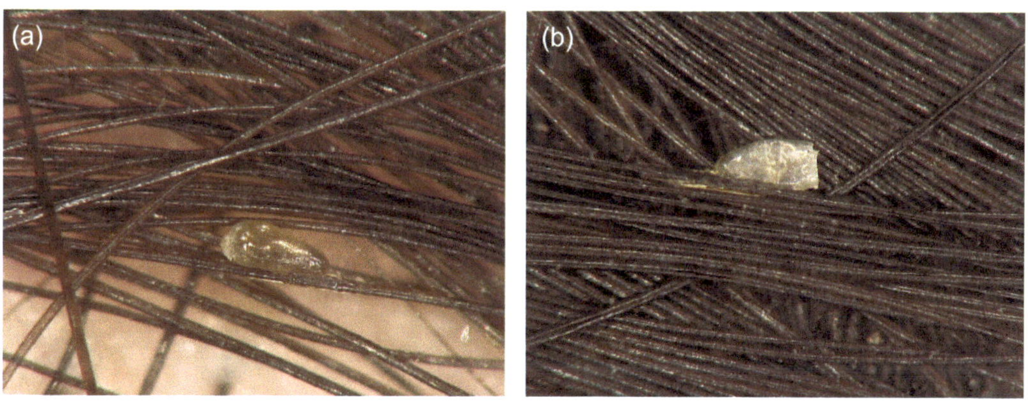

FIGURE 12.10 Pediculosis. ×50 Viable nit (a); ×50 empty harvested nit (b).

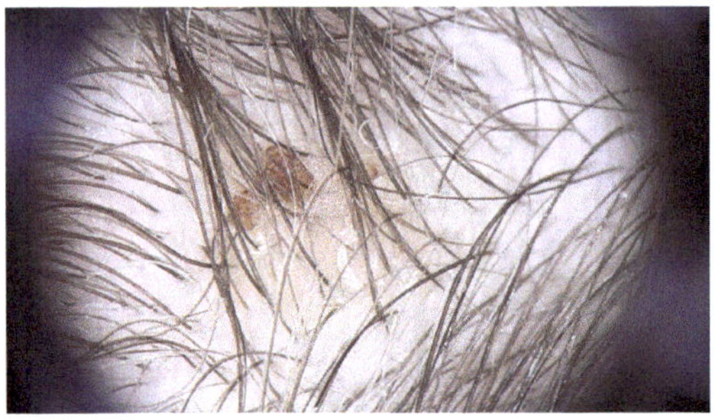

FIGURE 12.11 Scalp scabies. ×10 Delta-wing jet sign and jet contrail sign.

SUGGESTED READING

Doche I, Hordinsky MK, Valente NYS, Romiti R, Tosti A. Syphilitic alopecia: case reports and trichoscopic findings. *Skin Appendage Disord.* 2017;3(4):222–24.

Haliasos EC, Kerner M, Jaimes-Lopez N, Rudnicka L, Zalaudek I, Malvehy J, Hofmann-Wellenhof R, Braun RP, Marghoob AA. Dermoscopy for the pediatric dermatologist part I: dermoscopy of pediatric infectious and inflammatory skin lesions and hair disorders. *Pediatr Dermatol.* 2013;30(2):163–71.

Hughes R, Chiaverini C, Bahadoran P, Lacour JP. Corkscrew hair: a new dermoscopic sign for diagnosis of tinea capitis in black children. *Arch Dermatol.* 2011;147(3):355–6.

Khatu SS, Poojary SA, Nagpur NG. Nodules on the hair: a rare case of mixed piedra. *Int J Trichology.* 2013;5(4):220–3.

Lacarrubba F, Verzì AE, Micali G. Trichoscopy in the differential diagnosis of pseudonits. *Skin Appendage Disord.* 2019;5(3):142–45.

Piraccini BM, Broccoli A, Starace M, et al. Hair and scalp manifestations in secondary syphilis: epidemiology, clinical features and trichoscopy. *Dermatology.* 2015;231(2):171–76.

Verzì AE, Lacarrubba F, Dinotta F, Micali G. Dermatoscopy of parasitic and infectious disorders. *Dermatol Clin.* 2018;36(4):349–58.

13 Eyebrows and Eyelashes

EYEBROW LOSS (MADAROSIS) AND EYELASH LOSS (MILPHOSIS)

Main Causes

Inflammatory

- Alopecia areata
- Frontal fibrosing alopecia
- Discoid lupus erythematosus
- Psoriasis/seborrheic dermatitis
- Demodicosis
- Atopic dermatitis
- "Coup de sabre" scleroderma

Traumatic

- Post-injury
- Autoinduced—trichotillomania

Infectious

- Syphilis
- Leprosy
- Dermatophytosis
- Varicella Zoster virus

Drugs

- Chemotherapy/radiotherapy
- Selective estrogen receptor modulators/aromatase inhibitors

Neoplastic

- Folliculotropic mycosis fungoides

Endocrine

- Hypothyroidism

Genetic

- Keratosis follicularis spinulosa decalvans (see Chapter 7)
- Netherton's syndrome (see Chapter 6)
- Monilethrix (see Chapter 6)

Nutritional

- Zinc deficiency

Alopecia Areata (Figures 13.1, 13.2)

- Signs of active disease are less common due to the lower proportion of hairs in the anagen phase (10% compared to 85%).
- Difficulties in distinguishing hairs that have been plucked by the patients from broken hairs and black dots.

Dermoscopy

- Yellow dots
- Broken hairs
- Exclamation mark hairs (difficult to be found)
- Black dots
- Coudability (rare)

Frontal Fibrosing Alopecia (FFA) (Figures 13.3, 13.4)

Dermoscopy of Eyebrows

Often shows non-scarring features:

- Yellow dots
- Pinpoint white dots (in dark-skin phototypes)
- Black dots
- Hairs growing in different directions
- Broken hairs (rare)
- Peripilar casts (rare)
- Pili torti (rare)

The involvement of the eyelashes is more easily detected by dermoscopy than by clinical examination and might affect up to one-third of patients.

Dermoscopy of Eyelashes

- Visualization of the hair bulbs (upper eyelashes)
- Broken/dystrophic hairs
- Black dots
- Ingrown hairs
- Focal atrichia

DOI: 10.1201/9780429351433-13

Discoid Lupus Erythematosus (DLE) (Figure 13.5)

Scarring alopecia with erythema and scaling mainly affecting the lateral portions of the lower eyelid and eyelashes, either unilaterally or bilaterally.

Dermoscopy of Eyebrows

- Keratotic plugs
- Loss of follicular openings
- Peripilar casts

Eyelashes may be the sole area affected by DLE and the diagnosis can be challenging.

Dermoscopy of Eyelashes

- Red dots
- Telangiectasia, polymorphic and tortuous vessels
- Yellow dots
- Yellowish scales

Seborrheic Dermatitis/ Psoriasis (Figure 13.6)

Patients often complain of excessive shedding of eyebrows and eyelashes.

Dermoscopy of Eyebrows and Eyelashes

- Dermoscopy of pulled hairs shows telogen roots.
- Typical vascular abnormalities can be seen in the eyebrows: Arborizing vessels (seborrheic dermatitis), twisted capillary loops (psoriasis).
- Eyelashes may show tubular casts in seborrheic blepharitis.

Demodicosis (Figure 13.7)

- Causes itching blepharitis, most commonly located in the upper eyelash.
- Dermoscopy shows small casts surrounding the proximal shaft.
- *Demodex* mite can be visualized at high magnification (×70 or up).

Trichotillomania (Figure 13.8, 13.9)

- Eyebrows show irregular patches of hair loss with hairs broken at varying lengths.
- Trichotillomania typically spares the lower eyelashes, which are shorter and more difficult to grasp and pull out.

Dermoscopy of Eyebrows

- Broken hairs at different lengths
- Black dots
- Question mark hairs
- Tulip hairs
- Flame hairs

Dermoscopy of Eyelashes

- Broken hairs at different lengths

Dermatophytosis

Tinea faciei can also cause eyebrow involvement.

- Tinea blepharo-ciliaris typically affects eyelids, causing prominent erythema and swelling, and eyelashes, but does not involve the eyebrows.
- The main causative pathogens belong to: *Microsporum*, *Trichophyton*, or *Epidermophyton* spp.

Dermoscopy

- Comma hairs
- Corkscrew hairs
- Morse-code hairs
- Zigzag hairs
- Bent hairs
- Diffuse erythema/scaling
- Tubular structures (casts) encircling the eyelashes
- Interfollicular pustules in the eyelid

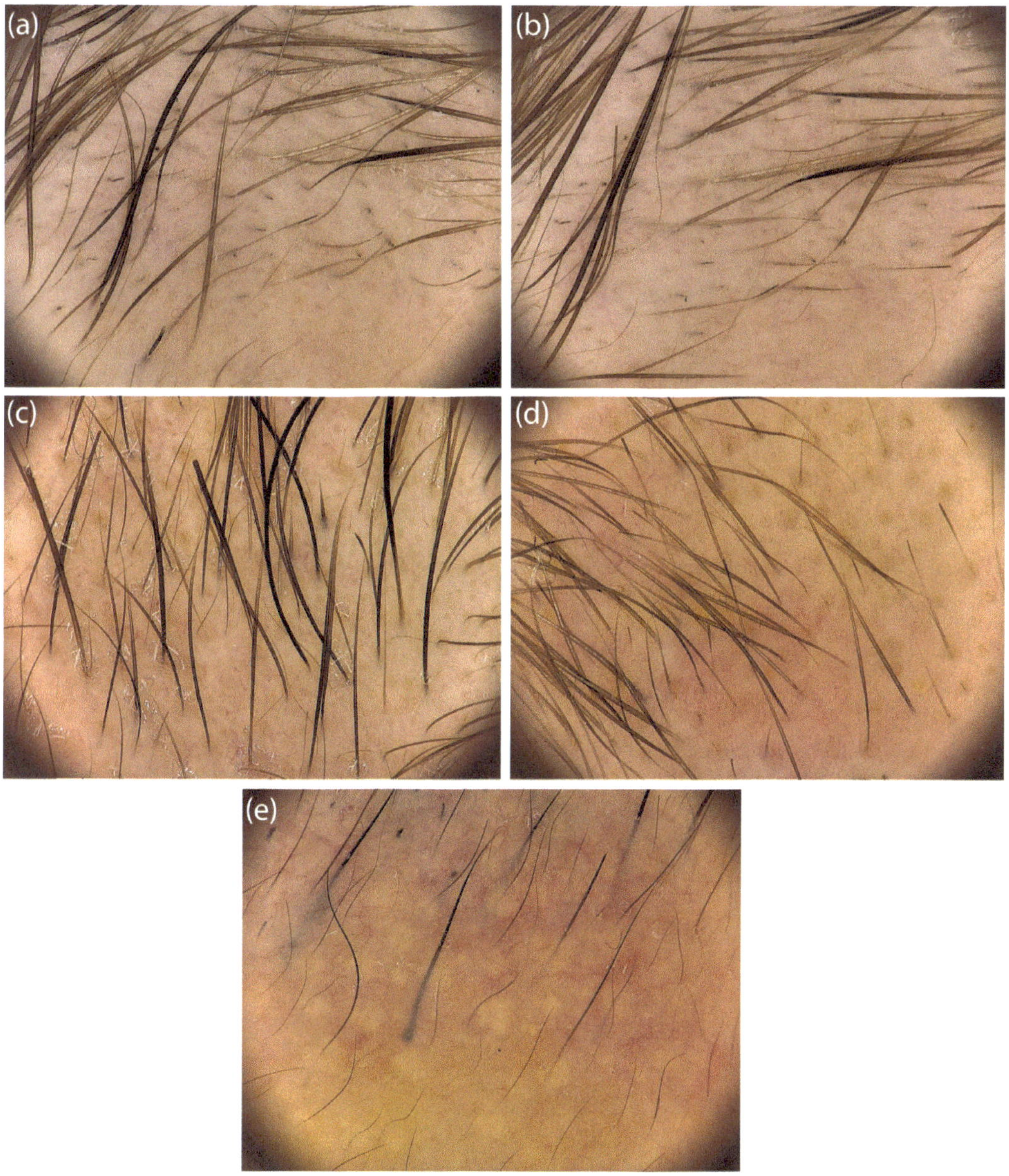

FIGURE 13.1 Alopecia areata eyebrows. ×20 Broken hairs and black dots (a); ×40 coudability (b); ×20 exclamation mark hair, short regrowing hairs, and yellow dots (c,d); ×50 broken hairs and atrophy with visualization of the roots due to repeated steroid injections (e).

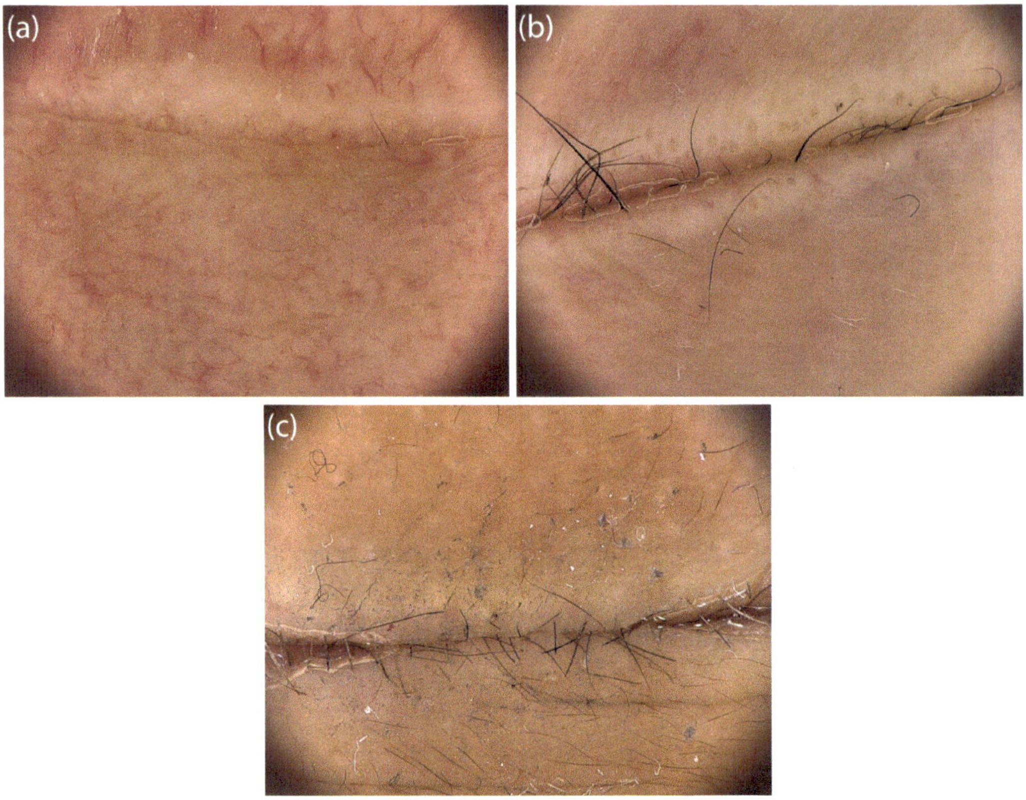

FIGURE 13.2 Alopecia areata of the eyelashes. ×50 Yellow dots (a); ×50 yellow dots, short regrowing hairs, and flame hairs (b); ×50 broken hairs of different length (c); evaluation can be difficult due to make-up.

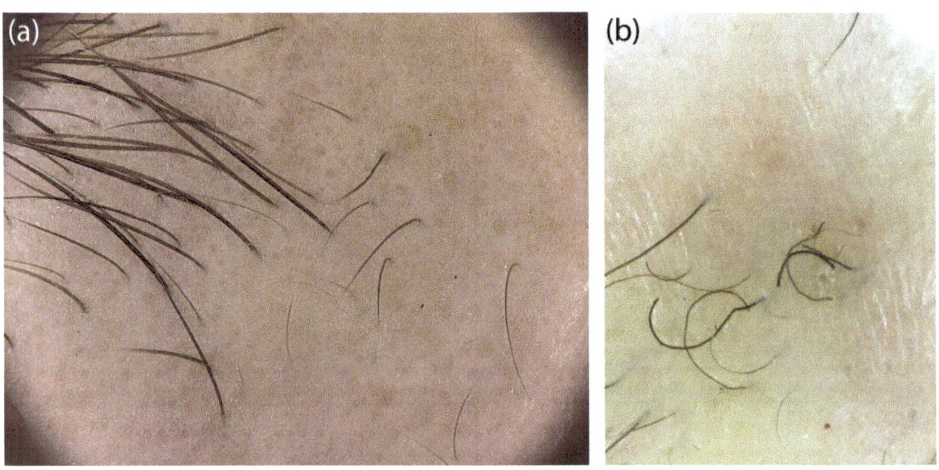

FIGURE 13.3 FFA. ×40 Eyebrows growing in different directions (a); ×50 loss of follicular openings, pili torti, and peripilar casts (b).

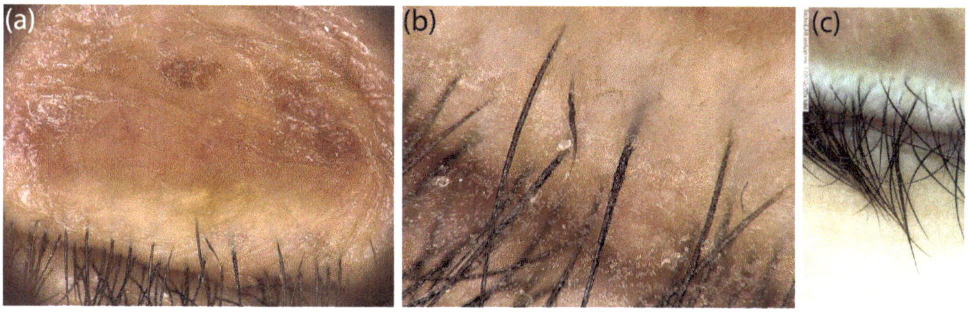

FIGURE 13.4 FFA. ×20 Dystrophic hair on the upper eyelashes (a); ×50 higher magnification (b); ×20 visualization of the hair roots in the upper eyelashes (c).

FIGURE 13.5 DLE. ×20 Keratotic plugs in discoid lupus affecting the eyebrows.

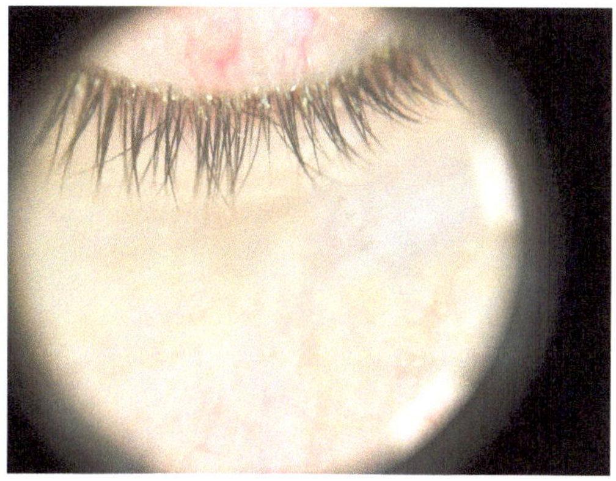

FIGURE 13.6 Seborrheic blepharitis. ×10 Yellowish tubular casts.

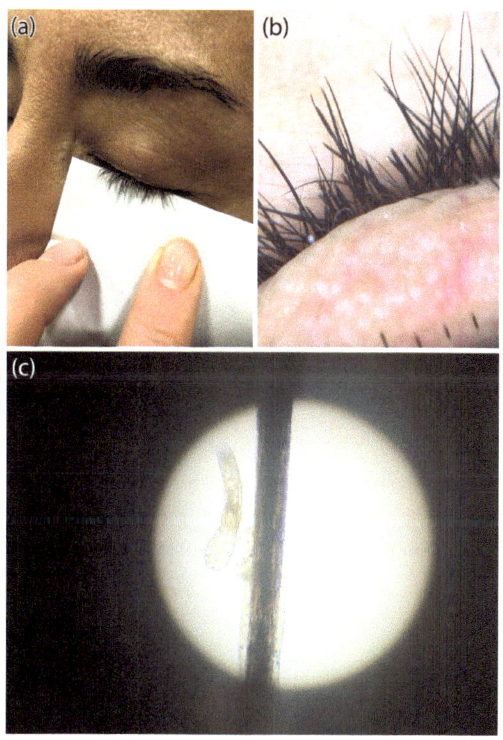

FIGURE 13.7 Demodicosis. A sheet of paper under the lashes makes dermoscopy examination easier (a); ×10 small white cast and breakage of the lashes due to scratching (b); *Demodex folliculorum* attached to the hair shaft under the microscope (c). (Courtesy of Dr. Lorena Lammoglia Ordiales).

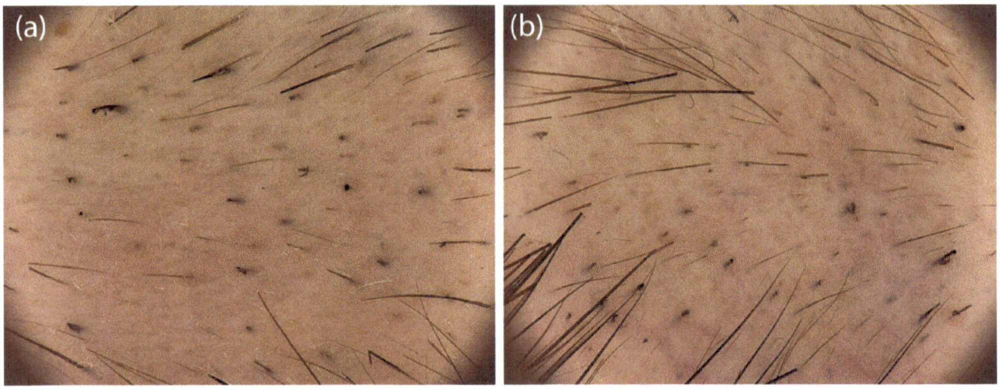

FIGURE 13.8 Trichotillomania of the eyebrows. ×20 Black dots, broken hairs, and question mark hair (a); ×20 broken, question mark, and flame hairs (b).

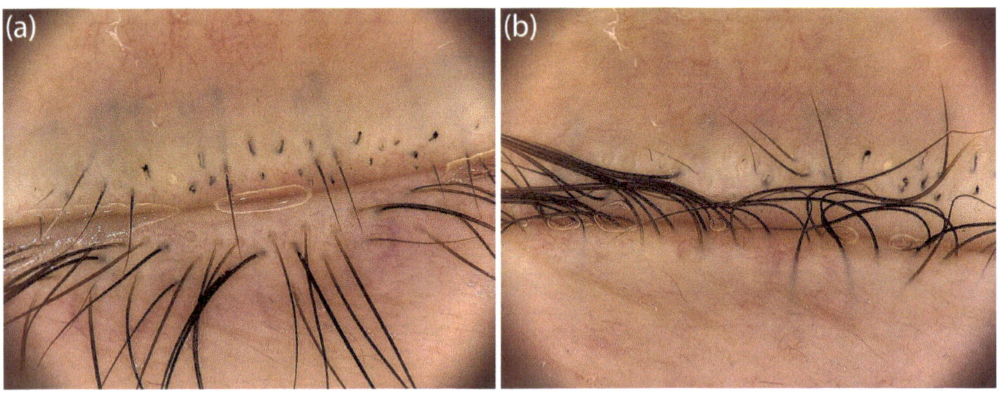

FIGURE 13.9 (a,b) Trichotillomania of the eyelashes. ×20 Multiple flame hairs and question mark limited to the upper eyelid.

SUGGESTED READING

Anzai A, Pirmez R, Vincenzi C, Fabbrocini G, Romiti R, Tosti A. Trichoscopy findings of frontal fibrosing alopecia on the eyebrows: a study of 151 cases. *J Am Acad Dermatol.* 2021;85(5):1130–34.

Cortez de Almeida RF, Ferreira BFM, Melo DF, Benez M, Vincenzi C, Starace M, Tosti A. Dermoscopic findings of discoid lupus erythematosus involving the eyelids. *Skin Appendage Disord.* 2022;8(5):424–26.

Nguyen B, Hu JK, Tosti A. Eyebrow and eyelash alopecia: a clinical review. *Am J Clin Dermatol.* 2023;24(1):55–67.

Salas-Callo CI, Tosti A, Stohmann D, Contarini P, Pirmez R. Eyelash involvement in frontal fibrosing alopecia: a prospective study. *J Am Acad Dermatol.* 2022;87(1):232–34.

Sławińska M, Jaworska K, Wyszomirski A, Rychlik K, Nowicki RJ, Sobjanek M. Videodermoscopy in the assessment of patients with ocular demodicosis. *Dermatol Pract Concept.* 2023;13(2).

Verzi AE, Lacarrubba F, Micali G. Trichoscopy of the eyelashes in tinea blepharo-ciliaris shows the full spectrum of tinea capitis features. *JAAD Case Rep.* 2020;6(7):661–62.

14 Body Hair Disorders

Inflammatory
- Keratosis pilaris
- Trichostasis spinulosa
- Eruptive vellus hair cysts
- Pseudofolliculitis
- Lichen planopilaris
- Alopecia areata
- Frontal fibrosing alopecia

Traumatic
- Rolled hairs
- Leg alopecia
- Trichotillomania

Infectious
- Trichomycosis palmellina
- Pediculosis pubis
- Tinea corporis

Tubular Structures Encircling Body Hairs
- Multiple myeloma
- Trichodysplasia spinulosa
- Demodicosis

Other
- Senescent alopecia
- Circle hairs

INFLAMMATORY

Keratosis Pilaris (Figure 14.1)

- Rough tiny erythematous papules typically located on the upper arms, thighs, cheeks, and buttocks.
- A scarring evolution may occur in ulerythema ophryogenes and keratosis follicularis spinulosa decalvans.

Dermoscopy

- Vellus hairs partially embedded into the horny layer.
- Vellus hairs can be single or merge as a group of two to three hairs.
- Perifollicular erythema in light phototypes.
- Perifollicular hyperpigmentation in dark-skin phototypes.
- Circle embedded hairs within the follicular openings.
- Keratotic plugs in the follicular ostia.

Trichostasis Spinulosa (Figure 14.2)

- Results from retention of 5 to 50 telogen vellus hairs within the follicle
- In elderly patients typically affects the nose with comedo-like lesions
- In young patients affects the trunk and upper arms with itchy, keratotic, tiny follicular papules

Dermoscopy

- More than six fine vellus hairs emerging from a dilated single follicle, encircled by a keratinous sheath

Eruptive Vellus Hair Cysts

- Typically appear in childhood or early adulthood
- Are characterized by flesh-colored or slightly hyperpigmented papules, ranging 1–4 mm in size, mainly clustered on the chest and abdomen

Dermoscopy

- Follicular opening on the top of the cyst.
- Embedded vellus hair is sometimes visible through the skin.
- Perifollicular hyperpigmentation/erythema can be seen according to the phototype.

DOI: 10.1201/9780429351433-14

Pseudofolliculitis (Figure 14.3)

- Papulo-pustular eruption mostly affecting the legs, groin, beard, and the nape area.
- Post-inflammatory hyperpigmentation is common.

Dermoscopy

Embedded hair shafts can have either a trans-follicular or an extrafollicular penetration:

- Trans-follicular penetration is typical of epilation practices and the embedding of the hair shaft occurs before its emergence.
- Extrafollicular penetration is typical of shaving; the hair re-enters within the epidermis 1–2 mm away from its emergence.

Lichen Planopilaris (Figure 14.4)

Lichen planus follicularis may occur in patients with lichen planopilaris/frontal fibrosing alopecia (FFA) with a diffuse eruption of follicular papules surrounding the body hairs; this is reversible with treatment.

Dermoscopy

- Peripilar casts
- Perifollicular erythema
- Broken hairs

Frontal Fibrosing Alopecia (Figure 14.5, 14.6)

- Limb involvement is very common.
- Axillary and pubic hairs can also be affected.
- Beard involvement is very common.
- Lichen follicularis can occur.
- In case of hairline recession in men, FFA of the beard is a clue to make the differential diagnosis with androgenetic alopecia.

Dermoscopy

- Loss of follicular openings
- Peripilar casts

Beard Dermoscopy

- Loss of follicular openings, can be difficult to see due to shaving
- Peripilar casts
- Diffuse/perifollicular erythema

TRAUMATIC

Rolled Hairs (Figures 14.7, 14.8)

- Dark hairs forming a perfect circle interspersed among normal hairs
- More common in hairy men, especially in friction prone areas

Dermoscopy

- Rolled circle hairs forming a complete ring

Leg Alopecia (Figure 14.9)

- Predominantly affects the lower extremities, particularly the anterolateral side of lower limb.
- Is characterized by well-defined or diffuse areas of reduced hair density without inflammatory changes.
- In most cases the condition is scarring.

Dermoscopy

- Broken hairs due to friction (few)
- Proximal trichorrhexis nodosa
- Loss of follicular openings

INFECTIOUS

Trichomycosis Palmellina (Figure 14.10)

- Superficial infection of axillary and pubic hairs caused by *Corynebacterium* spp.
- Dermoscopy shows yellowish/orange granular concretions that completely or partially surround the hair shaft.
- Not all the hairs are affected.

Pediculosis Pubis

Dermoscopy

- *Pthirus pubis* is characterized by a dorsoventrally flattened body and

crab-like appearance, typically clasping hair shafts with their claws or feeding by inserting mouth parts into the skin.
- Empty nits appear as tiny translucent white structures with a flattened end, firmly adherent to pubic hairs/eyelashes.
- Viable nits containing nymphs have an ovoid shape, are brown in color.
- Bluish-gray macules, corresponding to the parasite's bites for feeding, can be found in the interfollicular skin.

Tinea Corporis (Figure 14.11)

Dermoscopy

- Hair shaft abnormalities of the vellus hair include comma, broken, Morse-code, corkscrew, and zigzag hairs
- Tubular casts encircling the hair shaft
- Dotted vessels
- Follicular micro pustules

TUBULAR STRUCTURES ENCIRCLING BODY HAIRS

Multiple Myeloma

- Follicular keratotic spicules localized to the face, and especially to the nose, are a skin manifestation of multiple myeloma's paraproteinemia, and a possible marker of disease progression.
- They correspond to precipitated monoclonal proteins and may resolve with effective treatment.
- Eyelashes hair casts can also occur.

Dermoscopy

- Follicular keratotic spicules surrounding the vellus hairs
- Tubular casts encircling the eyelashes at their proximal base

Trichodysplasia Spinulosa (Figure 14.12)

Mainly affects immunocompromised individuals, and is caused by the trichodysplasia spinulosa-associated polyomavirus.

Clinical Features

Follicular keratotic spicules surrounding terminal and vellus hairs.

Dermoscopy

- Keratotic follicular spicules
- Dense linear jelly spicules encircling the terminal and vellus hairs for most of their length

Demodicosis

Dermoscopy

- Tubular jelly structures encircling the vellus hairs
- Enlarged follicular openings filled with round, grayish-brown plug, encircled by an erythematous halo
- Thin arborizing vessels and linear vessels

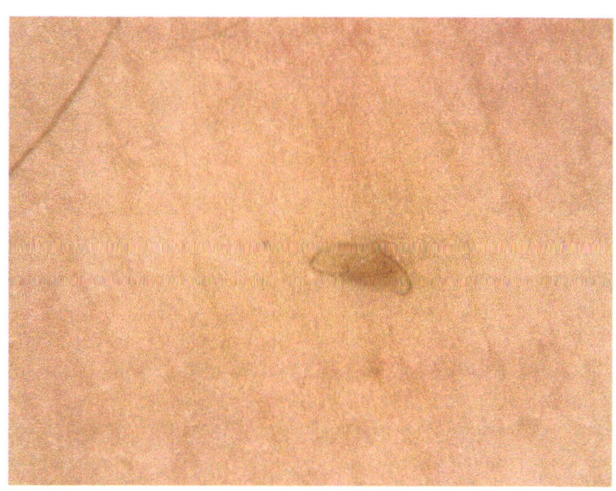

FIGURE 14.1 Keratosis pilaris. ×50 Keratotic papules with hair embedding and peripheral erythema.

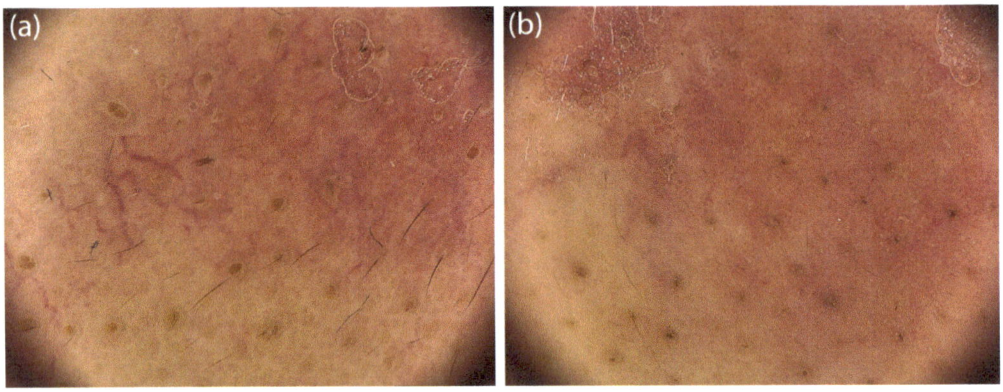

FIGURE 14.2 (a,b) Trichostasis spinulosa. ×20 Tufts of vellus hairs emerging from dilated openings and yellow-brown follicular plugs. Also note enlarged arborizing vessels due to associated rosacea.

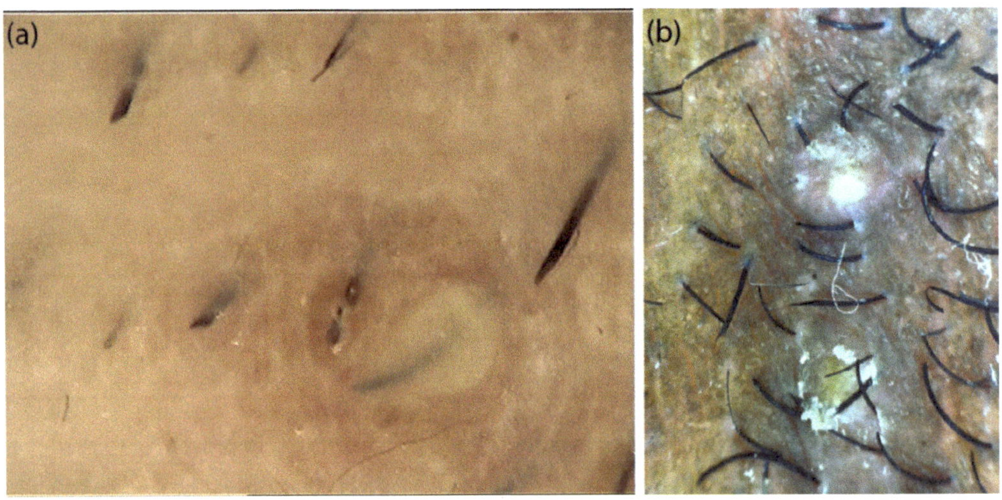

FIGURE 14.3 Pseudofolliculitis. ×50 Embedding of the hair shaft before its emergence from the skin (trans-follicular penetration) (a); ×50 extrafollicular penetration from shaving (b).

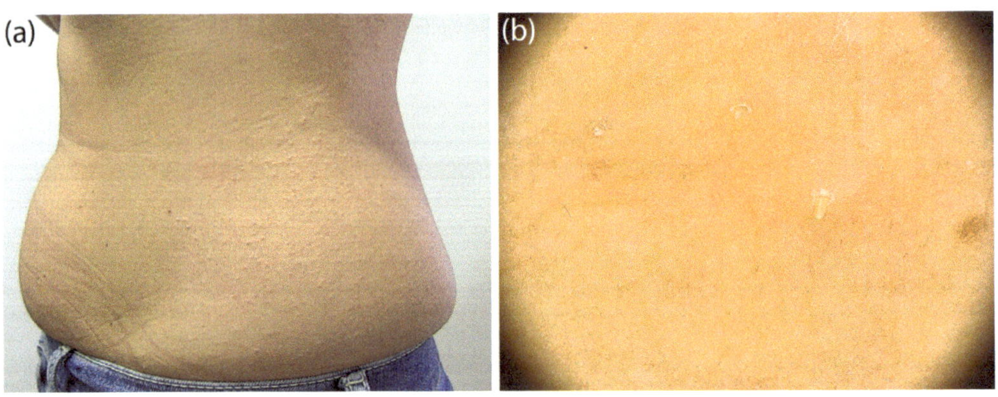

FIGURE 14.4 (a,b) Lichen follicularis. Clinical presentation: ×50 keratotic follicular spicules with a scaly rim.

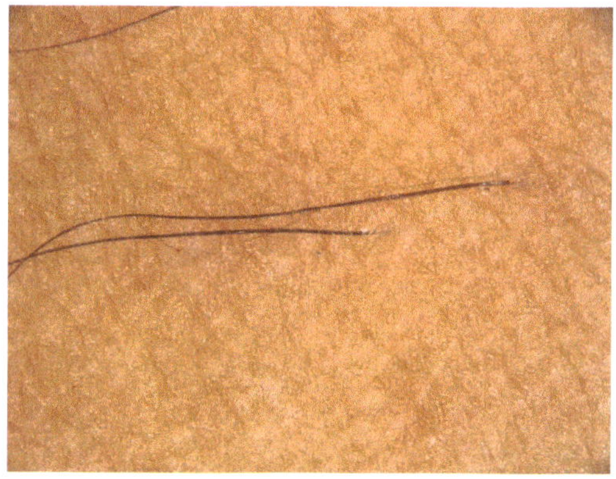

FIGURE 14.5 FFA of the limb. ×50 Loss of follicular openings and peripilar casts around the remaining hairs.

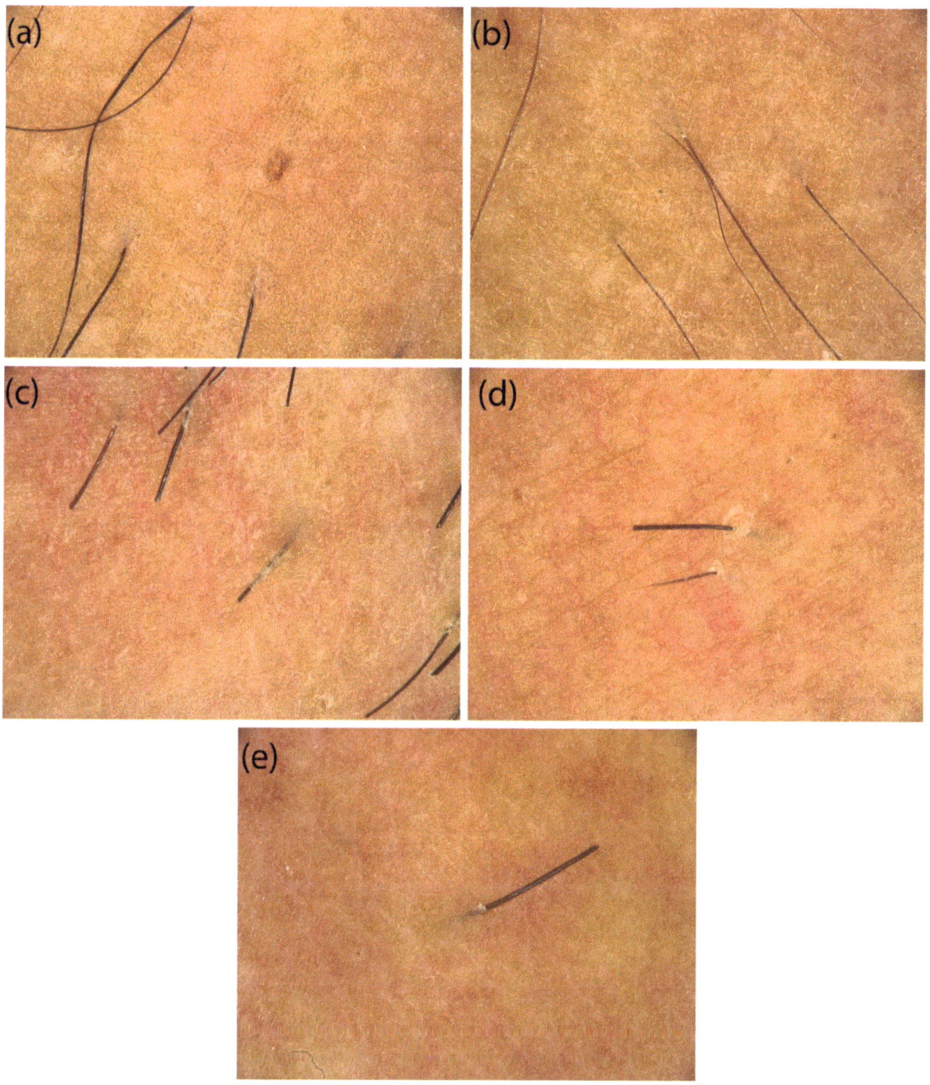

FIGURE 14.6 Lichen follicularis in FFA. ×50 Transparent emergences of the hairs and peripilar casts in the body (a,b); ×50 beard involvement with diffuse erythema, peripilar casts, and tubular casts (c); note that peripilar casts affect both a shaved terminal hair and a short regrowing hair (d); ×70 peripilar cast at high magnification (e).

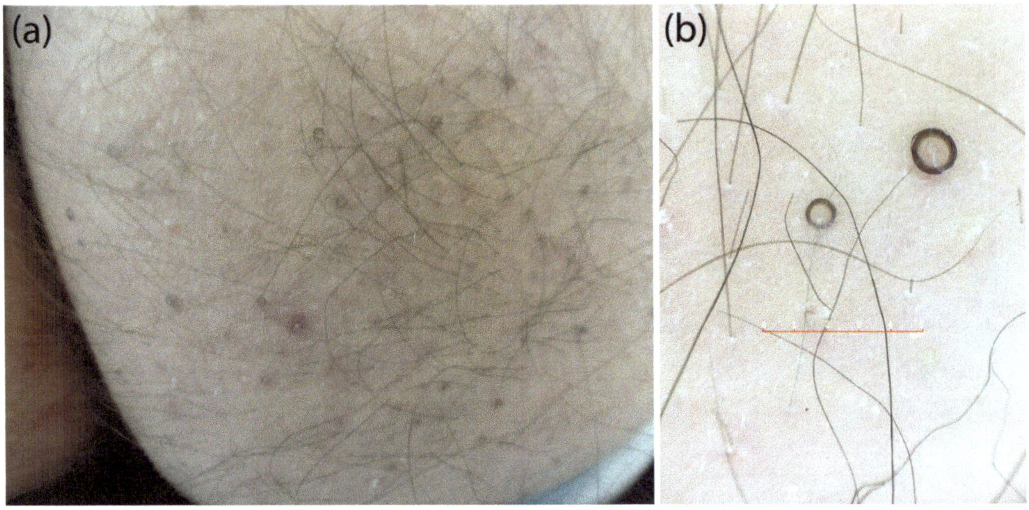

FIGURE 14.7 Rolled hair. Inflammatory papular lesions with twisted hairs interspersed between normal hairs (a); ×20 regularly twisted subcorneal hairs (b). (Courtesy of Dr. Martin Zaiac.)

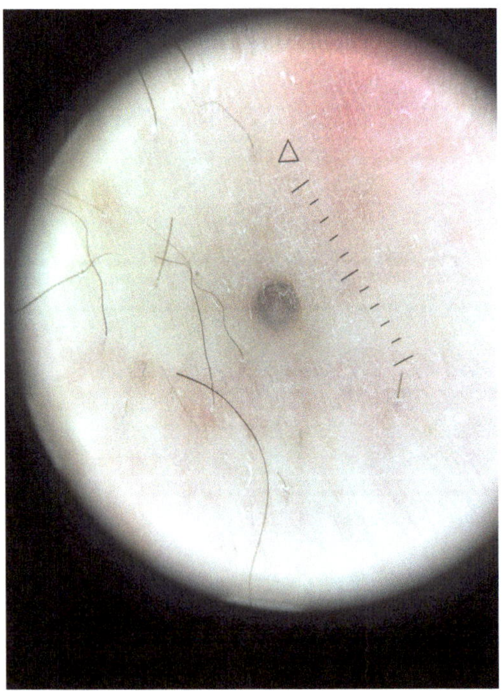

FIGURE 14.8 ×10 Rolled hair in the intergluteal area.

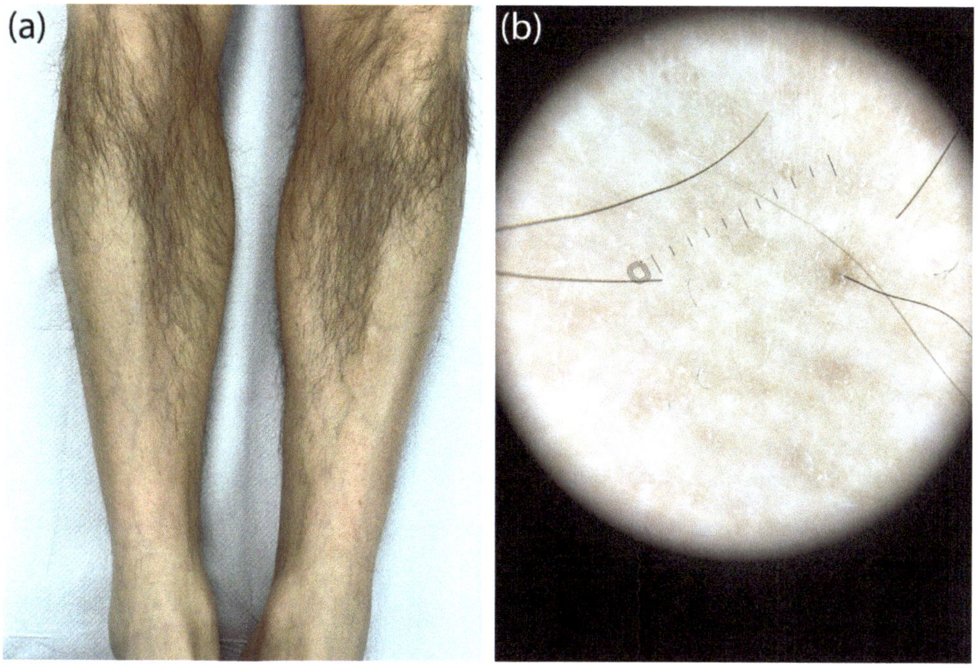

FIGURE 14.9 Leg alopecia. ×10 loss of follicular openings (a); note a subtle cast surrounding a remaining terminal hair (b).

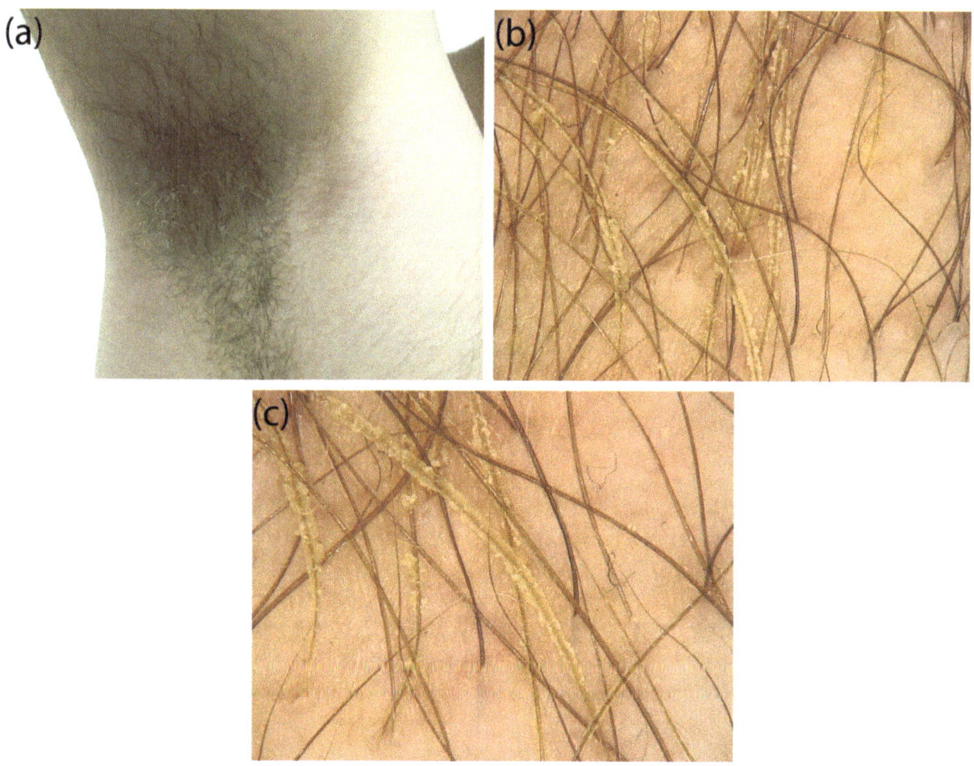

FIGURE 14.10 Trichomycosis palmellina. Infection of axillary area (a); ×20 yellowish granular concretions surrounding some of the axillary hairs (b); ×50 the waxy and yellowish aggregates partially or completely encircle the hair (c).

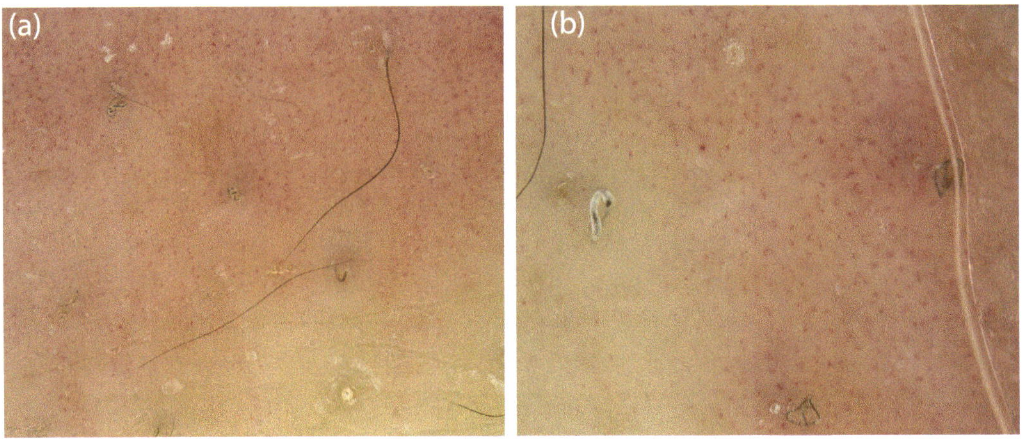

FIGURE 14.11 Tinea corporis: ×50 Comma and corkscrew hairs (a); ×50 note a tubular scale encircling the comma hair and dotted vessels (b).

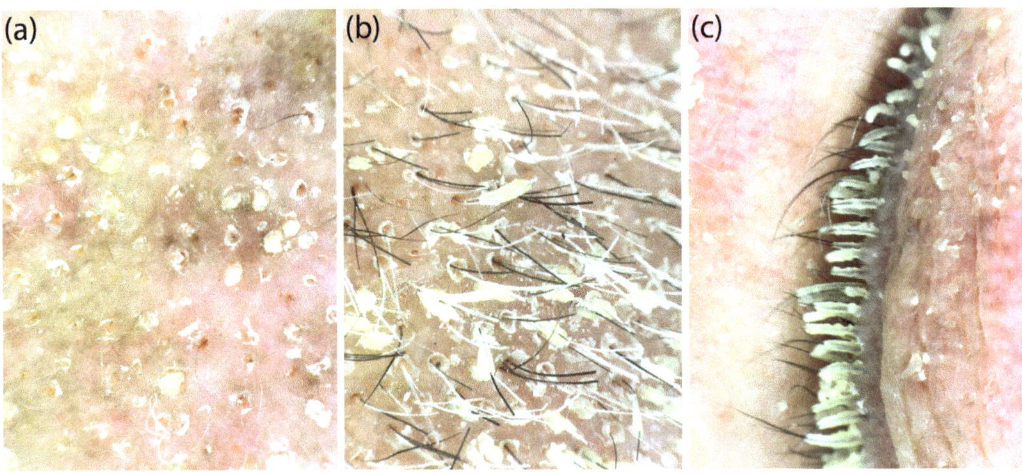

FIGURE 14.12 Trichodysplasia spinulosa. ×20 Keratotic plugs filling and emerging from the follicular ostia (a); ×20 jelly spicules encircling the terminal hairs (b); and ×20 the eyelashes (c).

SUGGESTED READING

Lacarrubba F, Misciali C, Gibilisco R, Micali G. Circle hairs: clinical, trichoscopic and histopathologic findings. *Int J Trichology.* 2013;5(4):211–3.

Panchaprateep R, Tanus A, Tosti A. Clinical, dermoscopic, and histopathologic features of body hair disorders. *J Am Acad Dermatol.* 2015;72(5):890–900.

Pozo L, Bowling J, Perrett CM, Bull R, Diaz-Cano SJ. Dermoscopy of trichostasis spinulosa. *Arch Dermatol.* 2008;144(8):1088.

Shakshouk H, Tosti A. Trichoscopy beyond scalp. A narrative review. *Int J Dermatol.* 2023;62(3):416–27.

Stonesifer CJ, Husain SA, Niedt GW, Gallitano SM. Dermatoscopy case of the month: trichodysplasia spinulosa. *JAAD Case Rep.* 2021;17:116–18.

15 Hair Root Evaluation

PULL TEST (FIGURES 15.1–15.7)

Pull Test Findings

- Telogen roots: Club-shaped and non-pigmented.
- Early telogen roots: With keratinous envelopes.
- Late telogen roots: Devoid of the sheaths.
- Anagen roots, pigmented rectangular distal end. Never extracted with pull test, except for scarring alopecias, pemphigus, and loose anagen hair syndrome (LAHS).
- Anagen roots obtained with the pull test in pemphigus can be stained with direct immunofluorescence for diagnostic purposes.
- Anagen roots with thickened sheaths are associated with scarring alopecias (mainly lichen planopilaris and folliculitis decalvans).
- Anagen roots without sheaths are associated with the loose anagen hair syndrome. The roots have a rectangular/conic-pointed or irregular shape and the cuticle may be ragged.
- Dystrophic anagen roots are detected at the pull test of acute anagen effluvium, including alopecia areata or chemotherapy alopecia. They have a pigmented, pencil point-like, or blunt brush-like shape. The shafts may also have irregular narrowings known as Pohl-Pinkus marks.
- Broken hair shafts due to trichorrhexis nodosa are common in African hairs and in patients with hair weathering.

See also Table 15.1.

TRICHOGRAM (FIGURES 15.8–15.10)

Dermoscopy-Assisted Trichogram

- A semi-invasive procedure performed by extracting a tuft of hairs with hemostatic forceps covered with a plastic/silicone tube to prevent the breakage of the hair shafts before the scalp level.
- Hairs are plucked and examined 5 cm from the root; they are collected on white/black paper and secured with tape before removing the forceps in order to align the roots.
- The extracted roots can be placed in a plastic envelope to be examined with the dermatoscope (envelope trichogram).
- The authors believe that this procedure is only necessary to prove the diagnosis of loose anagen hair syndrome (see Chapter 7).

DOI: 10.1201/9780429351433-15

TABLE 15.1
Dermoscopic Findings of Extracted Hairs in the Pull Test in Different Hair Disorders

Disease	Pull Test	Dermoscopy of Pulled Roots
LAHS	Often negative as hairs have already been extracted by minimal trauma	Anagen roots without sheaths
Short anagen	Often positive	Short hairs with pointed tips and telogen roots
Acute telogen effluvium	Positive	Telogen roots (in early, mature and late stages)
Lichen planopilaris	Positive in active lesions	Anagen roots with thickened sheaths
Folliculitis decalvans	Positive in active lesions	Anagen roots with thickened sheaths
Alopecia areata (as any other anagen effluvium)	Positive in active lesions	Dystrophic anagen roots Telogen roots in different stages
Alopecia areata incognito	Positive	Telogen roots in different stages
Psoriasis	Positive	Telogen roots (in chronic disease the majority are in late stage)
Hair weathering	Positive tug test	Broken hairs with trichorrhexis nodosa

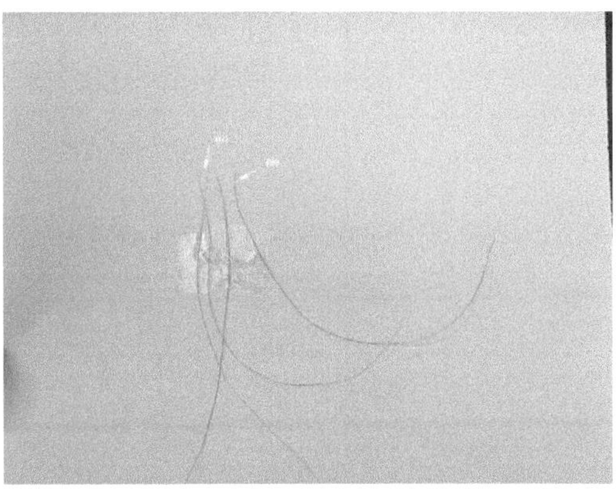

FIGURE 15.1 The pulled roots are placed on a piece of white paper (dark hairs) or black paper (blonde/white hairs) and fixed with tape in order for the roots to be aligned.

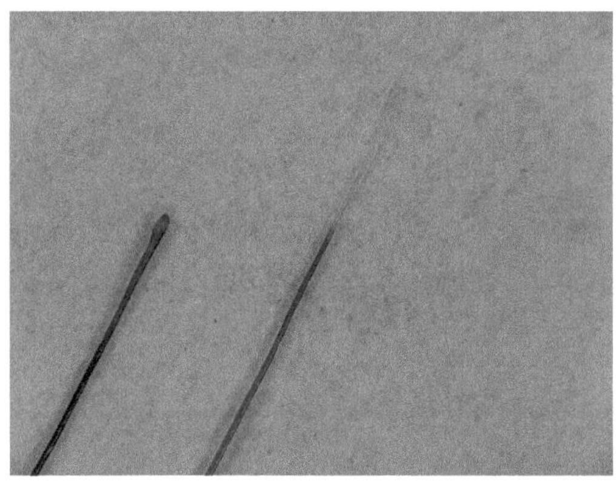

FIGURE 15.2 ×50 Telogen roots of a pigmented and non-pigmented hair shaft, showing a typical club shape.

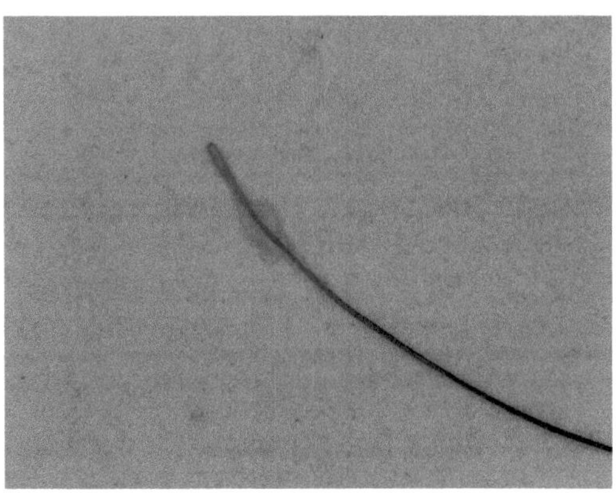

FIGURE 15.3 ×50 Early telogen hair shows the persistence of telogen sac.

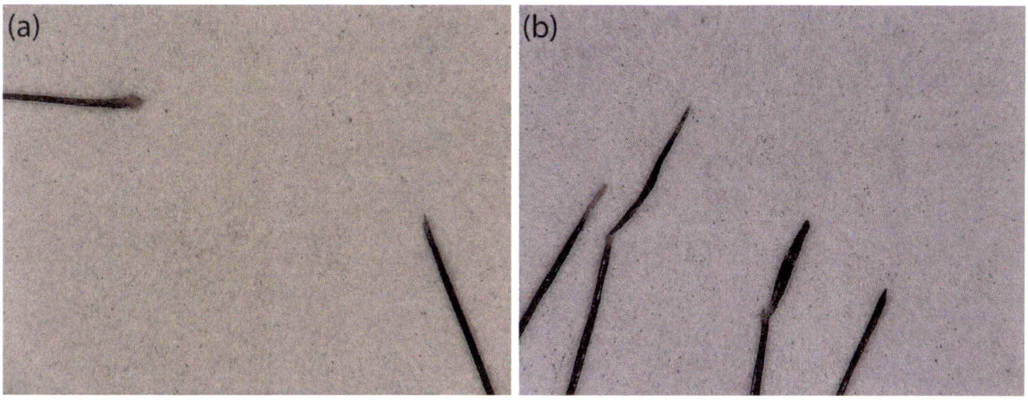

FIGURE 15.4 Pull test of alopecia areata. ×50 Telogen hair on the left and dystrophic anagen hair on the right (a); ×50 dystrophic roots showing constriction and irregularly shaped tip (b).

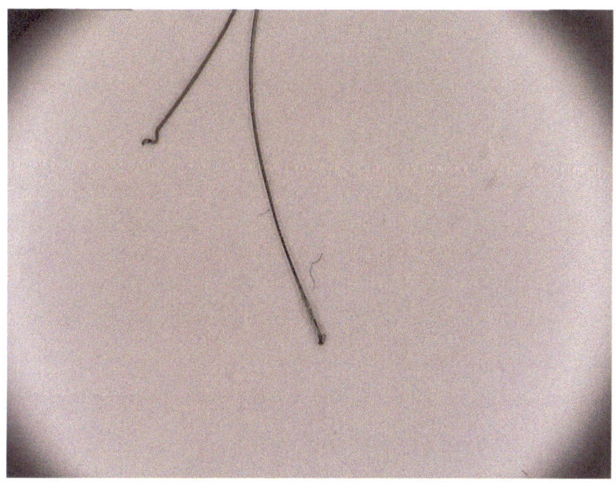

FIGURE 15.5 Loose anagen hair syndrome: pull test is often negative, but it can show anagen root without sheaths.

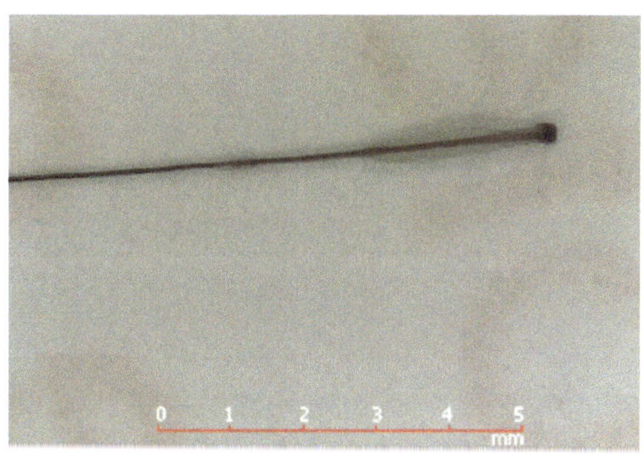

FIGURE 15.6 Pull test of lichen planopilaris. ×20 Anagen roots with thickened sheaths.

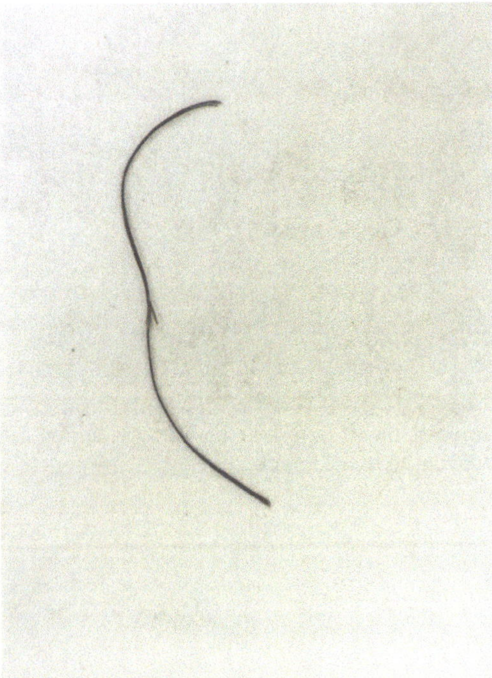

FIGURE 15.7 ×20 Broken hair shaft at the pull/tug test of trichorrhexis nodosa.

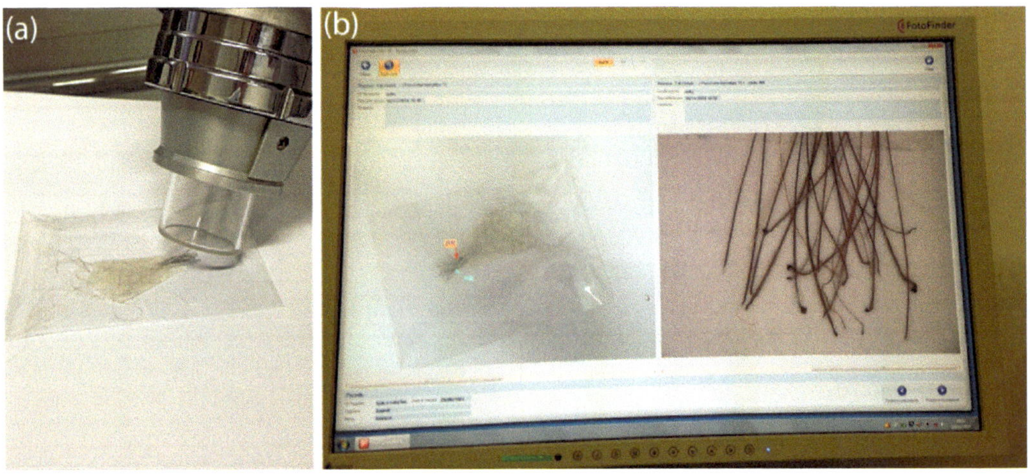

FIGURE 15.8 (a,b) Envelope trichogram. (Courtesy of Dr. Fernanda Torres.)

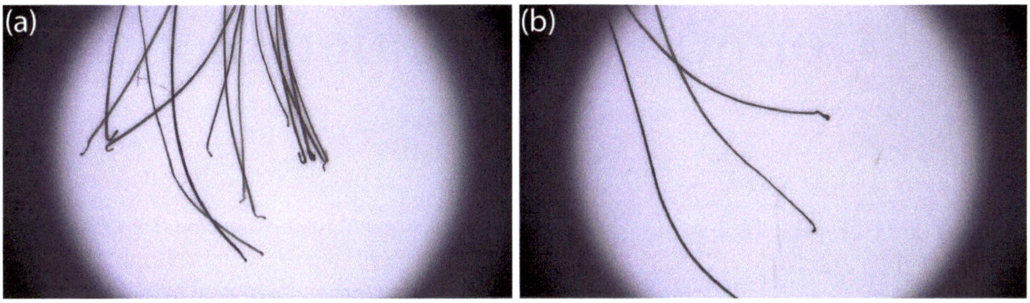

FIGURE 15.9 Loose anagen hair syndrome. ×20 Trichogram shows absence of telogen hairs and anagen hairs devoid of sheaths (a); ×50 note irregular shape of the roots (b).

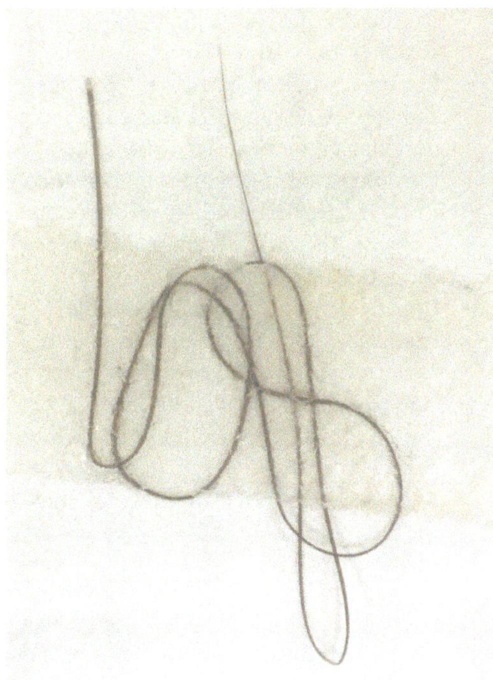

FIGURE 15.10 Short anagen hair syndrome. ×20 The short telogen hair has not been cut, as it presents a pointed tip.

SUGGESTED READING

Tsiogka A, Laimer M, Ahlgrimm-Siess V. Trichoscopy-assisted hair pull test: a helpful adjunct to trichoscopy for diagnosing and managing alopecias. *Australas J Dermatol.* 2021;62(4):e602–e605.

16 Dermoscopy-Guided Biopsies

BIOPSY SITE (TABLE 16.1 AND FIGURES 16.1–16.10)

- Utilizing dermoscopy for biopsy improves precise pathological diagnosis in scarring alopecias, with a success rate of 95%.
- Biopsies guided by dermoscopy facilitate dermoscopic-pathological correlations.
- For cicatricial alopecia, biopsy site should include typical features such as peripilar casts, pustular lesions, keratotic plugs, hair tufting, or red dots.
- In connective tissue diseases presenting with diffuse alopecia, biopsy sites should include abnormal vessels.
- In patchy alopecia with doubtful clinical diagnosis, biopsy should be taken at center of the patch to distinguish scarring from non-scarring alopecia.
- 2-mm dermoscopy guided biopsies can be considered when the alopecia affects cosmetic-sensitive areas, like the frontal hairline or the eyebrows in frontal fibrosing alopecia (FFA). These biopsies require a specific processing technique and a trained pathologist.
- 3-mm dermoscopy guided biopsies can be utilized in scarring alopecias, particularly fibrosing alopecia in a pattern distribution (FAPD), lichen planopilaris, and discoid lupus erythematosus, to reduce scar size.
- In non-scarring alopecia it is necessary to perform 4-mm dermoscopy-guided biopsies to allow the pathologist to perform hair counts.

TECHNIQUE

- The selected area is marked, encircled, and photographed with a dermoscope before the biopsy.
- A 2-, 3-, or 4-mm punch biopsy, angled parallel to hair exit from the skin and extending to subcutaneous fat, is recommended for preserving follicle structure and facilitating accurate sectioning.

TABLE 16.1
Optimal Site of Biopsy in Different Disorders

Disease	Biopsy Site
Scarring alopecias	
Lichen planopilaris	Tuft of hairs with peripilar casts
Frontal fibrosing alopecia	Terminal hairs with peripilar casts
Discoid lupus erythematosus	Keratotic plugs or red dots
Folliculitis decalvans	Tuft of hairs with peripilar casts
Central centrifugal cicatricial alopecia	Terminal hair surrounded by white-gray halos
Non-scarring alopecias	
Alopecia areata	Exclamation mark hairs, black dots, broken hairs, yellow dots, circle hairs
Alopecia areata incognito	Yellow dots, circle hairs, and short regrowing hairs of normal thickness
Androgenetic alopecia	Hair diameter diversity
Dissecting cellulitis	3D-yellow dots, black dots, keratotic plugs
Trichotillomania	Broken hairs, flame hairs, question mark hairs

DOI: 10.1201/9780429351433-16

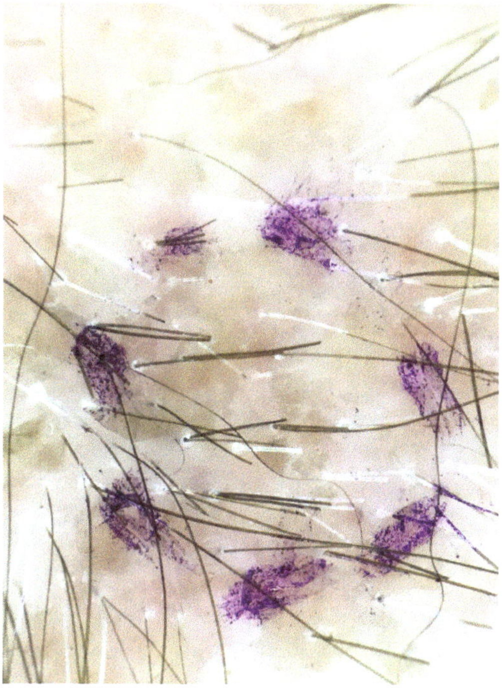

FIGURE 16.1 ×20 In lichen planopilaris and FAPD the biopsy site should include the peripilar cast.

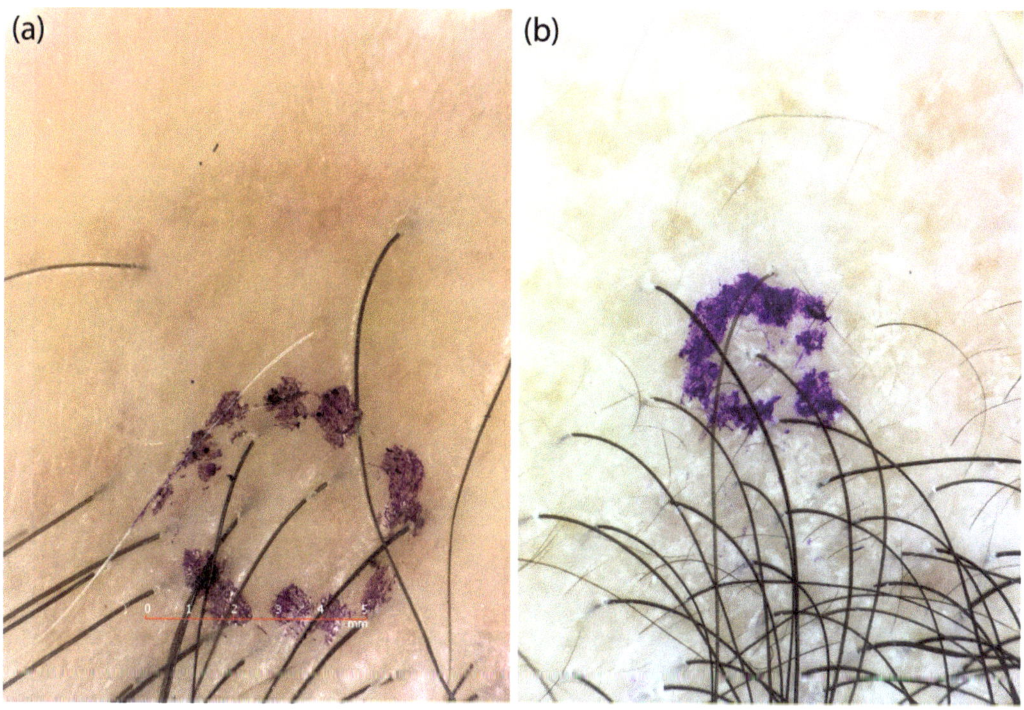

FIGURE 16.2 FFA. ×20 Biopsy site includes subtle peripilar casts. In this patient vellus hairs are preserved (a); the biopsy site includes a peripilar cast (b).

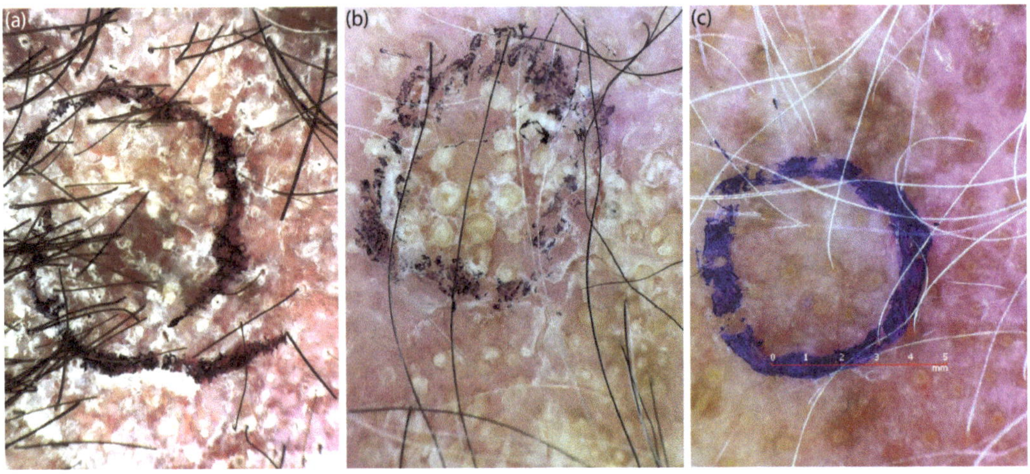

FIGURE 16.3 Discoid lupus erythematosus. ×20 The biopsy site is selected in an area with evident keratotic plugs (a,b) or red dots (c).

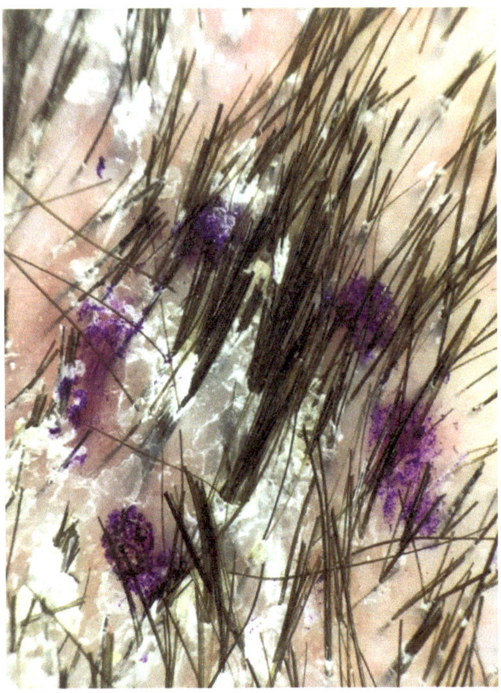

FIGURE 16.4 Folliculitis decalvans. ×20 Biopsy site includes tufts of hair surrounded by peripilar casts.

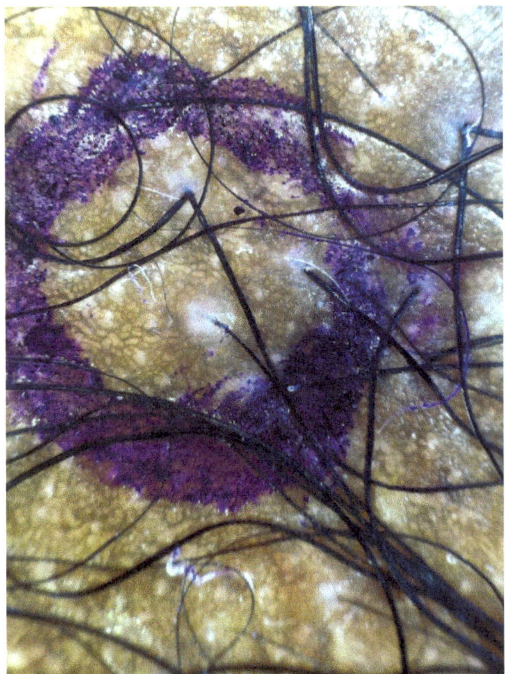

FIGURE 16.5 Central centrifugal cicatricial alopecia. ×20 The biopsy site is selected in an area with terminal hairs surrounded by white-gray halos.

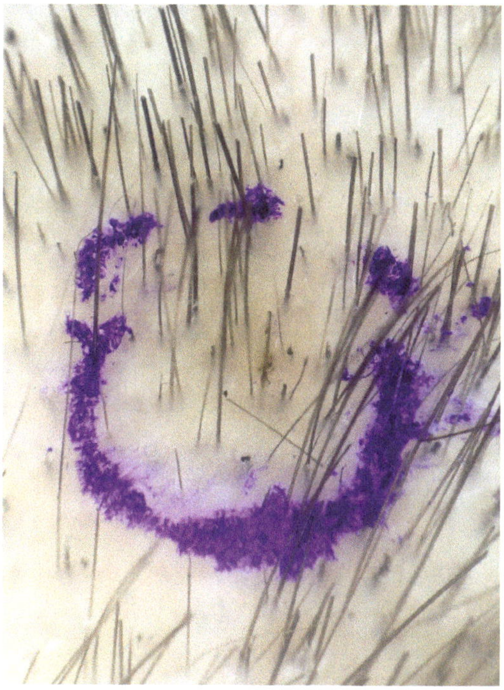

FIGURE 16.6 Trichotillomania. ×20 When differential is between alopecia areata and trichotillomania the biopsy site should include broken hairs.

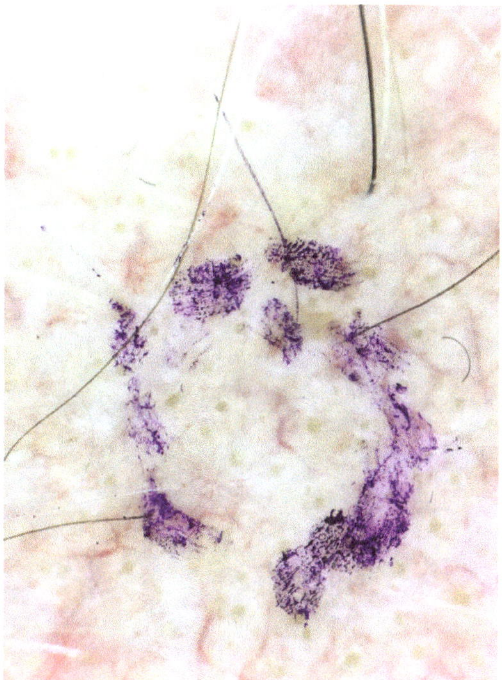

FIGURE 16.7 Scarring or not scarring? ×20 Biopsy was taken in area containing yellow dots. Final diagnosis was chronic alopecia areata, but clinical picture could also suggest scarring alopecia.

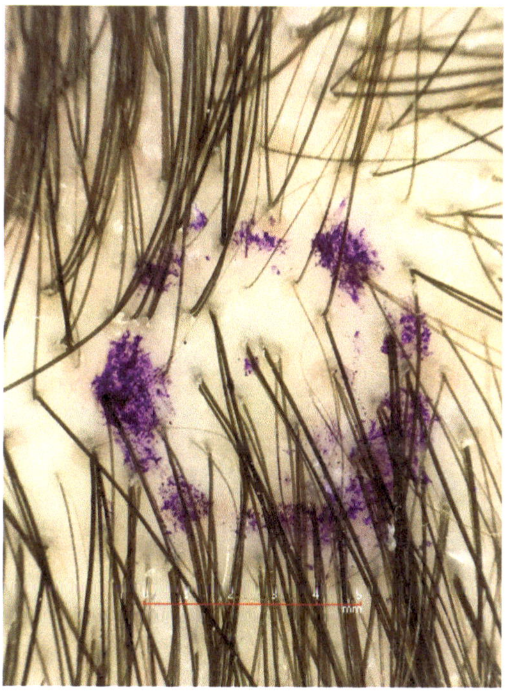

FIGURE 16.8 ×20 In androgenetic alopecia the biopsy site should include hair shaft variability.

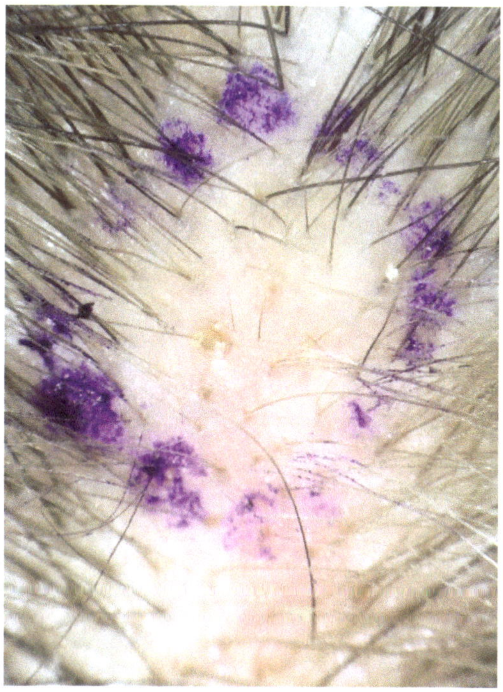

FIGURE 16.9 ×20 Dermoscopy-guided biopsy of a 3D yellow dot in early dissecting cellulitis.

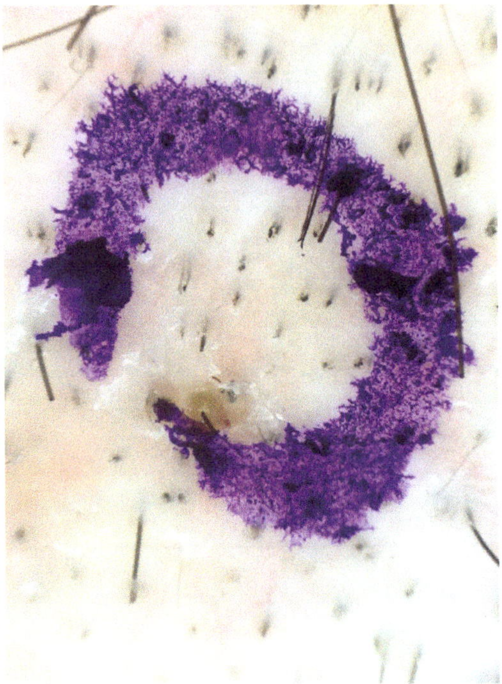

FIGURE 16.10 Trichotillomania. ×20 The biopsy site contains broken hairs and flame hairs.

SUGGESTED READING

Miteva M, Tosti A. Dermoscopy guided scalp biopsy in cicatricial alopecia. *J Eur Acad Dermatol Venereol*. 2013;27(10):1299–303.

Thompson CT, Tosti A. A method for more precise sampling of the scalp and eyebrows in frontal fibrosing alopecia. *J Am Acad Dermatol*. 2019;80(6):e155–e156.

17 Ex Vivo Dermoscopy on Biopsies

Dermoscopy of biopsy specimen ex vivo can optimize the processing of scalp horizontal sections as it helps in finding the correct level for bisection.

Specimens are laid horizontally over a piece of gauze and ×20 pictures are obtained with the dermatoscope lens pressed onto it. A transparent non-porous disposable plastic material (Parafilm®) is used to protect the lens of the dermatoscope from tissue contamination.

EX VIVO DERMOSCOPY ON SCALP BIOPSIES (FIGURES 17.1,17.2)

- The dermoepidermal junction appears as a slightly brownish wavy line.
- Correct level of bisection is 1–1.5 mm below this line.

EX VIVO DERMOSCOPY ON SLIDES (FIGURE 17.3)

- Measure specimen size.
- Establish if specimen needs to be reoriented.
- Evaluate the level of section (bulbar, isthmus, infundibular).

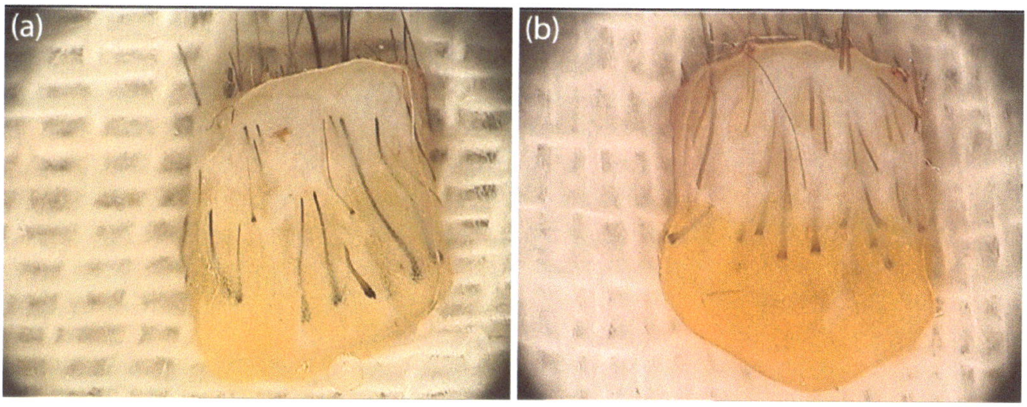

FIGURE 17.1 ×20 Ex vivo dermoscopy of a punch biopsy of androgenetic alopecia (a) and telogen effluvium (b).

DOI: 10.1201/9780429351433-17

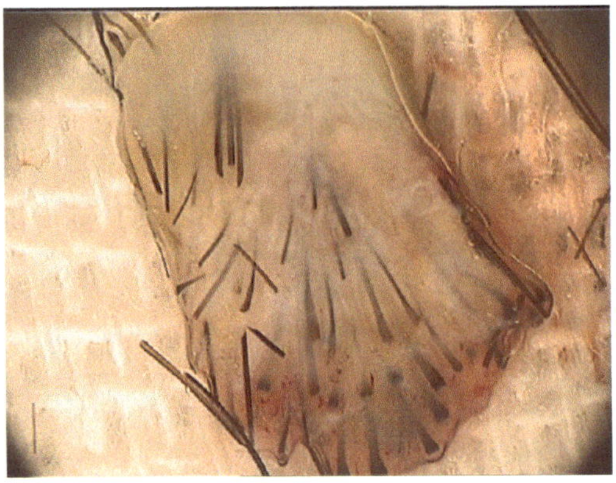

FIGURE 17.2 ×20 Ex vivo dermoscopy of a punch biopsy of folliculitis decalvans showing tufting in the dermis and hypodermis.

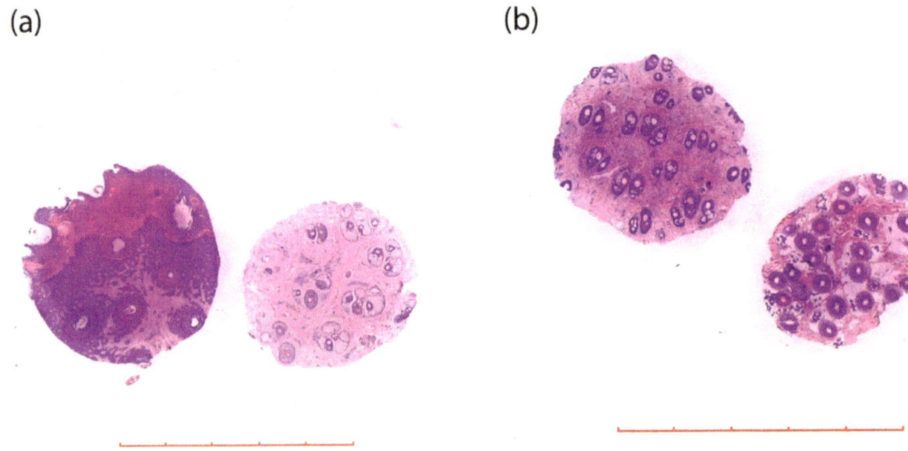

FIGURE 17.3 Ex vivo dermoscopy of glass slide. ×20 Specimen cut is oblique, it should be re-oriented for optimal evaluation (a); ×20 size and orientation are correct (b).

SUGGESTED READING

Miteva M, Lanuti E, Tosti A. Ex vivo dermatoscopy of scalp specimens and slides. *J Eur Acad Dermatol Venereol*. 2014;28(9):1214–8.

18 Teletrichoscopy

TECHNOLOGY (FIGURES 18.1–18.6)

- Incorporates smartphone applications and low-price trichoscopy instruments to connect to smartphones or laptops.
- Requires patient instructions for optimal image capturing.
- Teletrichoscopy can provide diagnoses of androgenetic alopecia, alopecia areata, telogen effluvium, scarring alopecias including folliculitis decalvans, dissecting cellulitis of the scalp, lichen planopilaris, frontal fibrosing alopecia. Rare scalp conditions such as loose anagen syndrome can also be diagnosed.
- The instrument can also be utilized to evaluate the roots of shed hairs.

Challenges and Considerations

- Information depends on the ability of the patient to take images from useful areas of the scalp.
- Images are captured at high magnification and do not provide an overall assessment of the scalp.
- Patients often become addicted to the instrument and take daily pictures of their own scalp.

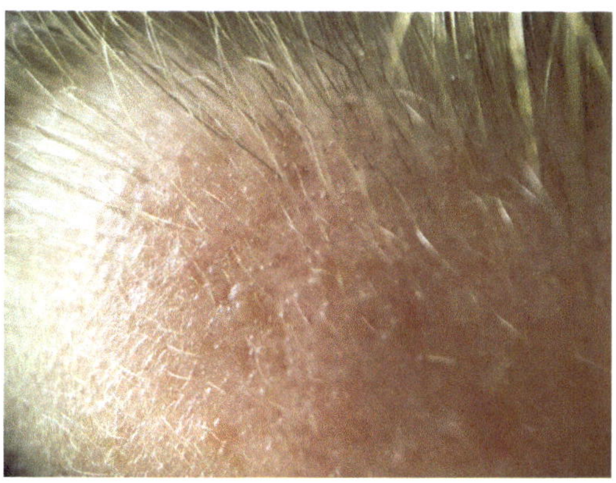

FIGURE 18.1 Image of hairline taken with a micro lens allows to evaluate presence of vellus hairs in a patient complaining of hairline recession.

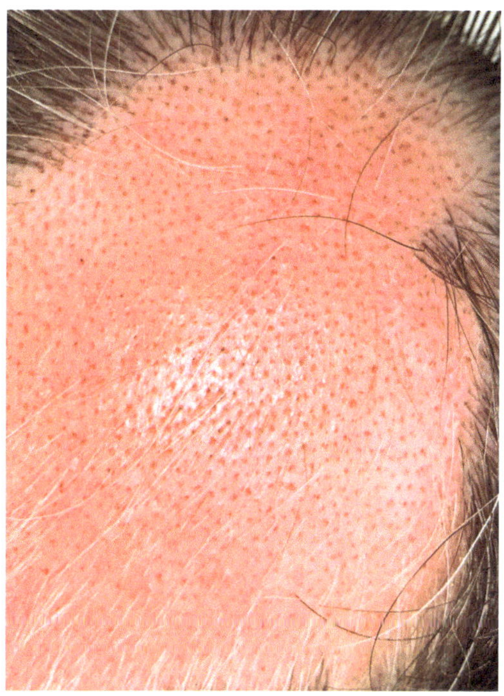

FIGURE 18.2 Alopecia areata. Image taken with a micro lens showing yellow dots and black dots.

DOI: 10.1201/9780429351433-18

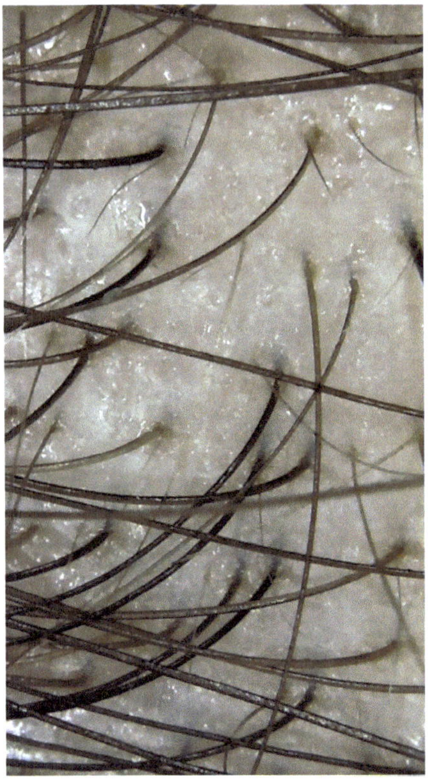

FIGURE 18.3 Telogen effluvium. Image taken with a microscope shows numerous upright short regrowing hairs.

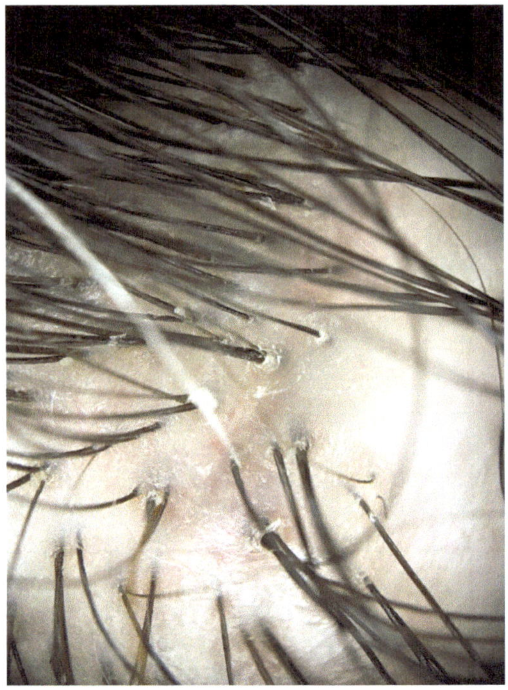

FIGURE 18.4 Peripilar casts and tufting suggesting LPP. Image taken with a microscope.

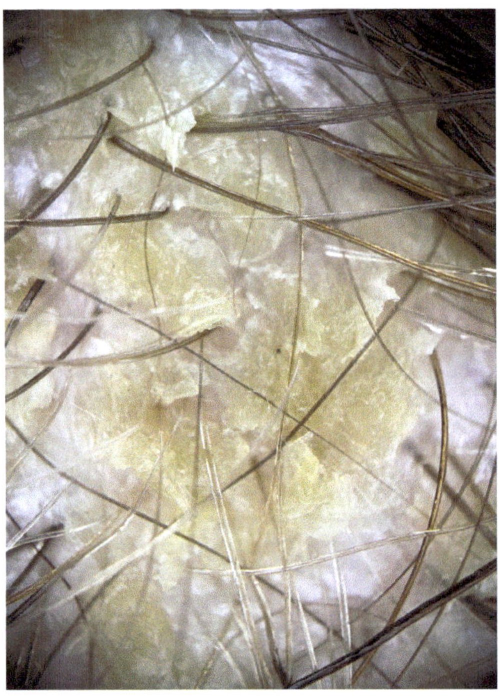

FIGURE 18.5 Thick white scales suggesting scalp psoriasis. Image taken with a microscope. Diagnosis confirmed at in-person follow-up.

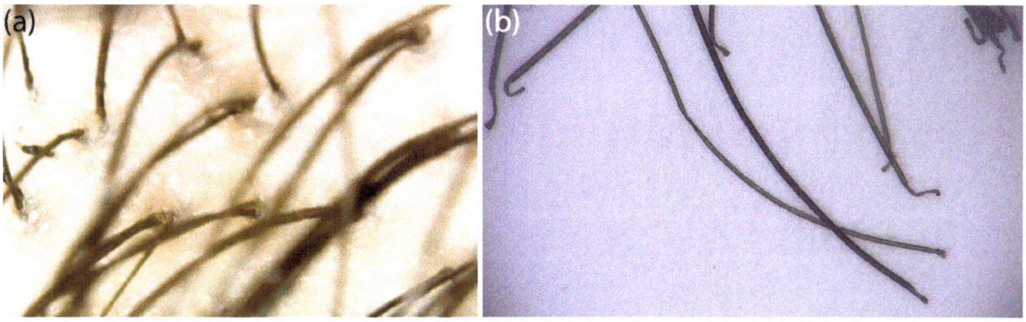

FIGURE 18.6 Loose anagen hair. Screenshot taken during tele-consultation showing rectangular structures in patient's image taken with a microscope (a); diagnosis confirmed by in-person evaluation: ×20 trichogram showing anagen hairs devoid of sheaths (b) (with permission from Lalama et al.).

SUGGESTED READING

Lalama MJ, Nguyen B, Peterson EL, Tosti A. Utility of teledermatology in the diagnosis of loose anagen syndrome. *Skin Appendage Disord.* 2023;9(2):137–40.

Maskan Bermudez N, Perez S, Nguyen B, Tosti A. Teledermatology in alopecia: a systematic review. *JAAD Int.* 2023;14:64–68.

Randolph M, Al-Alola A Tosti A. Diagnosis of hair disorders during the COVID-19 pandemic: an introduction to teletrichoscopy. *J Eur Acad Dermatol Venereol.* 2021;35(3):e167–e168.

19 Dermoscopy in Hair Transplantation

DONOR AREA

- Before transplantation: Follicular density in the donor area can be objectively evaluated using automated software such as TrichoLab or HairMetrix.
- After transplantation: Erythema, folliculitis, red dots, interfollicular crusts. Black dots and dystrophic short hairs may be present when follicular units are transected but not completely excised. A few months after the procedure, interfollicular white dots may appear corresponding to the scars from extracted follicular units.

RECIPIENT AREA

- Shows signs of anagen effluvium due to the stress of transplantation that injures the anagen follicles inducing an anagen arrest. The amount of these signs depends on the severity of transplant-induced damage to the follicles.

See further Figures 19.1–19.5.

DERMOSCOPY

Transitory Signs

- Folliculitis and crusts.
- Sparse black dots.
- Broken hairs, with a proximal thin hypopigmented shaft and distal thickened pigmented tip. Their tips are often slightly bent.
- The shape of the distal tip may be tulipoid or fusiform.
- The distal tip can occasionally be frayed.
- All hairs of the same follicular unit may be broken, sometimes at different levels.
- Short hairs with a sharp tip, corresponding to transplanted shaved hairs.
- Keratotic plug containing broken bent and twisted shafts.

Persistent Signs

- Whitish peripilar halo around transplanted follicular units.
- Pili torti.
- Frontal hairline devoid of terminal hairs with intermediate thickness; this may give the impression of frontal fibrosing alopecia, but vellus hairs are present.

DOI: 10.1201/9780429351433-19

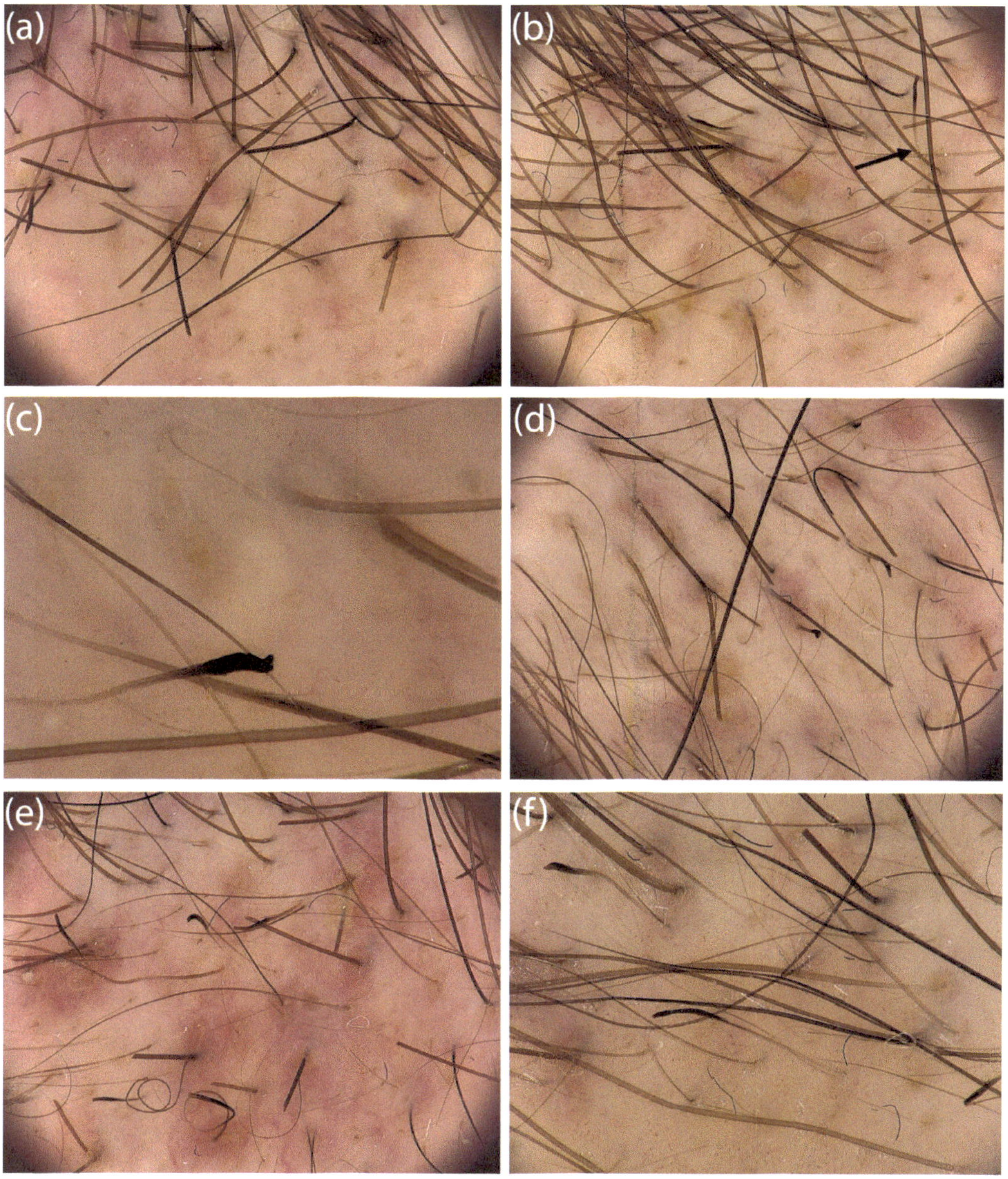

FIGURE 19.1 Recipient area. ×20 Short growing transplanted hair with a shaved tip. Also note a dystrophic hair (a); ×20 broken hair with a hypopigmented base and hyperpigmented thickened tip (arrow) (b); ×50 higher magnification of a broken hair (c); ×20 dystrophic hairs of different length and a typical bent broken hair (d); ×20 diffuse erythema, transplanted regrowing hairs with shaved tips and multiple dystrophic hairs, including the broken hairs with distal thickened tips (e); ×40 higher magnification of broken hair with hypopigmented base (f).

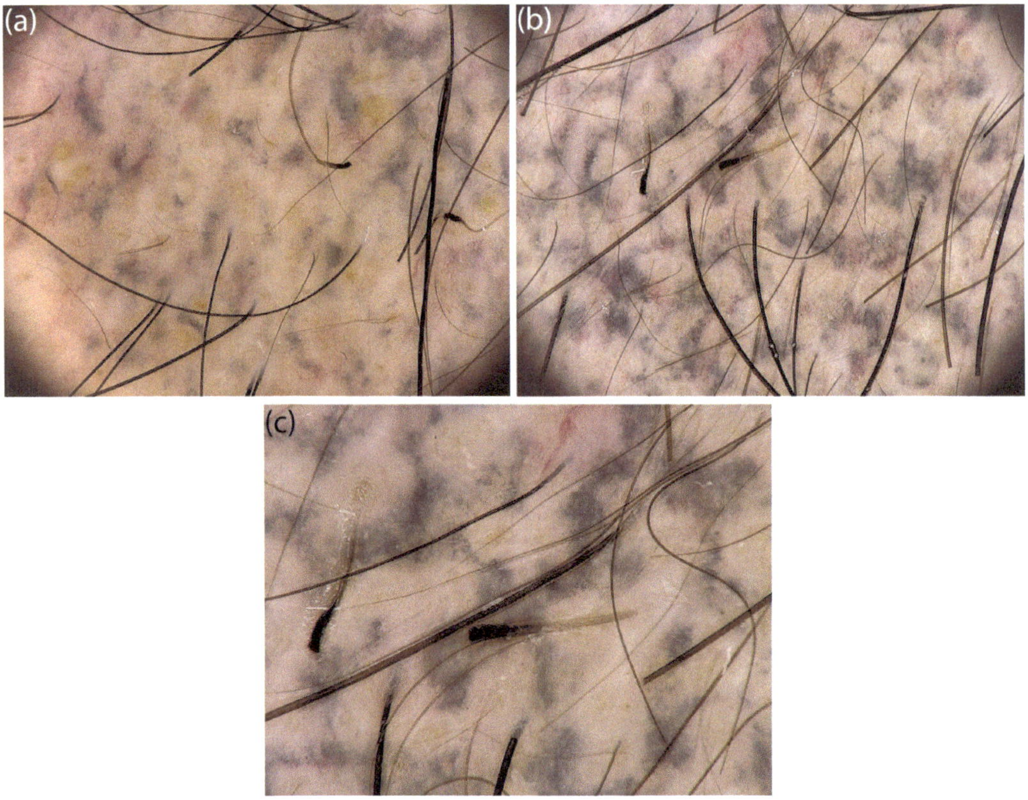

FIGURE 19.2 Hair transplantation in a patient with tricho-pigmentation. ×20 Hair shafts with shaved tips, and dystrophic hairs (a); ×50 dystrophic hairs with a dark tip and a hypopigmented base (b); ×70 higher magnification showing the contrast between the pigmented tip and the hypopigmented proximal portion (c).

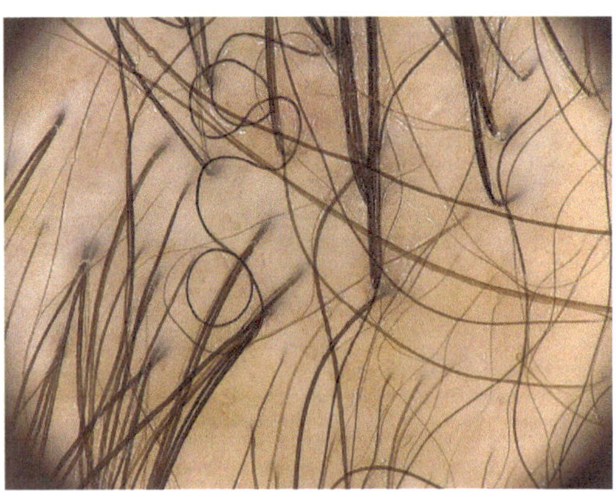

FIGURE 19.3 ×20 Pili torti are occasionally found even years after transplant.

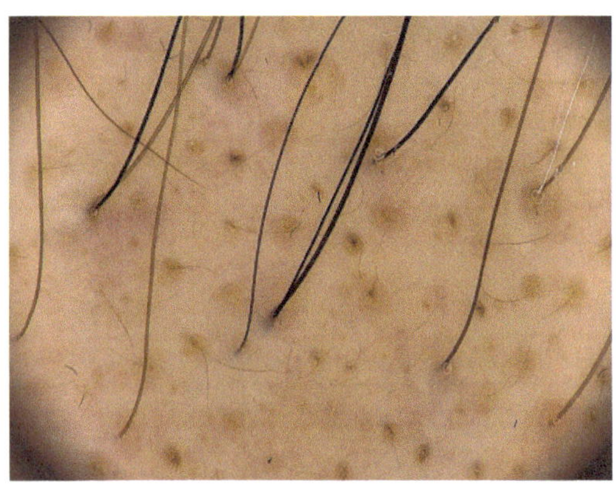

FIGURE 19.4 ×20 Transplanted hairline may resemble the hairline of frontal fibrosing alopecia, but vellus hairs are preserved.

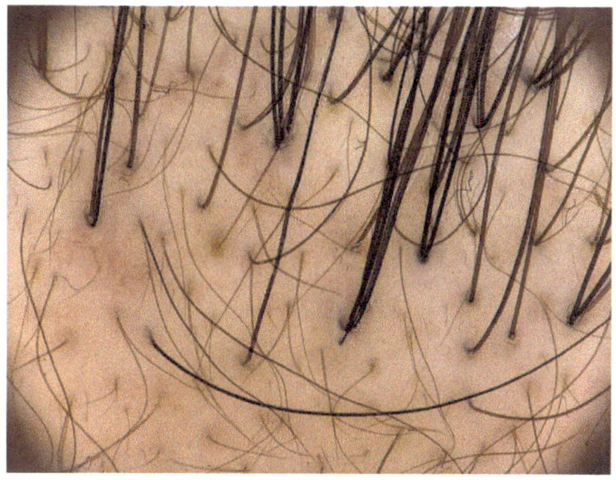

FIGURE 19.5 Dermoscopy one year after transplantation. ×20 The transplanted follicular units have a whitish peripilar halo and can be easily recognized.

SUGGESTED READING

Contin LA, Santos Júnior JB, Machado CJ, Rocha VB. Normal trichoscopic findings after hair transplantation in androgenetic alopecia: a prospective case series. *Skin Appendage Disord.* 2023;9(5):361–65.

Issa NT, Tosti A. Trichoscopy for the hair transplant surgeon-assessing for mimickers of androgenetic alopecia and preoperative evaluation of donor site area. *Indian J Plast Surg.* 2021;54(4):393–98.

20 Artifacts

Artifacts are common and should be distinguished by trichoscopy signs of hair disorders.

- They may affect the scalp or the hair shaft and can be due to staining or deposits.
- Some artifacts can be due to deposits under the skin surface.

STAINING

Scalp Surface

- Follicular staining
- Perifollicular staining
- Interfollicular staining

Under the Scalp Surface

- Dermal staining

Hair Shaft

- Color changes
- Deposits (pseudocasts)

SCALP SURFACE

Follicular Staining (Figures 20.1–20.3)

- Can be due to permanent dyes that are not properly removed on the day of coloring.
- Anthralin also typically causes follicular staining (black-brown dots).
- Follicular staining should not be confused with black dots.

Perifollicular Staining (Figure 20.4)

- Permanent dyes can color the contour of follicular openings. Sometimes the openings present a double ring of staining, possibly due to staining of the periphery of the upper infundibulum in addition to the perifollicular epidermis.

Interfollicular Staining (Figure 20.5)

- Permanent and semipermanent dyes often cause patchy irregular brown-black staining of the interfollicular scalp.
- Henna can cause diffuse or patchy red-orange staining of the interfollicular scalp.

UNDER THE SCALP SURFACE

Dermal Staining (Figures 20.6, 20.7)

- The most common cause is micropigmentation, utilized for cosmetic purposes.
- Micropigmentation causes black-brown irregular dots of different size.
- Traumatic tattoos can also cause dermal staining.

Deposits

- Deposits can be due to environmental particles, camouflage products, cosmetic or drug residues, textile fibers, and shaft fragments.
- Patients with Morgellons disease or other delusional parasitosis may often point to scalp deposits as proofs of their condition.

Perifollicular Deposits (Figure 20.8)

- Residues of products applied on the scalp may accumulate around hair emergences, simulating peripilar casts. However, they are usually associated with interfollicular deposits.
- In patients with lichen planopilaris, it may be difficult to discriminate between active disease and scalp residues.
- Artifacts from water bubbles are often seen in oily scalps and can simulate peripilar sign/halos.

Interfollicular Deposits (Figures 20.9–20.13)

- Environmental particles present as dots of different size and shape and

DOI: 10.1201/9780429351433-20

are most commonly seen in children or elderly.

- Textile fibers are often found on the scalp of patients wearing hats, particularly alopecia areata patients. They may be confused with short bent hairs.
- Hair shaft fragments are usually detected on the scalp of patients who had recently had their hair cut and may persist after several shampoos; they should not be confused with broken hairs.
- Residues of products applied on the scalp such as topical steroids or minoxidil can mimic seborrheic dermatitis or scalp psoriasis. In case of scarring alopecia, should not be confused with signs of activity.
- Camouflage powders appear as granulate brown-black deposits.
- Camouflage fibers often persist on the scalp despite repetitive shampoos and can resemble broken hairs.

Dermal Deposits (Figure 20.14)

- Repeated injections of steroids cause whitish slightly elevated structureless and lobulated areas.
- These can be seen both in the follicular and interfollicular scalp.

HAIR SHAFT

Color Changes

- White hairs are more difficult to be evaluated by dermoscopy as they reflect light.
- It is therefore advisable to recommend patients to dye their hairs before the consultation.
- Hair dyes do not color all the shafts and about 15% of the hairs remain white after proper permanent dyeing. The proximal portion of the white hair shaft also often remains unstained.
- The hair cortex often presents as multiple non-pigmented tubular cavities that should not be confused with bubble hairs or pili annulati. This finding is more evident in white hairs, due to their transparent color.

Deposits (Figures 20.15, 20.16)

- Hair sprays and gels cause deposits on the hair shaft.
- Their surface can be granular or very smooth and waxy.
- Topical minoxidil can cause granular deposits on the shaft.

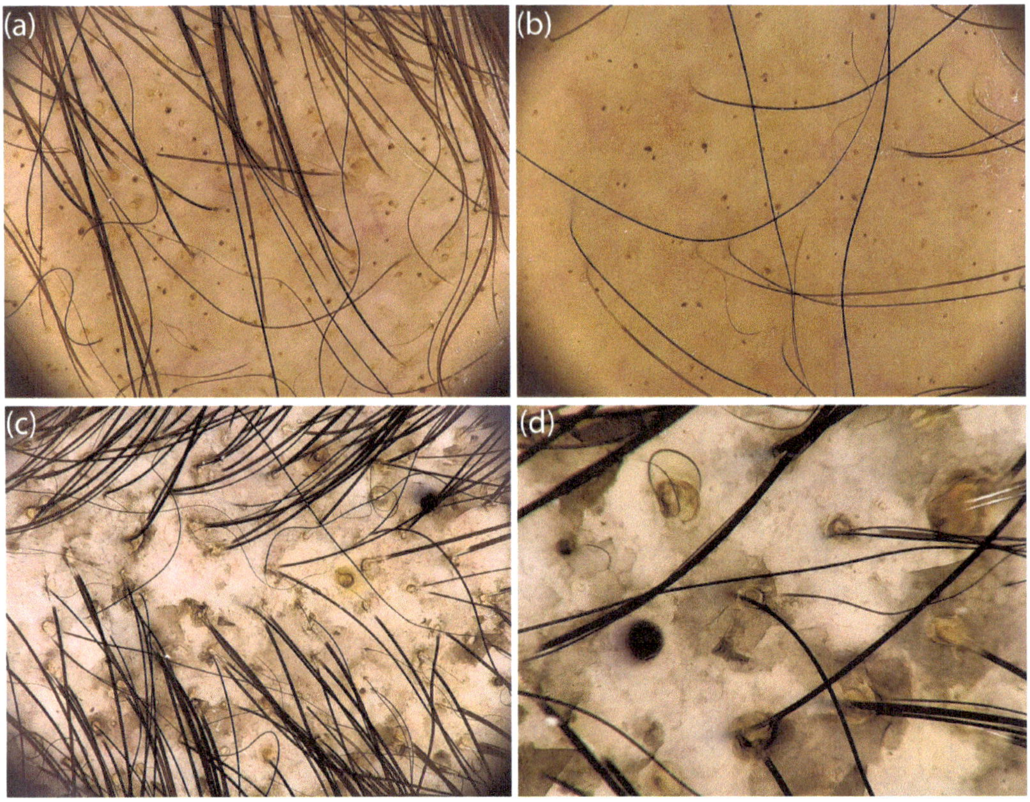

FIGURE 20.1 Hair dyes. ×20 Follicular staining after a permanent dye in a patient with alopecia areata, note that not all follicles are penetrated by the hair dye; don't confuse with black dots (a); ×50 high magnification (b); ×20 (c) and ×50 (d) follicular and interfollicular staining from permanent hair dye.

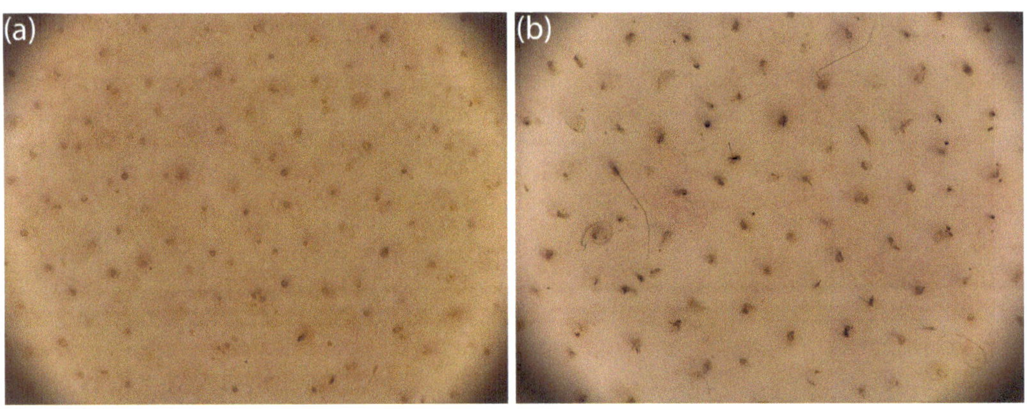

FIGURE 20.2 Anthralin. ×20 Brownish follicular staining due to anthralin in alopecia totalis (a); ×20 brown-black deposits in active alopecia areata; don't confuse with black dots (b).

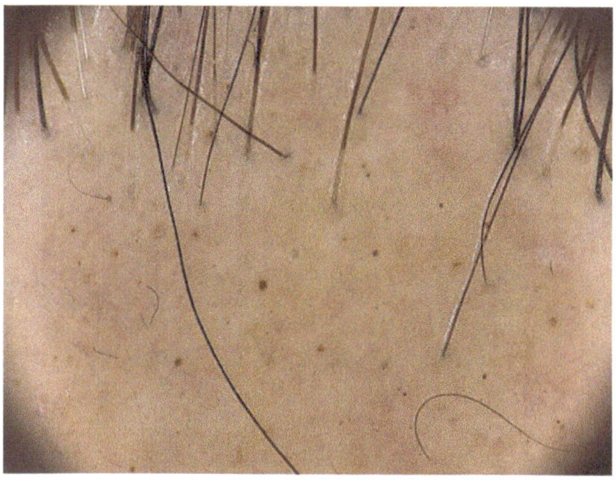

FIGURE 20.3 ×20 Follicular staining from hair dye in frontal fibrosing alopecia.

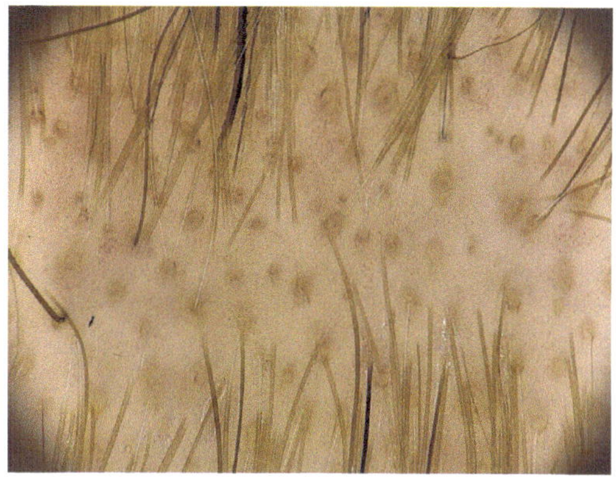

FIGURE 20.4 ×20 Perifollicular staining from hair dye resembling peripilar sign.

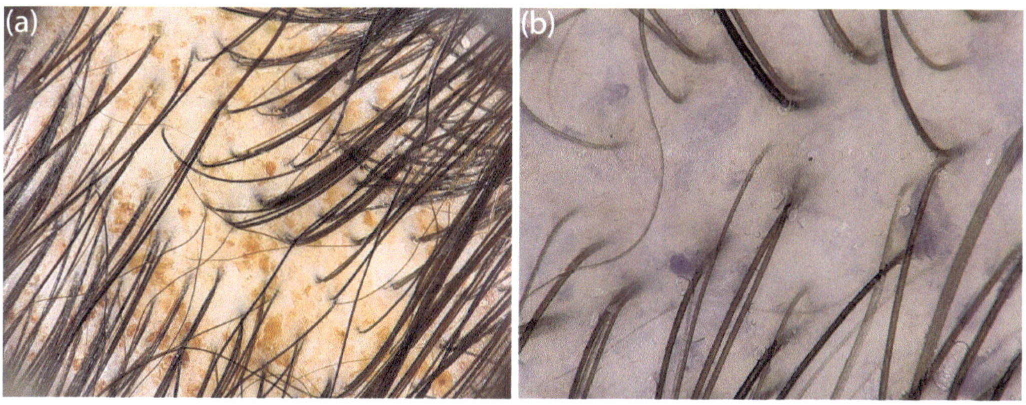

FIGURE 20.5 Hair dyes. ×20 Orange interfollicular staining due to semipermanent dyes (a); ×50 blue staining from semipermanent dye (b).

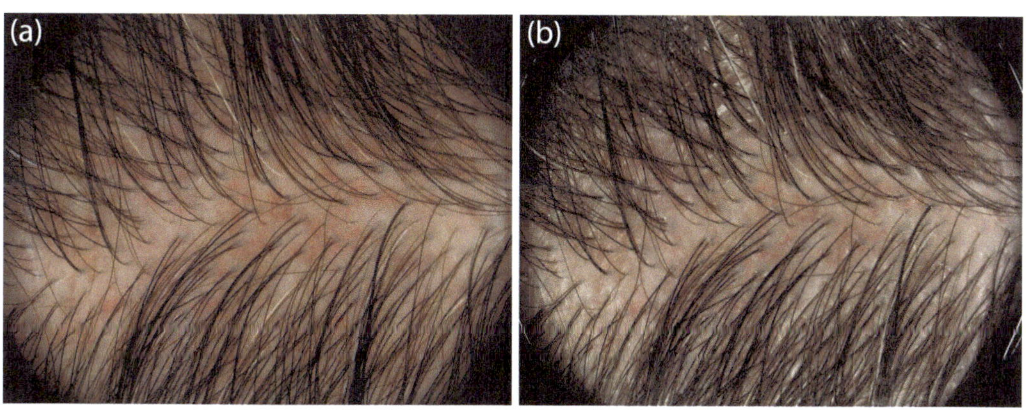

FIGURE 20.6 ×20 Reddish scalp staining due to faded micropigmentation (a,b); note the staining is homogeneous and should not be confused with vessels.

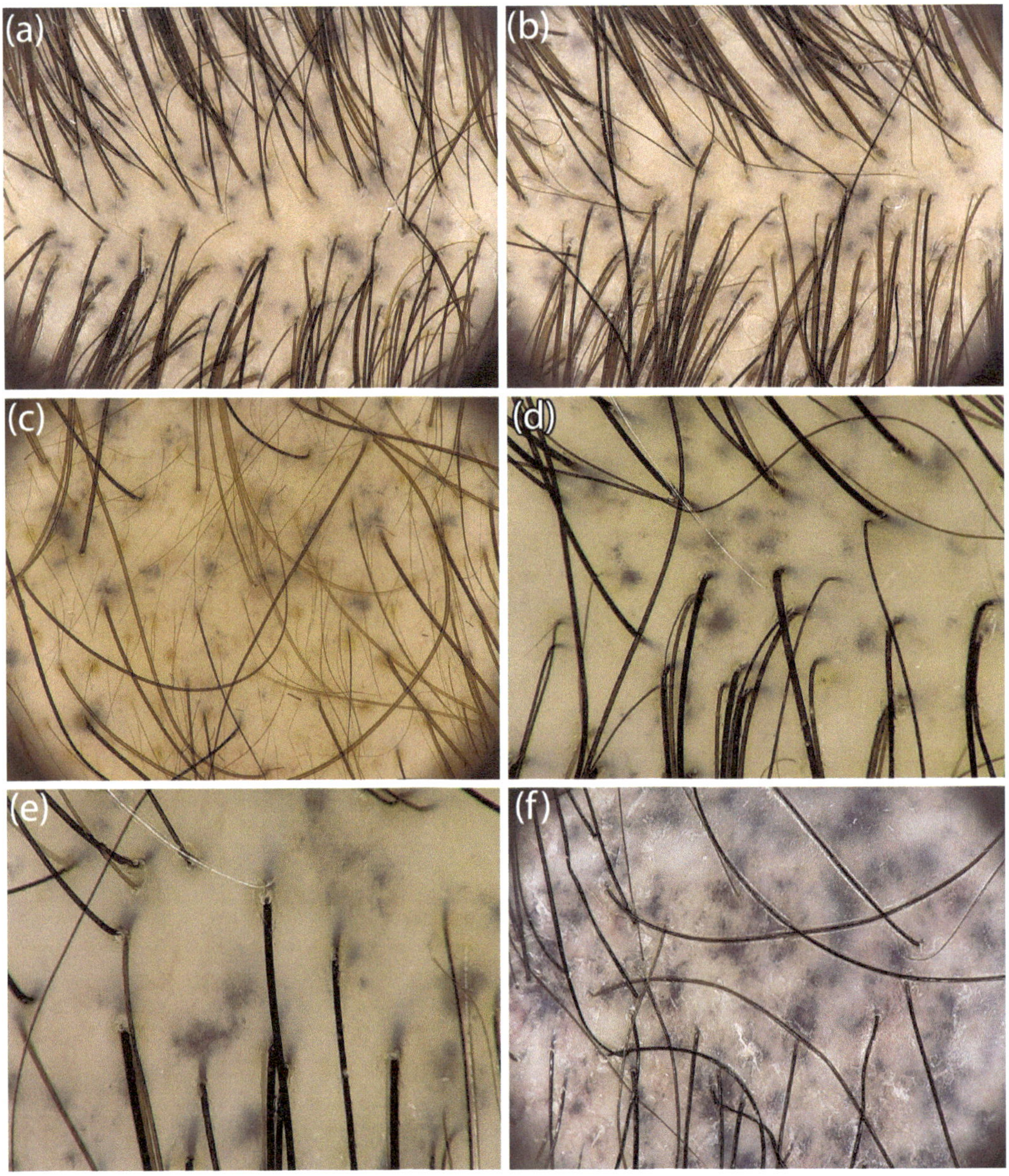

FIGURE 20.7 Micropigmentation. ×20 Small black dots between follicular units (a,b); ×40 dots are of different shape and size (c); ×50 (d) and ×70 (e) note granular diffusion of the pigment at high magnification; ×20 irregular black dots in scarring alopecia (f).

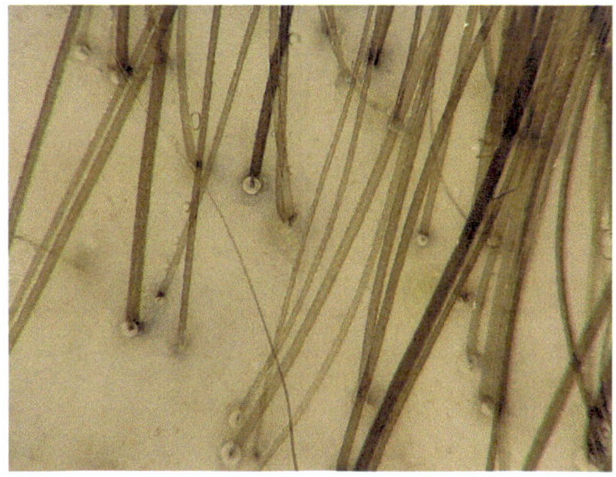

FIGURE 20.8 ×20 Water bubbles.

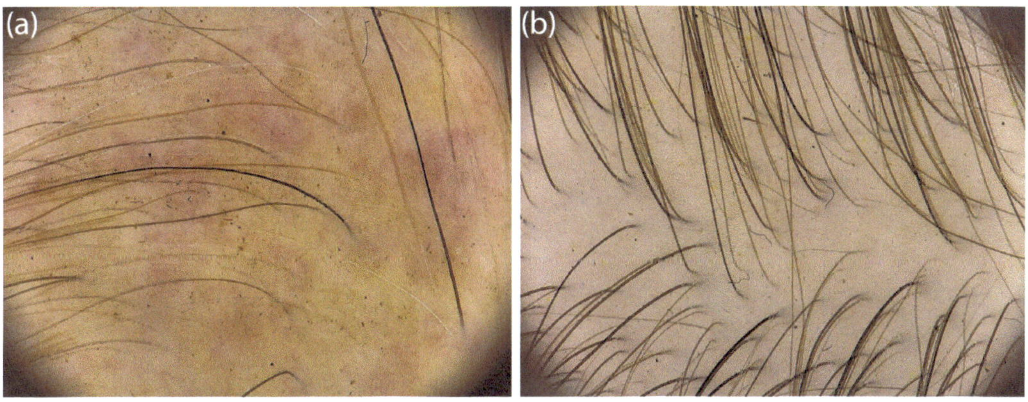

FIGURE 20.9 ×20 Dirty scalp in an elderly patient (a); and ×20 in a child with alopecia areata (b).

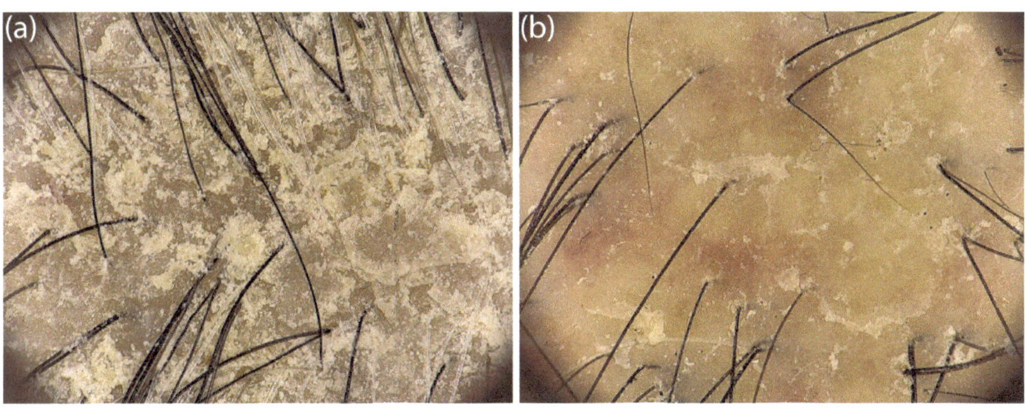

FIGURE 20.10 ×20 Granular residues of topical minoxidil in non-scarring (a) and scarring alopecia (b).

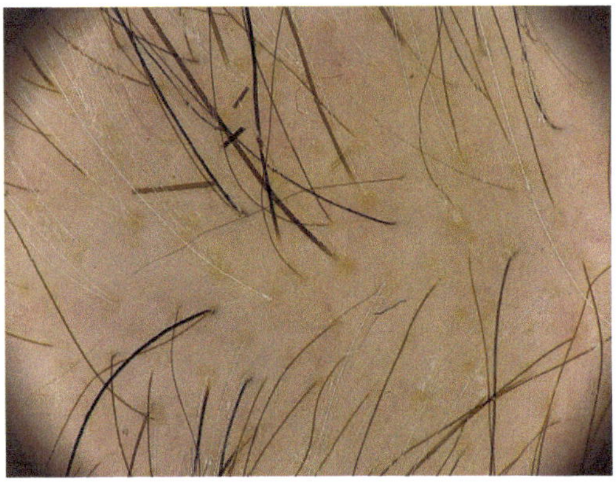

FIGURE 20.11 ×20 Hair shaft fragments after haircut.

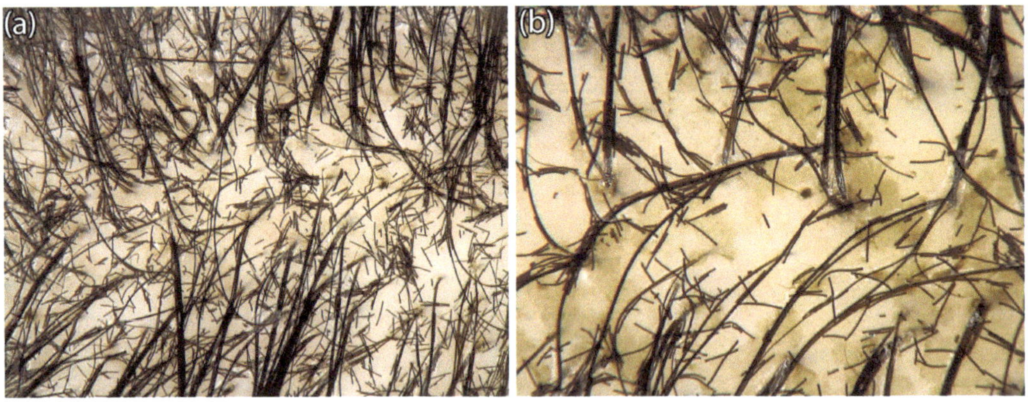

FIGURE 20.12 ×20 Interfollicular deposits from hair fibers (a); ×50 note that hair fibers have different lengths (b).

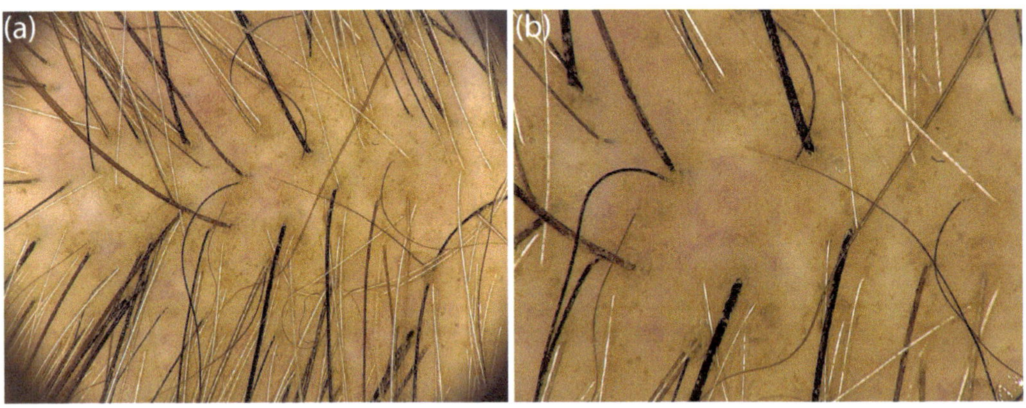

FIGURE 20.13 ×20 Interfollicular brownish granular deposits from hair powder (a); ×50 note that powder also deposits on proximal shafts (b).

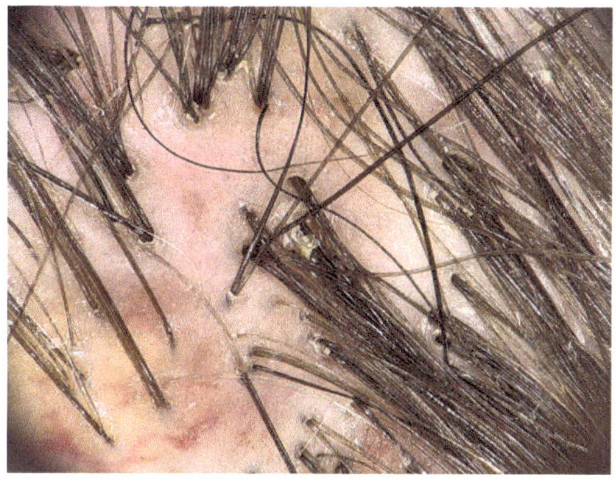

FIGURE 20.14 ×20 White structureless areas due to dermal deposit of steroids in a patient with folliculitis decalvans.

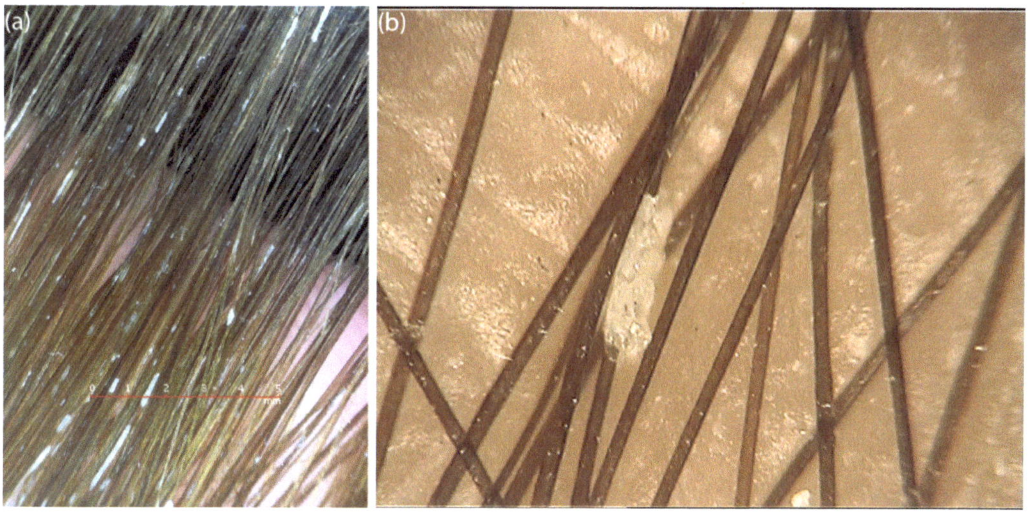

FIGURE 20.15 ×20 Hair spray deposits presenting as multiple tubular structures encircling the hair shafts (a); ×70 note the waxy appearance at high magnification; differently from white piedra the hair shaft is not visible through the deposits (b).

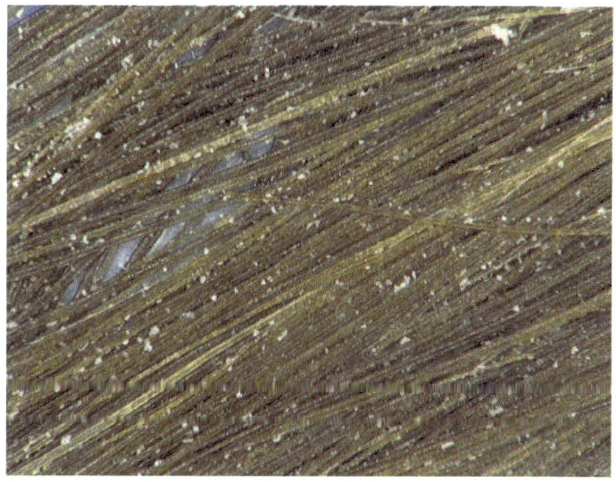

FIGURE 20.16 ×20 Multiple granular small residues of topical minoxidil on the hair shaft surface.

SUGGESTED READING

Angra K, LaSenna CE, Nichols AJ, Tosti A. Hair dye: a trichoscopy pitfall. *J Am Acad Dermatol.* 2015;72(4):e101–2.

Doche I, Vincenzi C, Tosti A. Casts and pseudocasts. *J Am Acad Dermatol.* 2016;75(4):e147–8.

Nguyen B, Mervis JS, Romanelli P, Tosti A. Scalp Micropigmentation: a clinicopathologic correlation. *Skin Appendage Disord.* 2022;8(5):412–4.

21 Dermoscopy of Shaved Scalp

GENERAL PRINCIPLES

- Shaving prevents evaluation of broken hairs.
- Shaving prevents the detection of abnormalities that involve the hair shaft, including coudability, pseudo-monilethrix, and circle hairs.
- Congenital hair shaft disorders are not visible in a shaved area.
- If shaving is not at scalp level, telogen hairs can be distinguished as they appear as black dots/flame hairs at skin level since they are not growing.
- It is therefore possible to identify telogen hairs within a follicular unit.
- If shaving is not perfect the tip of the shaft can look frayed and be misdiagnosed as trichorrhexis nodosa.
- Mosaic pigmentation due to sun exposure is evident in most cases.

See Figures 21.1–21.7 and Table 21.1.

Androgenetic Alopecia

- Hair shaft variability is clearly visible.
- When shaving is not at scalp level, anagen hairs have different thickness with miniaturized hairs being of shorter length and lighter color.
- Short regrowing anagen hairs may have normal or reduced thickness.
- Telogen hairs resemble black dots/flame hairs.
- In androgenetic alopecia of closely shaved scalp, telogen terminal and miniaturized hairs look like black dots of different size. Variability can be detected comparing the thickness of the emerging shafts that correspond to the anagen hairs.
- The number of terminal growing anagen hairs is highly variable depending on the scalp region.
- Yellow dots are usually sparse and contain black dots.
- Vascular abnormalities including twisted capillary loops and arborizing vessels are clearly visible.
- Differential diagnosis with alopecia areata can be difficult.

Alopecia Areata

- The presence of patches devoid of anagen hairs with yellow dots and without black dots is suggestive of alopecia areata.
- The presence of grouped white anagen hairs is suggestive for alopecia areata.

Scarring Alopecia

- Loss of follicular openings is evident.
- Vascular abnormalities indicative of connective tissue disorders can be the only clue.
- Inflammatory signs such as peripilar casts and keratotic plugs are visible.

DOI: 10.1201/9780429351433-21

TABLE 21.1
Trichoscopic Patterns Seen in the Shaved Scalp

Disease	AGA	Anagen Effluvium*
Black dots	Most show different size, as correspond to shaved telogen hairs of different thickness	Usually same size, corresponding to broken hairs below the scalp level
Yellow dots	Scattered, may contain black dots of different thickness	Clustered, usually containing black dots of the same size
Empty follicles	Yes	Yes
Flame hairs	Yes, corresponding to shaved thin hairs	Yes, corresponding to broken hairs just above the scalp level
Hair shaft variability	Diffuse, and visible also in the black dots	Clustered

*Alopecia areata, pressure alopecia, dissecting cellulitis of the scalp, chemotherapy/radiotherapy alopecia

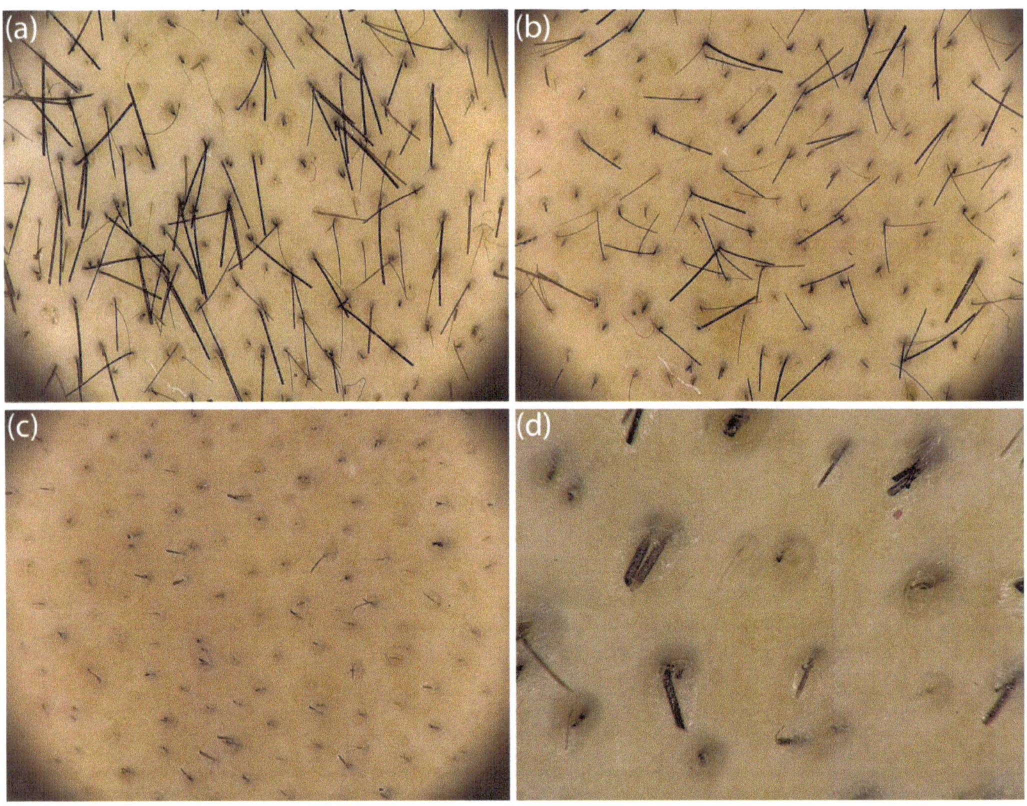

FIGURE 21.1 Androgenetic alopecia. ×20 Telogen hairs appearing as black dots or flame/like hairs in contrast with anagen hair that are shaved a few centimeters above scalp level (a); ×20 differential diagnosis with alopecia areata is very difficult (b); particularly on the areas with severe miniaturization (c); ×70 black dots due to telogen hairs in contrast with the anagen hair with the shaved tip (d).

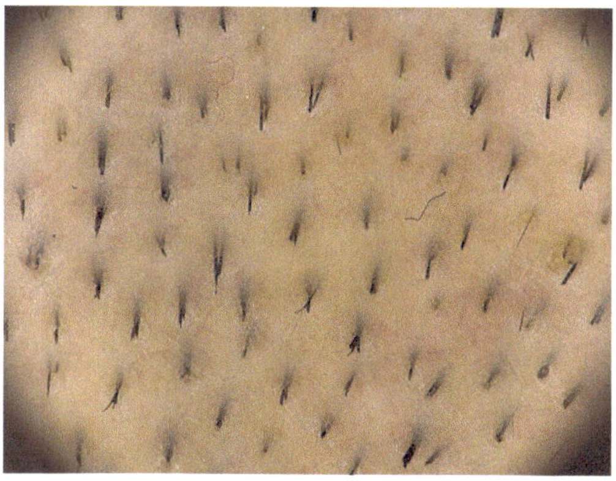

FIGURE 21.2 ×40 Frayed tips due to imperfect shaving.

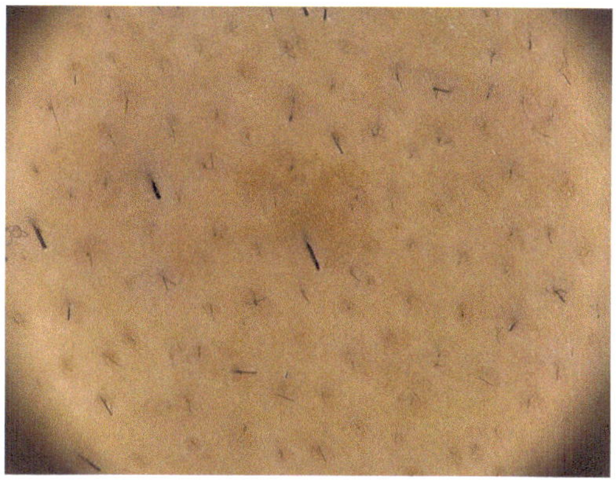

FIGURE 21.3 ×40 Severe androgenetic alopecia, very thin hairs are not shaved and have a tip, also note pigmented network due to sun exposure.

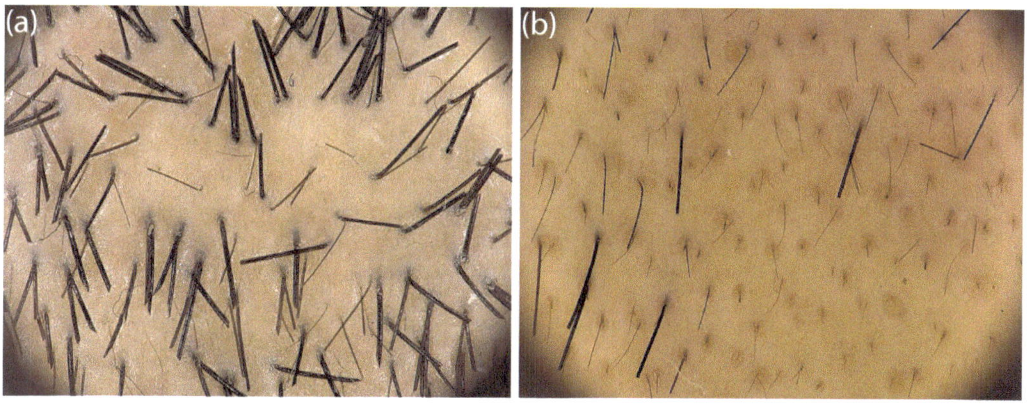

FIGURE 21.4 Androgenetic alopecia. ×20 Mild disease is easily diagnosed (a); ×20 severe disease can be difficult to distinguish from alopecia areata (b).

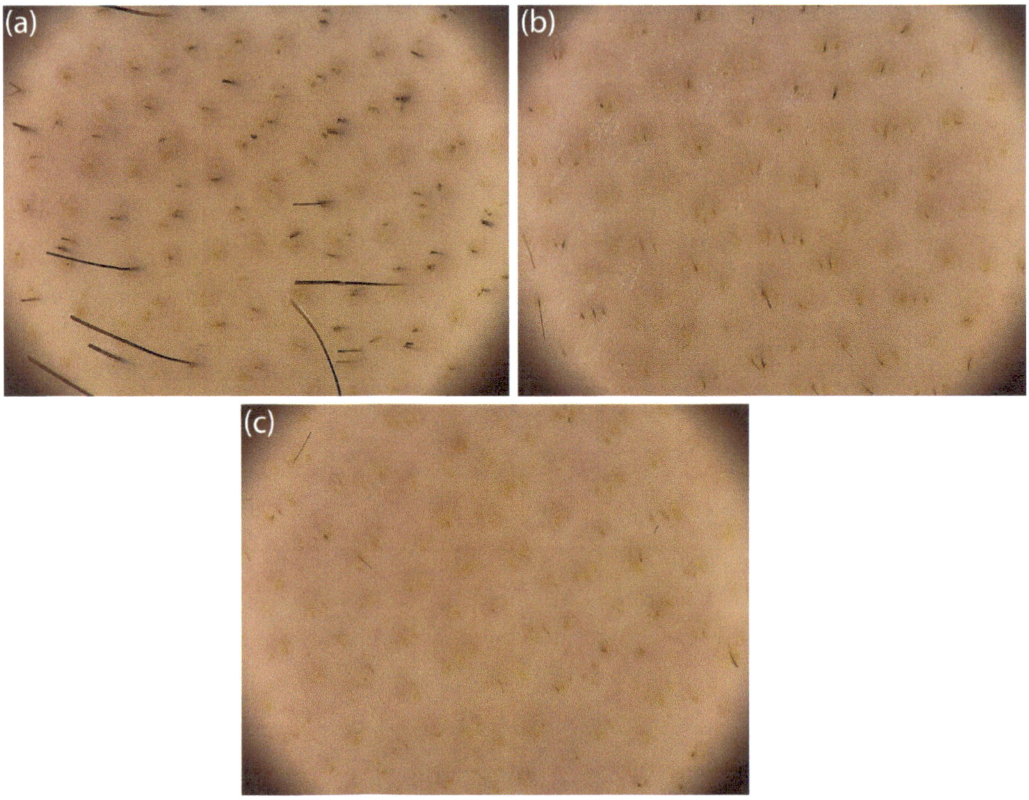

FIGURE 21.5 Alopecia areata. ×20 Active areas can be difficult to distinguish from advanced AGA (a); ×20 (b) and ×40 (c) looking at the whole scalp may detect typical features such as diffuse yellow dots.

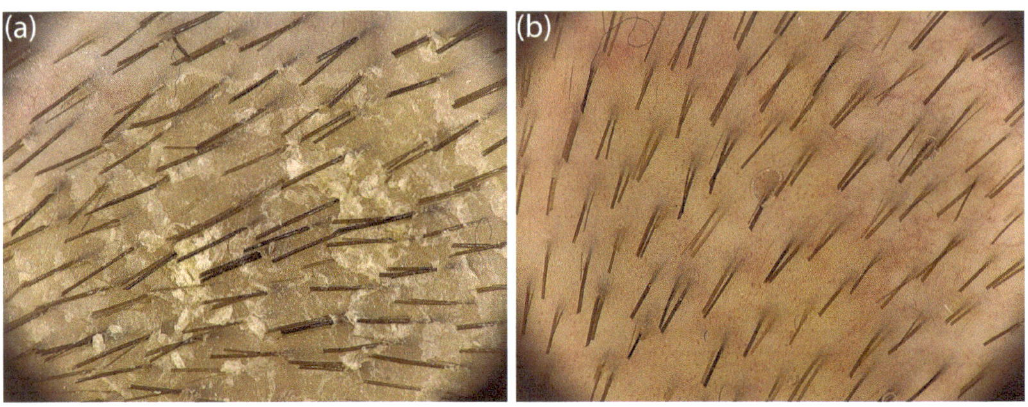

FIGURE 21.6 Scalp psoriasis shaving can act as Koebner phenomenon. ×50 Scales obscure the vascular pattern that should be searched in adjacent areas (a); ×40 note typical vascular pattern (b).

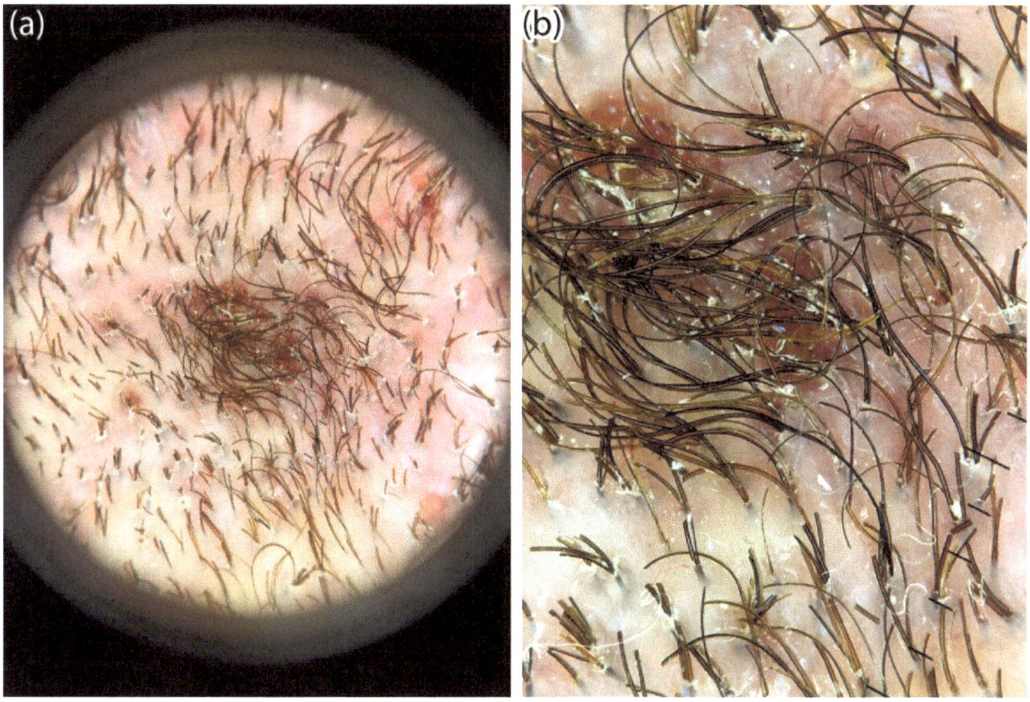

FIGURE 21.7 Folliculitis decalvans. ×10 Tufting and crusting (a); ×40 shaving is not very close in areas of crusting that also show pustular exudation (b).

22 Scalp Tumors

Scalp tumors can be melanocytic, such as nevi and melanomas, or non-melanocytic, including basal cell carcinomas (BCCs), squamous cell carcinomas, vascular tumors like pyogenic granuloma, and, rarely, adnexal tumors.

NEVI (FIGURE 22.1)

- Common in younger individuals (<30 years).
- Dermoscopic patterns: Exhibit either a globular or network pattern, distinctively accompanied by central or perifollicular hypopigmentation, a hallmark of benignity in scalp lesions.
- The typical network consists of thickened, brown pigmented lines around hair follicles, but without asymmetric pigmented hair follicles, rhomboidal structures, or annular–granular structures.
- Central hypopigmentation (Eclipse Nevus): Common, especially in younger individuals, with a clear zone around the hair follicle.

MELANOMA (FIGURES 22.2–22.4)

Predominantly found in males with androgenetic alopecia older than 65 years, and with significant sun damage.

Often diagnosed at a later stage due to the challenging location, leading to a poorer prognosis compared to melanomas located elsewhere.

Thin Melanomas (<1 mm)

a) Atypical pseudo network: Characterized by asymmetric pigmented hair follicular openings, rhomboidal structures, annular–granular structures, or black dots within the hair follicle, indicating destruction of hair follicles.
b) Diffuse/multifocal hypopigmentation: More prevalent in melanoma in situ, indicating areas lighter than the pigmentation of the lesion, often spread out or multifocal, contrasting with the centralized hypopigmentation seen in nevi.
c) Atypical network/pseudo network and regression.

Advanced Melanomas (>1 mm)

- Blue-white veil, unspecific patterns, and irregular black blotches or dots, indicating more aggressive disease progression.

BASAL CELL CARCINOMA (FIGURES 22.5–22.9)

More common in sun-exposed scalp, can also affect scalp areas with normal hair density. May affect scalp with scarring alopecia and even be misdiagnosed as a scarring alopecia.

Dermoscopy

- Arborizing vessels: Large, branching blood vessels more prominent in non-pigmented BCC and very well seen in the scalp due to thinner dermis.
- Leaf-like areas and blue-gray ovoid nests.

SQUAMOUS CELL CARCINOMA (FIGURE 22.9)

- Keratin scales: Thick and yellow, indicative of keratin production.
- Ulceration: Can appear as erosions or crusted areas.
- Vascular patterns: The appearance of dotted or linear-irregular vessels, which is a critical feature to consider for excision in non-pigmented tumors on the scalp.

DOI: 10.1201/9780429351433-22

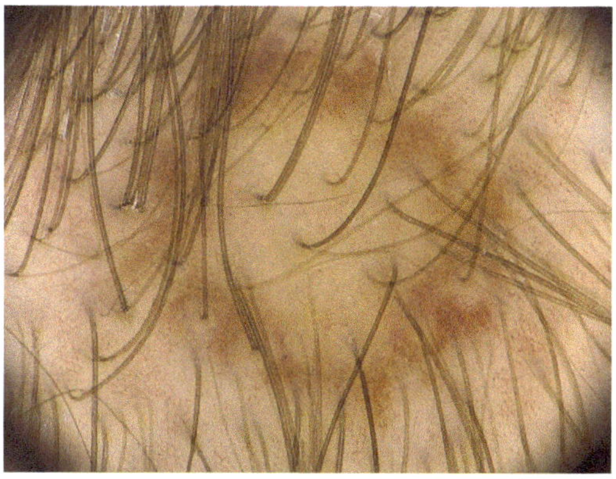

FIGURE 22.1 ×40 Eclipse nevus of the scalp with typical central hypopigmentation.

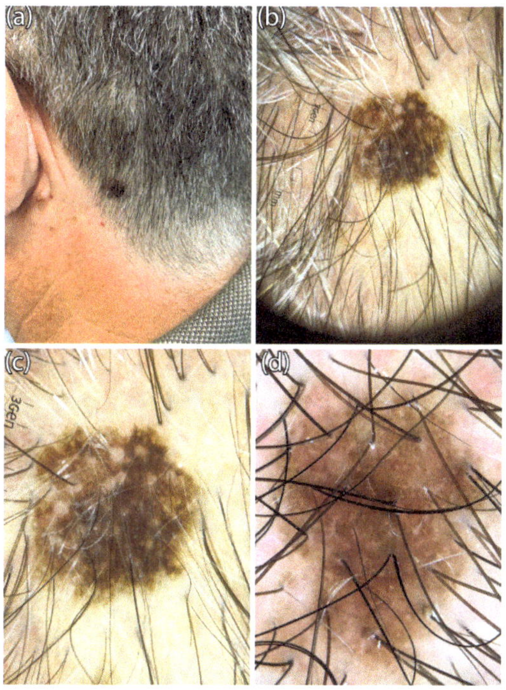

FIGURE 22.2 Melanoma in sun-protected scalp (a); ×10 atypical pseudo network and multifocal hypopigmentation (b); ×20 higher magnification (c) (Courtesy of Dr. Francesco Savoia); ×10 different lesion showing atypical pseudo network and multifocal hypopigmentation (d).

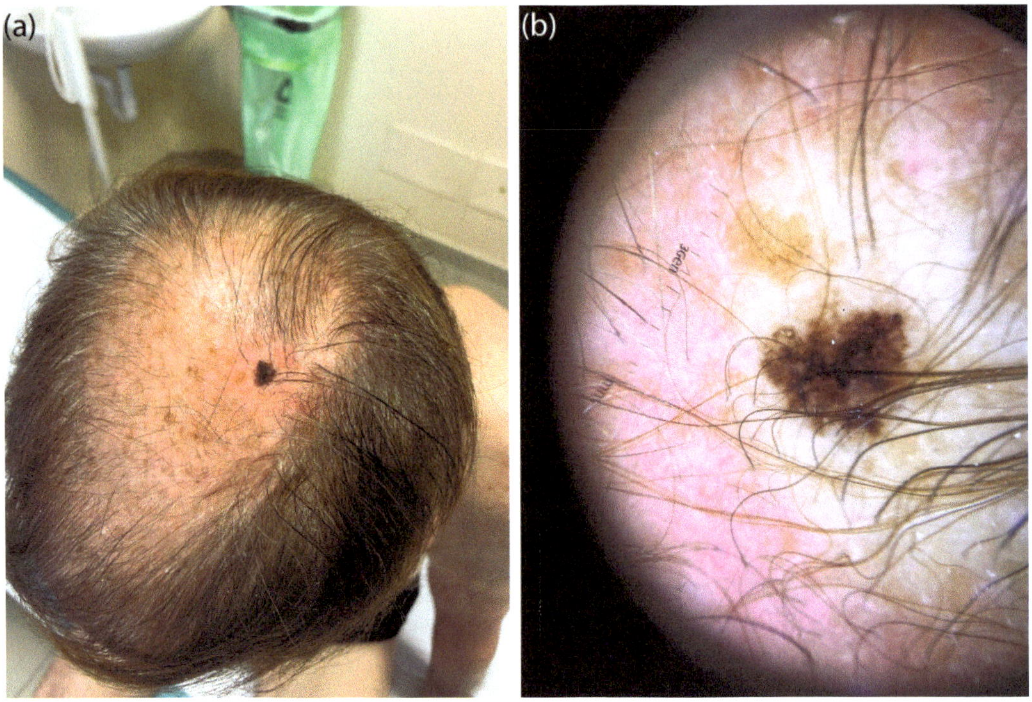

FIGURE 22.3 Melanoma in sun-exposed scalp (a); ×10 black rhomboidal structure, peripheric dots, irregular streaks (b). (Courtesy of Dr. Francesco Savoia.)

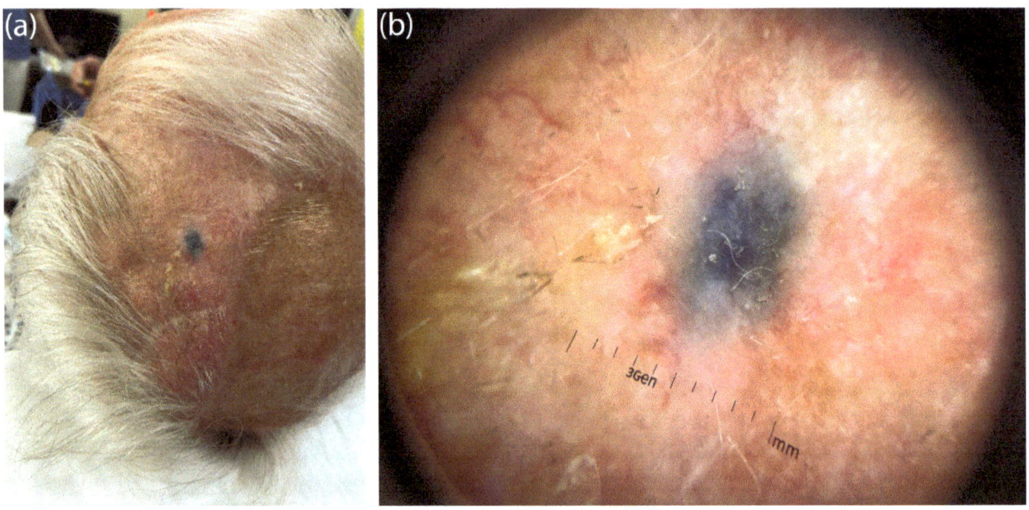

FIGURE 22.4 Scalp metastases of melanoma (a); ×10 homogeneous diffuse monochromatic blue-gray pigmentation (b). (Courtesy of Dr. Francesco Savoia.)

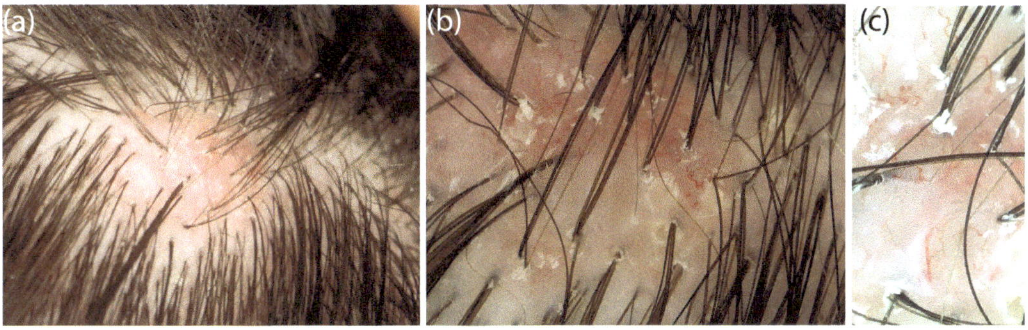

FIGURE 22.5 Nodular basal cell carcinoma presenting as erythematous nodular lesion in a woman without alopecia (a); ×20 large branching vessels (b); ×50 more visible at high magnification (c).

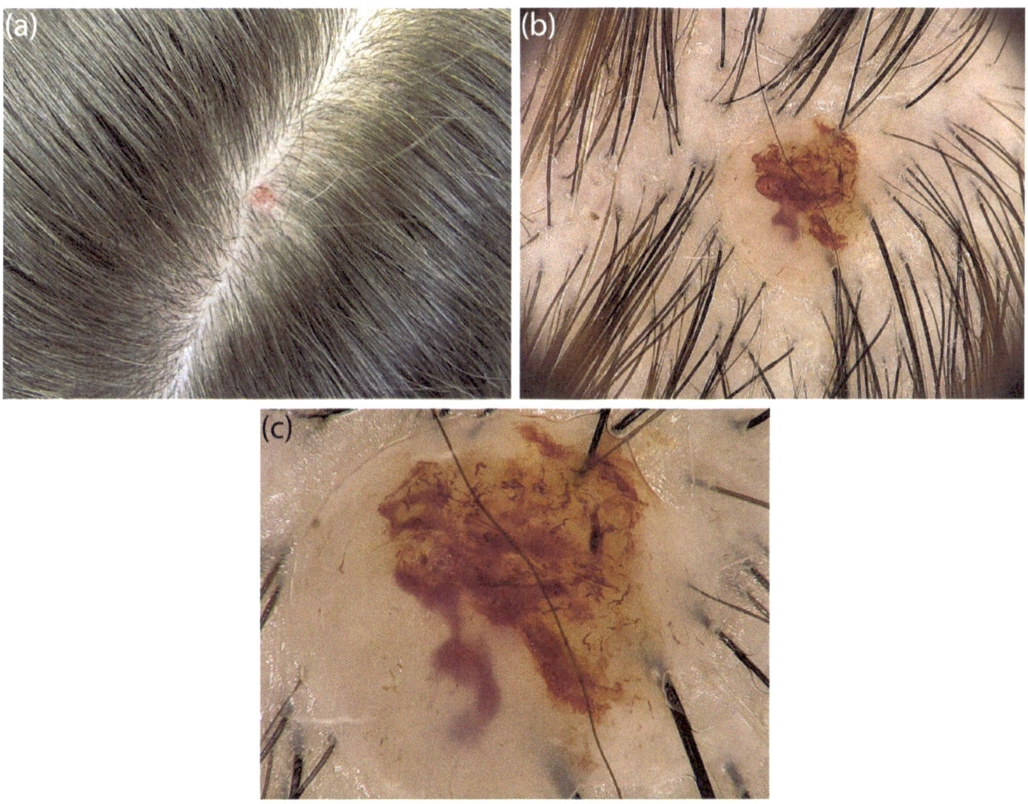

FIGURE 22.6 Nodular basal cell carcinoma presenting as erythematous nodular lesion in a woman with mild androgenetic alopecia (a); ×20 large branching vessels (b); ×70 high magnification (c).

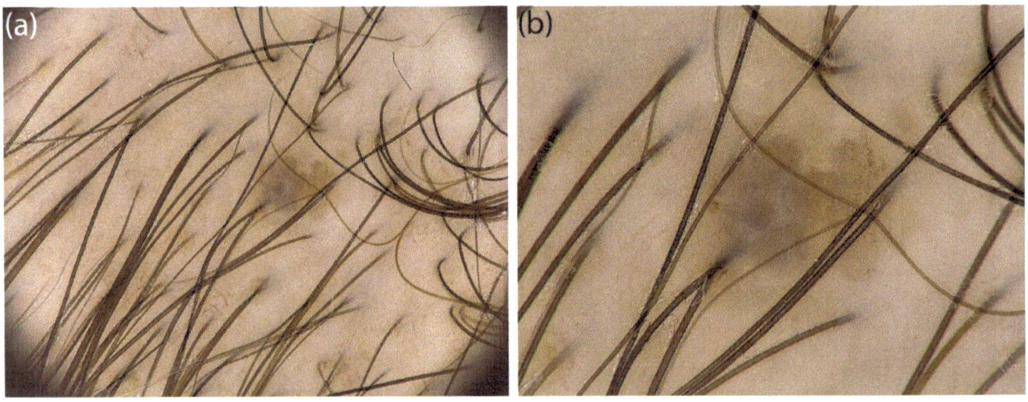

FIGURE 22.7 Basal cell carcinoma. (a) and (b) ×20, ×40 Leaf-like areas and blue-gray ovoid nests.

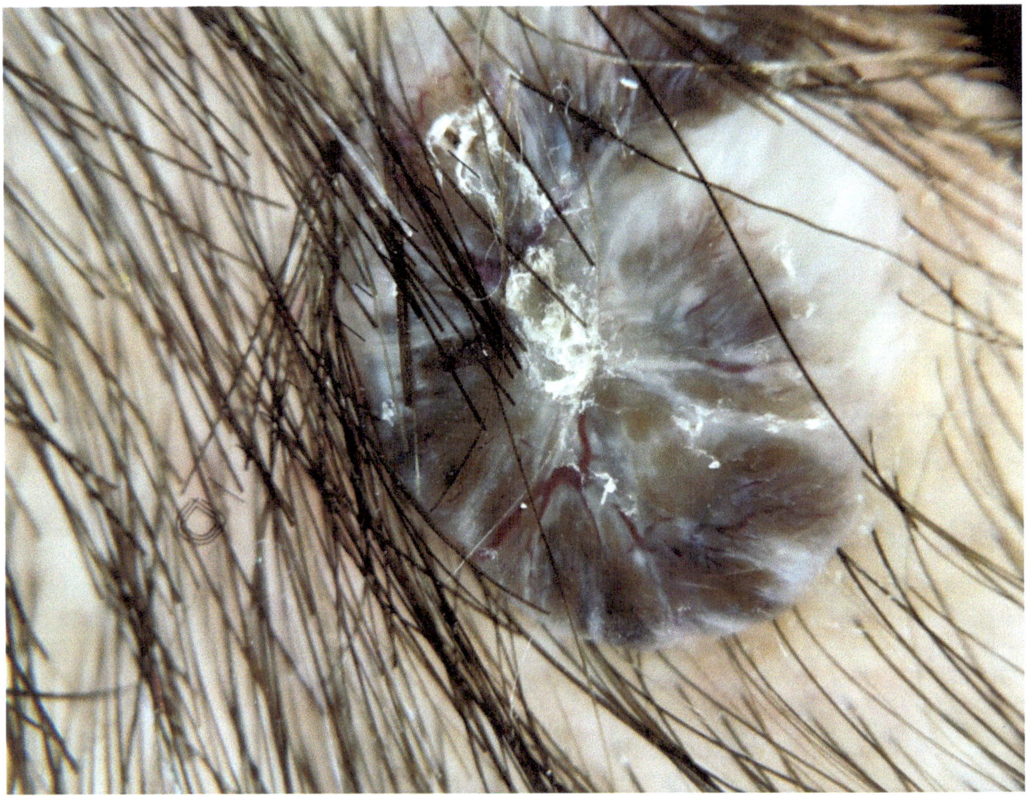

FIGURE 22.8 Pigmented basal cell carcinoma ×10.

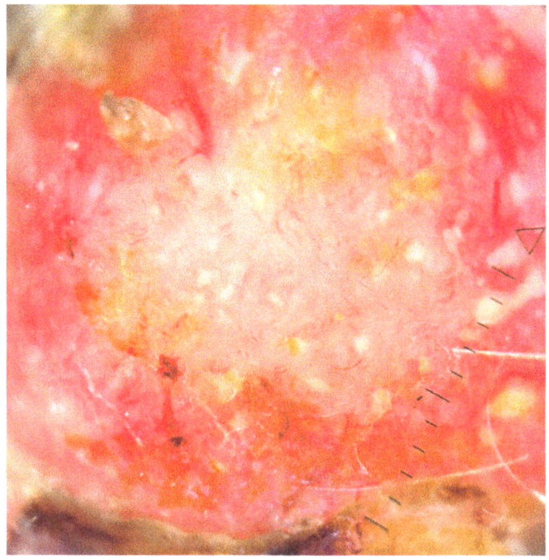

FIGURE 22.9 Squamous cell carcinoma. ×10 Keratin scales, ulceration, and linear irregular vessels.

SUGGESTED READING

Avilés-Izquierdo JA, Ciudad-Blanco C, Sánchez-Herrero A, Mateos-Mayo A, Nieto-Benito LM, Rodríguez-Lomba E. Dermoscopy of cutaneous melanoma metastases: a color-based pattern classification. *J Dermatol.* 2019;46(7):564–69.

Regio Pereira A, Hirata S, Pietkiewicz P, Menzies SW, Brancaccio G, Collgros H, Argenziano G, Lo SN, Ahmed T, Pampena R, Longo C, Guitera P. Dermoscopy of lentiginous melanomas and equivocal benign pigmented macules of the scalp: a case-control multicentric study. *Dermatology.* 2024;240(1):132–41.

Serraino D, di Meo N, Zalaudek I. Dermoscopic features of face and scalp basal and squamous cell carcinomas according to clinical histopathologic characteristics and anatomical location. *J Eur Acad Dermatol Venereol.* 2021;35(3):e237–e239.

Torres F, Fabbrocini G, Hirata SH, Yamada S, De Vita V, Annunziata MC, Tosti A. Dermoscopy of scalp melanoma: report of three cases. *Cancers (Basel).* 2010;2(3):1597–601.

23 Dermoscopy of the Nail Plate

Polarized dermoscopy without an interface solution can be utilized with good results. Non-polarized dermoscopy of the nail plate requires the use of a gel (ultrasound gel) due to the convex shape of the nail plate. This gel will fill the gap between the convex nail surface and the handheld or videodermoscopy device.

NORMAL NAIL (FIGURES 23.1–23.3)

- The cuticle is transparent and smooth
- The lunula is whitish with a semicircular shape and is usually visible only in a few nails. Abnormal lunula shape is seen in nail tumors, onychotillomania, and nail patella syndrome.
- The onychodermal band is visible as a transversal reddish semicircular area in the distal nail bed that follows the shape of the nail plate edge. At high magnification it is characterized by the presence of multiple fine parallel linear capillaries.

LEUKONYCHIA (FIGURES 23.4–23.6)

- True leukonychia: Irregular white spots, macules, and transverse lines with a normal nail plate surface. Color does not fade with pressure.
- Pseudo-leukonychia: Irregular white/yellowish spots with fine scales and a granular nail plate surface.
- Apparent leukonychia: Often more visible at naked eye than at dermoscopy. Color fades with pressure.

NAIL PLATE PIGMENTATION (FIGURE 23.7)

- Proximal margin of the pigmentation follows the shape of the proximal nail fold when exogeneous.
- Proximal margin of the pigmentation follows the shape of the lunula when endogenous.

SPLINTER HEMORRHAGES (FIGURES 23.8–23.10)

- Splinter hemorrhages appear as irregular purple-red longitudinal lines with multiple constrictions.
- They are seen through the distal nail plate in inflammatory, fungal, and traumatic conditions.
- They are seen along the whole nail in certain tumors (onychomatricoma and onychopapilloma) and in systemic amyloidosis.
- They involve the proximal nail in bacterial endocarditis, anti-phospholipid syndrome, and altitude syndrome.

SURFACE ALTERATIONS (FIGURES 23.11, 23.12)

- Longitudinal groove (furrow): Can be regular, often due to fibrokeratomas, or irregular and wavy, typically caused by myxoid pseudocysts.
- Beau's lines: Dermoscopy can better assess the depth and width of these transverse depressions that run horizontally across the nail plate.
- Onychomadesis: Dermoscopy shows a complete detachment of the nail plate from the proximal nail fold, often starting as a horizontal line near the cuticle.
- Longitudinal ridging: Multiple longitudinal striations.
- Onychorrhexis: Longitudinal striations are associated with longitudinal fissures of the nail plate.
- Splitting: Longitudinal fissure. Dermoscopy may enhance the detection of a growing mass beneath the fissure.
- Pitting: See Chapter 26.
- Trachyonychia: See Chapter 26.
- Fissuring/ridging: See Chapter 26.

DOI: 10.1201/9780429351433-23

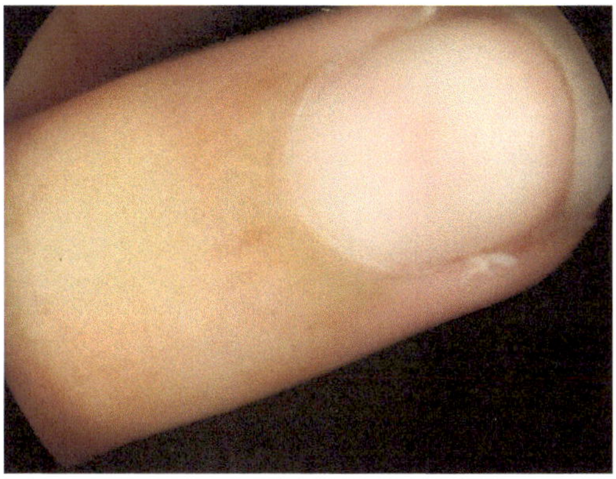

FIGURE 23.1 ×20 The nail cuticle is transparent and firmly attached to the nail plate. The lunula has a semicircular shape. In skin of color the proximal nail fold is pigmented.

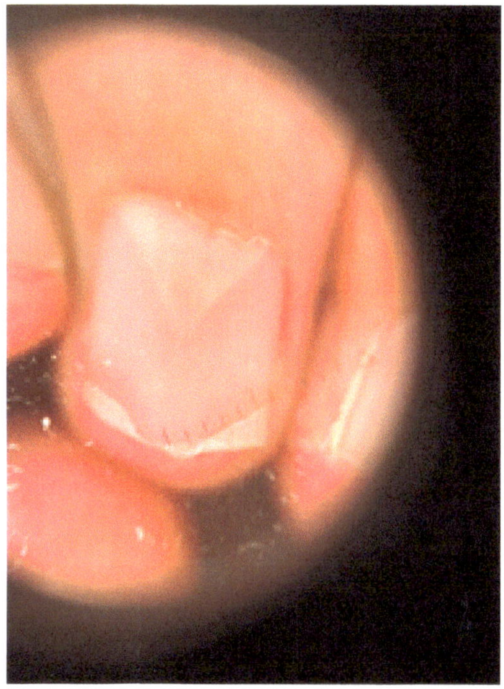

FIGURE 23.2 ×10 Triangular lunula in nail-patella syndrome.

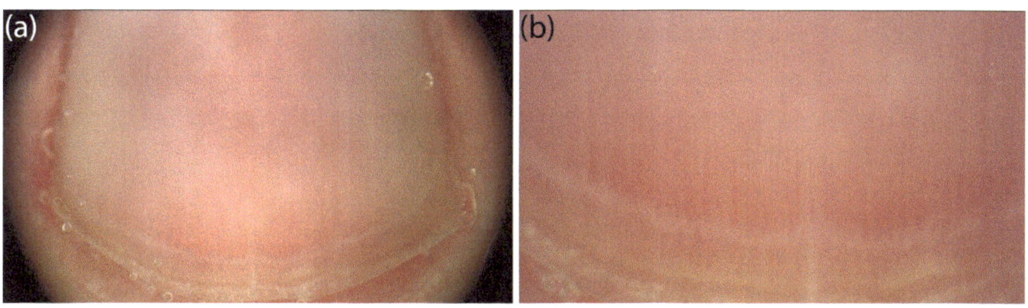

FIGURE 23.3 ×20 (a), ×50 (b) Onychodermal band showing multiple longitudinally oriented parallel linear capillaries.

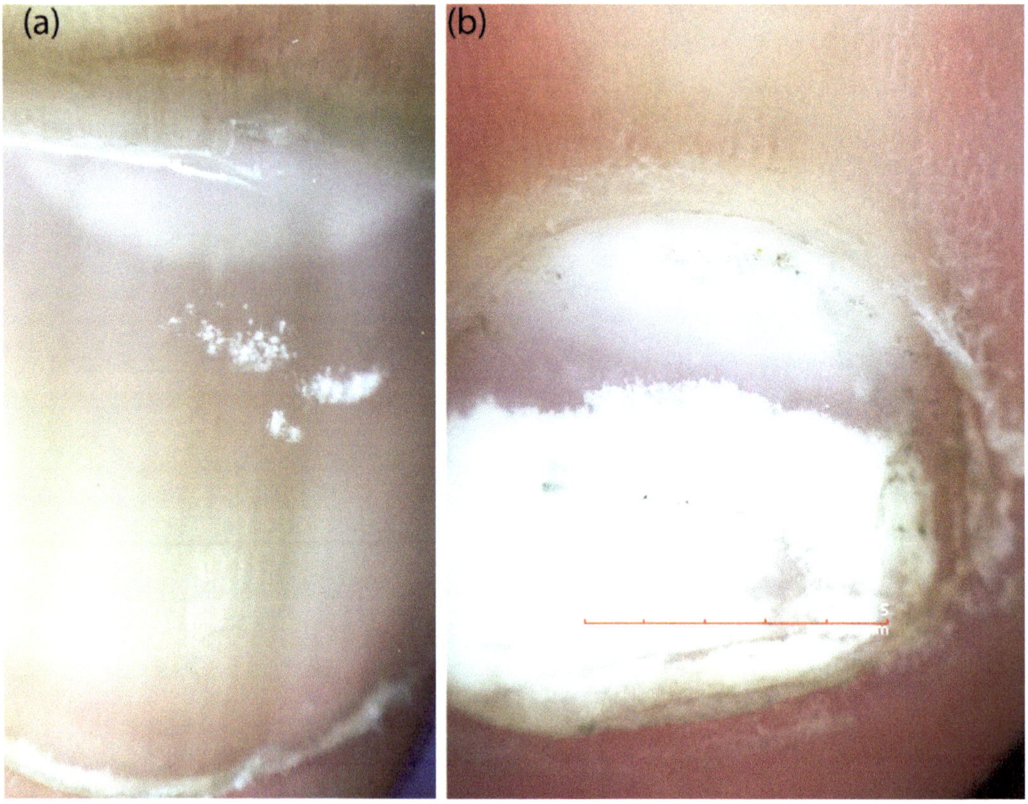

FIGURE 23.4 ×20 Punctate leukonychia (a); ×20 subtotal leukonychia (b).

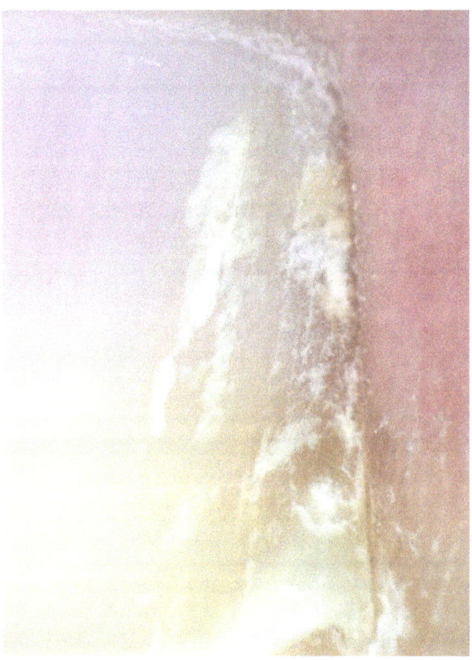

FIGURE 23.5 ×20 Pseudo leukonychia in white superficial onychomycosis: white/yellowish spots with granular scaling.

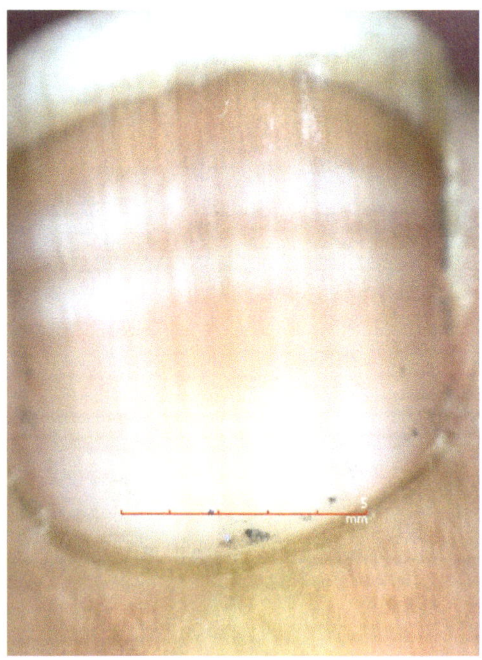

FIGURE 23.6 ×20 Apparent transverse leukonychia (Muehrcke's lines) in a patient undergoing chemotherapy.

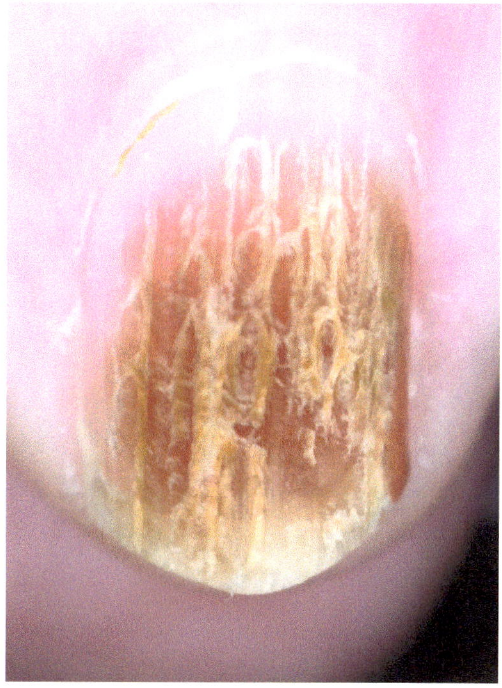

FIGURE 23.7 ×20 Exogenous pigmentation following the shape of the proximal nail fold. Also note keratin degranulation of the superficial nail plate.

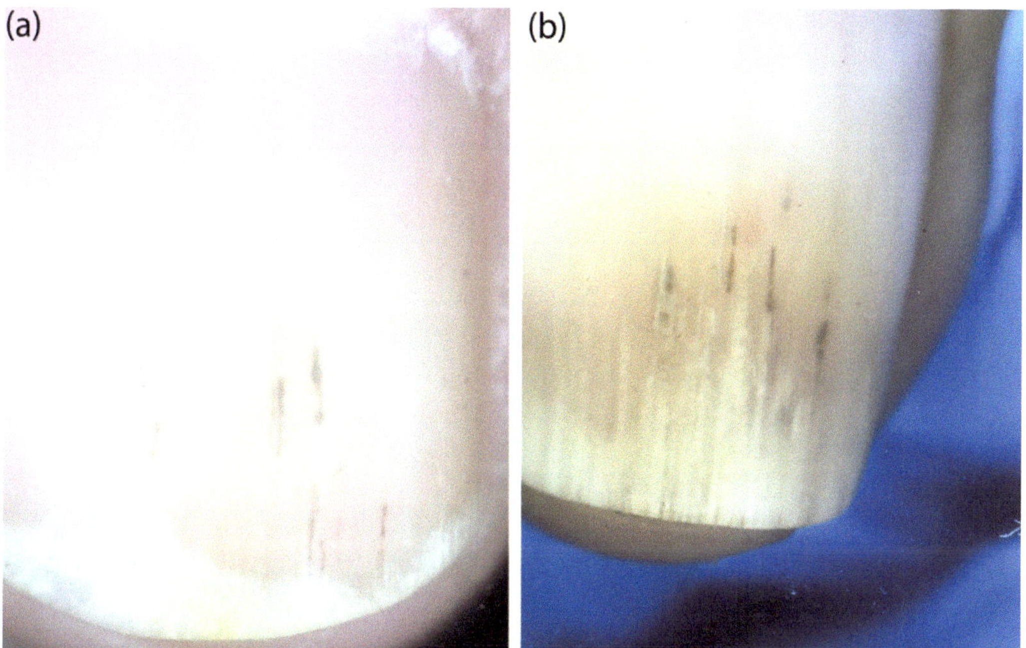

FIGURE 23.8 ×20 Splinter hemorrhages in psoriasis (a) and onychomycosis (b).

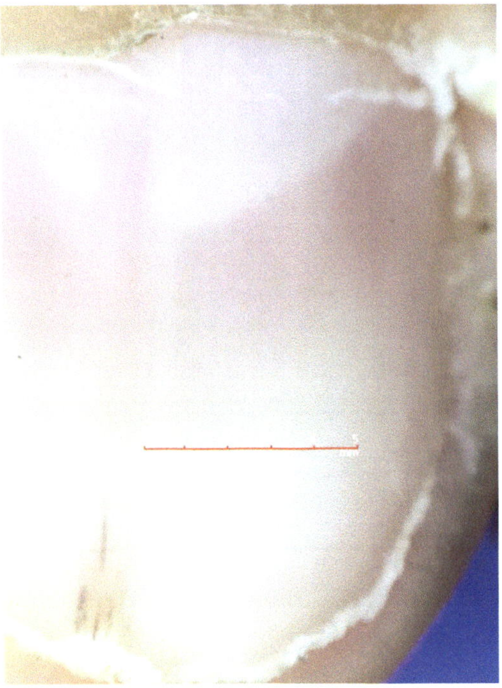

FIGURE 23.9 ×20 Splinter hemorrhages localized within the band of erytronychia in onychopapilloma.

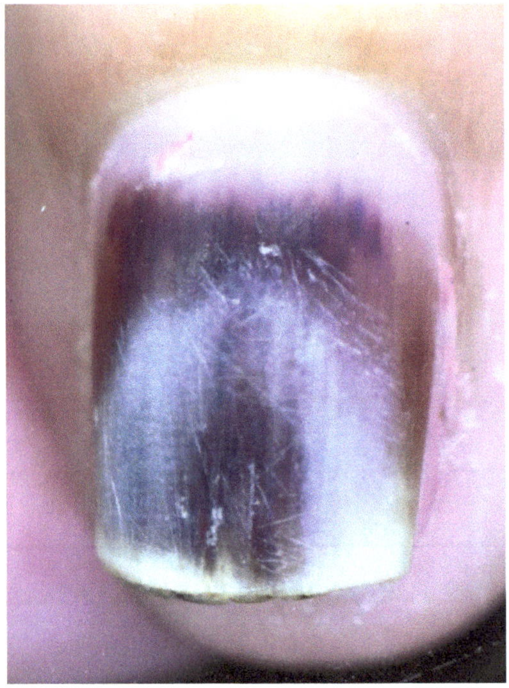

FIGURE 23.10 ×20 Hemorrhagic onycholysis. Note the presence of splinter hemorrhages in the proximal area.

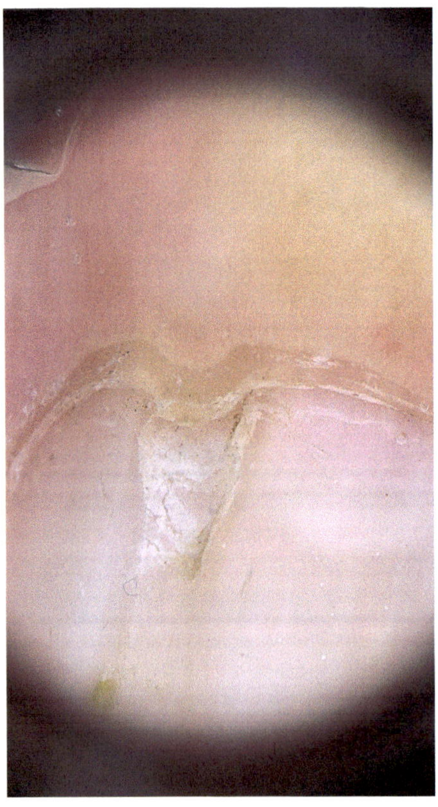

FIGURE 23.11 ×20 Longitudinal groove due to a myxoid cyst.

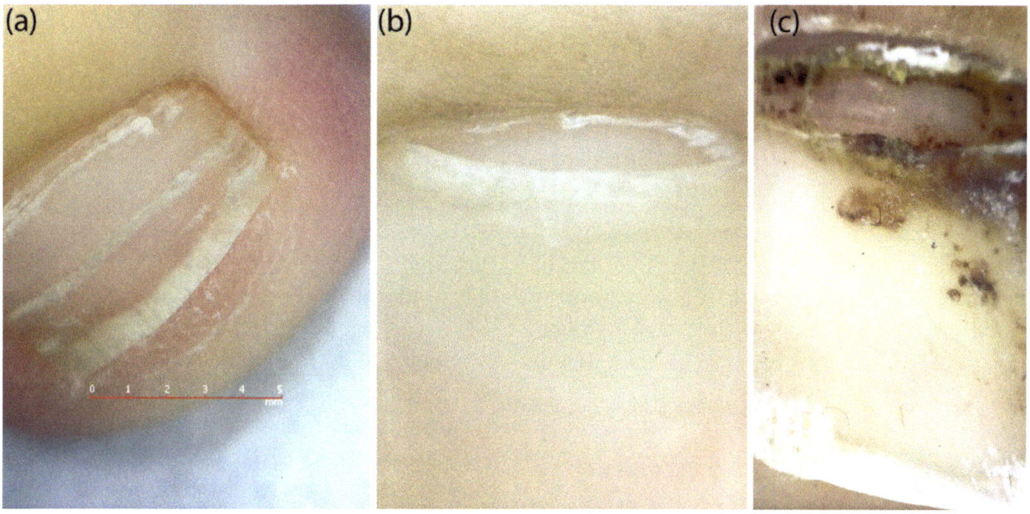

FIGURE 23.12 ×20 Beau line (a); ×20 onychomadesis of the proximal nail plate, note the complete detachment of the nail plate from the proximal nail fold (b); ×20 presence of peripheral dusky red dots indicates a traumatic cause (c).

SUGGESTED READING

Haenssle HA, Blum A, Hofmann-Wellenhof R, Kreusch J, Stolz W, Argenziano G, Zalaudek I, Brehmer F. When all you have is a dermatoscope- start looking at the nails. *Dermatol Pract Concept.* 2014;4(4):11–20.

Lencastre A, Lamas A, Sá D, Tosti A. Onychoscopy. *Clin Dermatol.* 2013;31(5):587–93.

Piraccini BM, Bruni F, Starace M. Dermoscopy of non-skin cancer nail disorders. *Dermatol Ther.* 2012;25(6):594–602.

Starace M, Rapparini L, Quadrelli F, Cedirian S, Pampaloni F, Piraccini BM. When onychoscopy makes the difference in a longitudinal furrow on the nail plate: myxoid pseudocyst versus ungual fibrokeratoma. *J Eur Acad Dermatol Venereol.* 2024;38(10):e861–e862.

24 Dermoscopy of the Proximal Nail Fold

Examination of the proximal nail fold can be performed with non-polarized dermoscopy using water or alcohol as interface solution. Polarized devices can also be utilized in this area.

DERMOSCOPY OF THE PROXIMAL NAIL FOLD (FIGURES 24.1–24.3)

- In normal subject capillary loops are thin, parallel, and longitudinally oriented.
- Connective tissue disorders: Capillary enlargement and loss.
- Pigmentation is very common in people of color.
- Periungual pigmentation: Pseudo-Hutchinson's vs. Hutchinson's sign, see Chapter 31.

Proximal nail fold dermoscopy is very important in the diagnosis and follow-up of connective tissue disorders. In normal conditions, the proximal nail fold capillaries flow parallel to the skin surface and each capillary vessel resembles a hairpin, being formed by two arms that make a distal convex loop. They have a regular distribution even with large intra/inter-individual variability. However, capillary loss and giant capillaries are not seen in normal pattern. In connective tissue disorders vessels are enlarged and tortuous, and the cuticle often shows small hemorrhages and infarcts (see Chapter 33).

Dermoscopy is useful to evaluate pigmentation of the periungual tissues as it easily distinguishes Hutchinson's sign from pseudo-Hutchinson's sign, where the cuticle looks pigmented as the underlying pigmentation is seen by transparency.

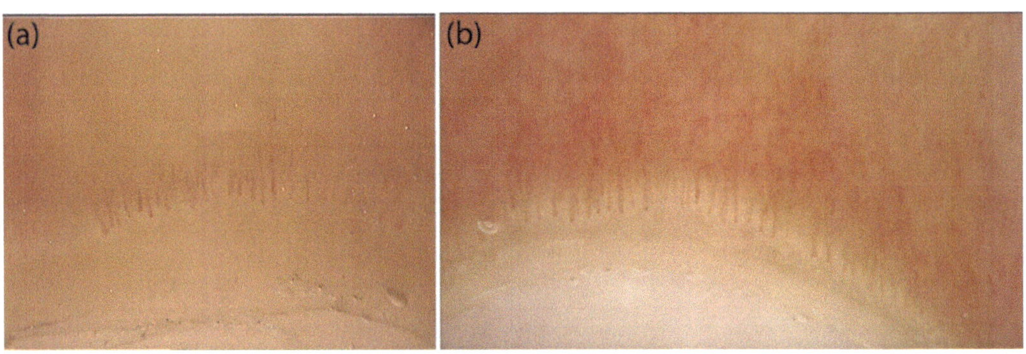

FIGURE 24.1 ×20 Dermoscopy of the proximal nail fold. In normal subjects, proximal nail fold capillaries are uniform in morphology and are homogeneously distributed in small loops above the cuticle (a). ×40 Some capillaries can be enlarged (b).

DOI: 10.1201/9780429351433-24

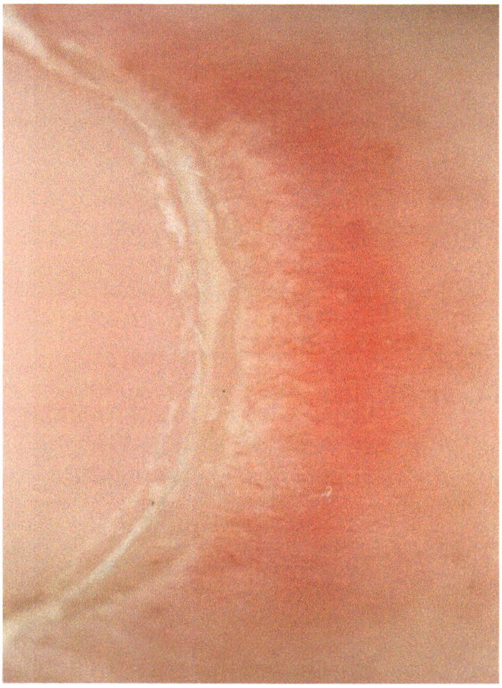

FIGURE 24.2 ×20 Capillary enlargement with giant capillaries and avascular areas in connective tissue diseases.

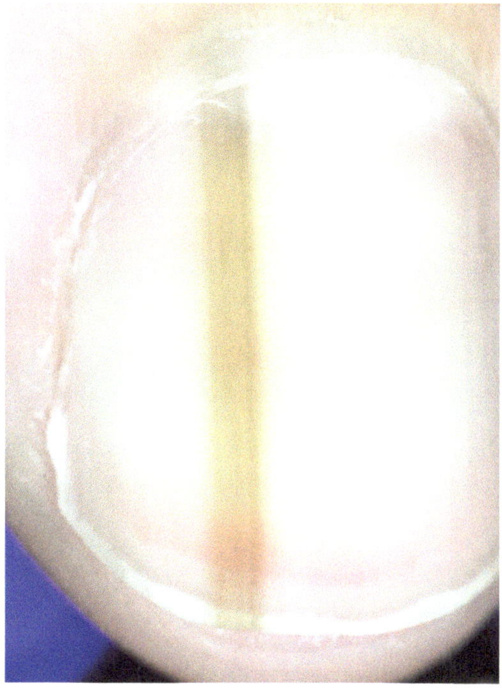

FIGURE 24.3 ×20 Pseudo-Hutchinson's sign. The pigmented band is seen through the transparent cuticle. This is seen even with pale bands.

SUGGESTED READING

Lencastre A, Lamas A, Sá D, Tosti A. Onychoscopy. *Clin Dermatol*. 2013;31(5):587–93.

Piraccini BM, Alessandrini A, Starace M. Onychoscopy: dermoscopy of the nails. *Dermatol Clin*. 2018;36(4):431–38.

Starace M, Alessandrini A, Piraccini BM. Dermoscopy of the nail unit. *Dermatol Clin*. 2021;39(2):293–304.

25 The Free Edge and the Hyponychium

DERMOSCOPY OF THE NAIL PLATE FREE EDGE (FIGURES 25.1–25.4)

Thickness

Dermoscopy can be utilized to detect nail thickening, which can be diffuse or localized.

- Onychopapilloma
- Onychomatricoma
- Pincer nails
- Psoriasis
- Onychomycosis

Shape

Overcurvature

- Pincer nails: The distal margin is very thickened and overcurved, and encircles the entire nail bed. The subungual area can be filled with entrapped scales.

Concave Shape

- Koilonychia

Color

Brown-Black

Longitudinal melanonychia

- Pigmentation localized in the upper portion of the nail plate edge: Indicates pigment is produced in the proximal nail matrix.
- Pigmentation localized in the lower portion of the nail plate edge: Indicates pigment is produced in the distal nail matrix.
- Full thickness pigmentation: Indicates pigment is produced by the whole nail matrix.

Red Purple

- Splinter hemorrhages: Spotty dots.

Yellow/White

- Onychomycosis/psoriasis/trauma: Often associated with thickening.

DERMOSCOPY OF THE HYPONYCHIUM (FIGURES 25.5–25.8)

Capillaries

- Normal capillaries: Presents as a regular pool of small red dots because of their perpendicular arrangement to the skin (each red dot observed represents the top of one capillary loop).
- Irregular/dilated capillaries: In psoriasis at high magnification (×50) dermoscopy shows characteristic coiled and twisted capillary loops.

Pigmentation

- Hutchinson's sign: The pigmentation typically follows the parallel ridge pattern characterized by accentuated pigmentation in the deep intermediate ridges, with or without obliteration of the eccrine gland ducts (see Chapter 31).
- Pseudo-Hutchinson's sign: Linear pigmentation across the skin marks (see Chapter 31).
- Pigmented dots: Of different size and shades of color, ranging from light brown to black, can be visible in the hyponychium in nevi (see Chapter 31).

DOI: 10.1201/9780429351433-25

Collarette

- Refers to a thin band of loosened keratin extending beyond the edge of a well-defined skin lesion, and is commonly observed in exostosis, fibrokeratoma, or pyogenic granuloma

Pterygium Inversum Unguis/ Distal Pterygium

- Disappearance of the subungual space seen in scleroderma or after acrylic manicure

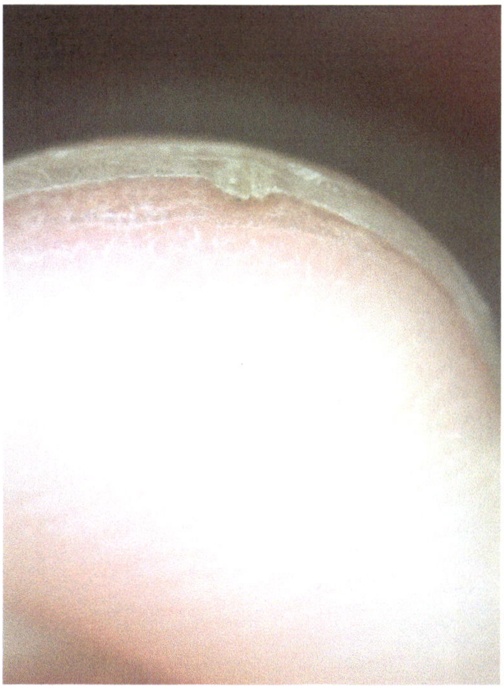

FIGURE 25.1 ×20 Onychopapilloma. Note localized thickening due to a keratotic mass at free edge in correspondence with the band.

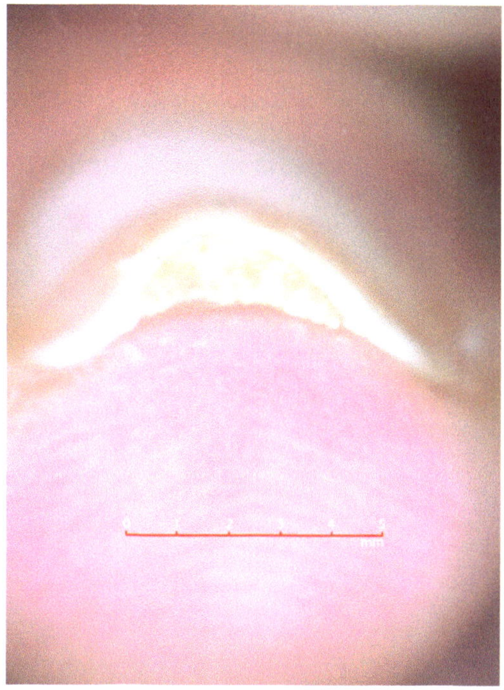

FIGURE 25.2 ×20 Onychomatricoma. Thickening of the free margin with multiple holes (honeycomb pattern).

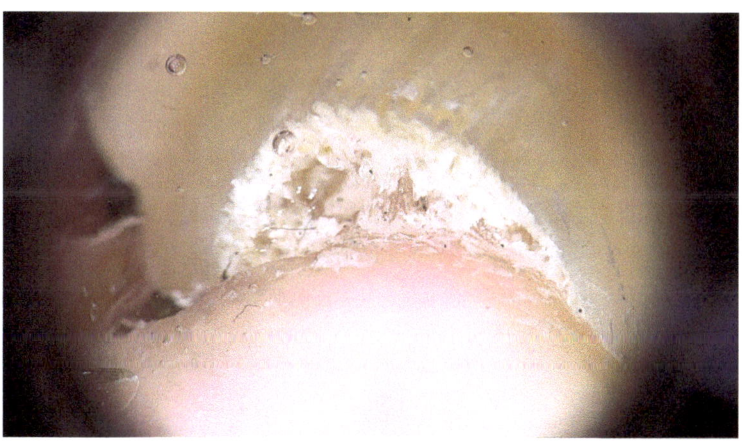

FIGURE 25.3 ×50 Onychomycosis. Diffuse thickening with whitish scales and multiple gaps (ruined appearance).

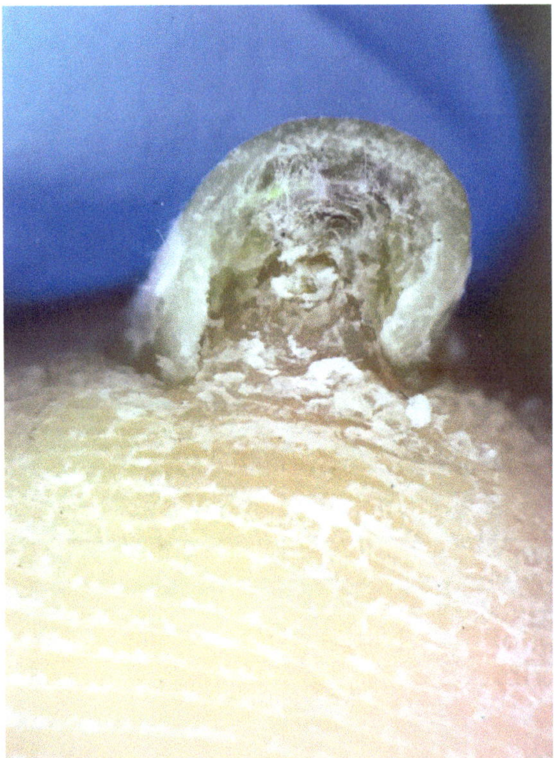

FIGURE 25.4 ×20 Pincer nail. Distal nail plate thickening and hypercurvature with nail bed constriction. Also note diffuse scaling.

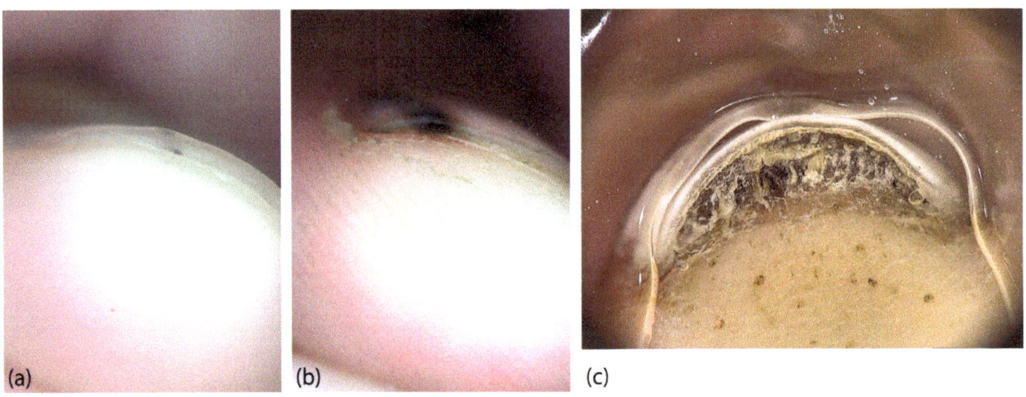

FIGURE 25.5 ×20 Dermoscopy of the distal edge: pigmentation in the ventral nail plate indicates that the lesion is located in the distal matrix (a); pigmentation of the entire nail thickness indicates a lesion of the whole matrix (b). Hemorrhages below the nail plate in hemorrhagic onycholysis: note that the nail plate is not pigmented but the subungual space contains multiple purple lakes (c).

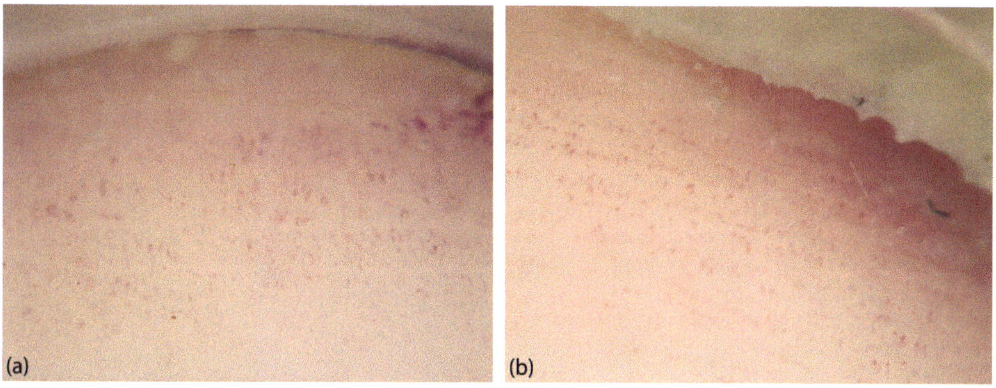

FIGURE 25.6 (a,b) ×50 Coiled twisted capillaries in nail psoriasis.

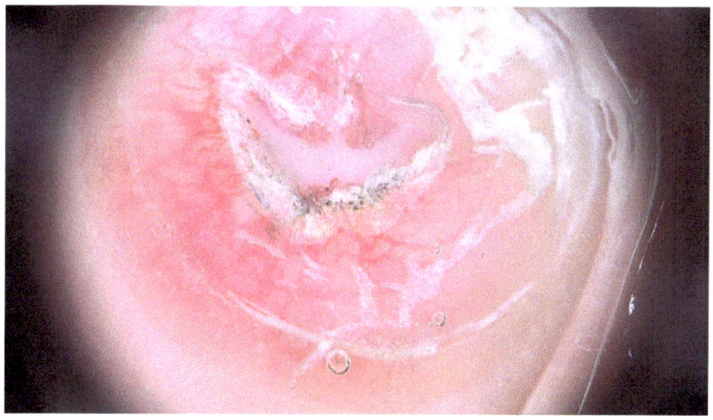

FIGURE 25.7 ×50 Collarette in exostosis. Linear white circle limiting the boundaries between the tumor and the surrounding tissue.

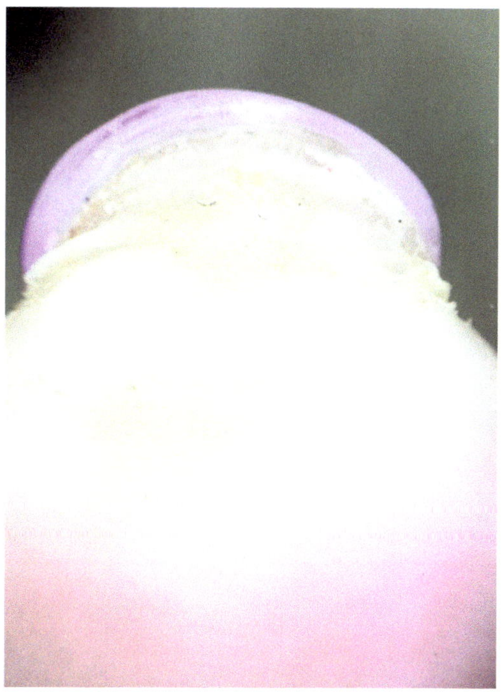

FIGURE 25.8 ×20 Pterygium inversum. The distal space is obliterated by tissue with overlying scales.

SUGGESTED READING

Iorizzo M, Dahdah M, Vincenzi C, Tosti A. Videodermoscopy of the hyponychium in nail bed psoriasis. *J Am Acad Dermatol.* 2008;58(4):714–5.

Iorizzo M, Starace M, Di Altobrando A, Alessandrini A, Veneziano L, Piraccini BM. The value of dermoscopy of the nail plate free edge and hyponychium. *J Eur Acad Dermatol Venereol.* 2021;35(12):2361–6.

Navarro Campoamor L. Frontal examination of the distal nail unit. *Actas Dermosifiliogr.* 2024;115(2):159–67.

Ocampo-Garza J, Jacomini Sobral P, Mendes Bretas J, Matana D, Tosti A. Dermoscopic technique for the evaluation of the nail unit. *J Am Acad Dermatol.* 2021;85(2). https://doi.org/10.1016/j.jaad.2017.10.019

Tosti A, Schneider SL, Ramirez-Quizon MN, Zaiac M, Miteva M. Clinical, dermoscopic, and pathologic features of onychopapilloma: a review of 47 cases. *J Am Acad Dermatol.* 2016;74(3):521–6.

26 Inflammatory Nail Disorders

NAIL PSORIASIS (FIGURES 26.1–26.5)

Dermoscopy helps to enhance the detection of most nail changes and allows to visualize vascular abnormalities that are important for diagnosis.

- Pitting is better evaluated with dry dermoscopy as whitish scales partially filling and surrounding multiple, irregularly distributed depressions. Pits located in the proximal nail plate contain more scales, as these are progressively shed with microtrauma.
- Leukonychia: Spotted opaque white areas with normal nail surface.
- Nail crumbling: Brittle and fragmented yellowish nail plate.
- Oil drop/salmon patches: Yellow-orange translucent areas visible through the nail plate, resembling an oil drop. They can surround the onycholytic nail plate or be isolated in the central/lateral part of the nail.
- Subungual hyperkeratosis: It is more common in the toenails and appears as accumulation of scales under the nail plate; in psoriasis the scales are white and compact as opposed to onychomycosis where the scales are yellowish and loose.
- Splinter hemorrhages: Single or multiple red to purple linear or filamentous lines, mostly localized in the distal nail bed. Areas of dilations and restrictions, as well as color variations from bright red to purple within the same line are common.
- Dilated and tortuous capillaries in the onychodermal band.
- Red spots in the lunula: Can also be seen in alopecia areata and lichen planus (mottled lunula).
- Twisted capillary loops in the hyponychium are a useful diagnostic sign that can only be seen at high magnification (×40 or more). Appear as irregularly distributed, dilated, tortuous capillaries, similar to those seen on the scalp. They are also seen in Hallopeau's acrodermatitis.

ACRODERMATITIS CONTINUA OF HALLOPEAU (FIGURE 26.6)

This primarily affects the periungual and subungual areas of one or few nails.

Dermoscopy

- Single or multiple yellow/greenish pustules in the nail bed and nail folds. They can be seen through the cuticle and cause onycholytic spots that may coalesce into larger areas.
- Yellowish crumbling and disruption of the nail plate with periungual erythema.
- Twisted enlarged capillaries in the hyponychium.

PARAKERATOSIS PUSTOLOSA (FIGURE 26.7)

This primarily affects children and is limited to one digit in most cases.

Dermoscopy

- Periungual erythema and crusting
- Nail bed pustules and yellowish scaling
- Partial or complete loss of the nail plate

DOI: 10.1201/9780429351433-26

NAIL LICHEN PLANUS (FIGURES 26.8, 26.9)

Dermoscopy is very useful to distinguish pterygium from nail plate destruction seen in onychotillomania.

- Longitudinal fissuring: Fissures vary in depth and are associated with longitudinal scaling with detachment of multiple layers of the nail plate in severe cases.
- Red dots in the lunula (mottled lunula).
- Pterygium: The skin projecting from the proximal nail fold shows irregular erythema or pigmentation. There is complete absence of the proximal sulcus. The nail plate is absent in the area underlying the pterygium, but it can be partially or totally present distally. On the lateral margins, the nail plate can be normal or show longitudinal fissuring.
- Wickham striae in the periungual tissue.
- Subungual hyperkeratosis.
- Melanonychia with homogeneous gray-brown color.

LICHEN STRIATUS OF THE NAIL UNIT (FIGURE 26.10)

This primarily affects children and more frequently occurs isolated and limited to one nail.

- Irregular longitudinal fissures of different depth limited to one side of the nail plate.
- Skin papules: When present, show reticular whitish lines with fine scales.

ALOPECIA AREATA (FIGURES 26.11, 26.12)

- Pitting: Pits are small, regularly distributed and contain small scales, which are often detectable also in the distal plate.
- Leukonychia: The white-opaque spots are very small and regularly distributed. They differ from pits because the nail plate is preserved and lacks scales.
- Trachyonychia: The nail roughness is due to superficial scaling of the nail plate, where there are multiple spotty areas or multiple thin parallel longitudinal furrows filled with scales.
- Red spots in the lunula (mottled lunula): The lunula shows multiple irregular red spots.

ALLERGIC CONTACT DERMATITIS OF THE NAILS (FIGURES 26.13, 26.14)

Predominantly affects women who make frequent use of artificial nails or nail salon workers due to occupational exposures.

Dermoscopy

- Onycholysis with severe compact subungual hyperkeratosis.
- Yellowish vesicles: Due to spongiosis, may be occasionally found in periungual skin.

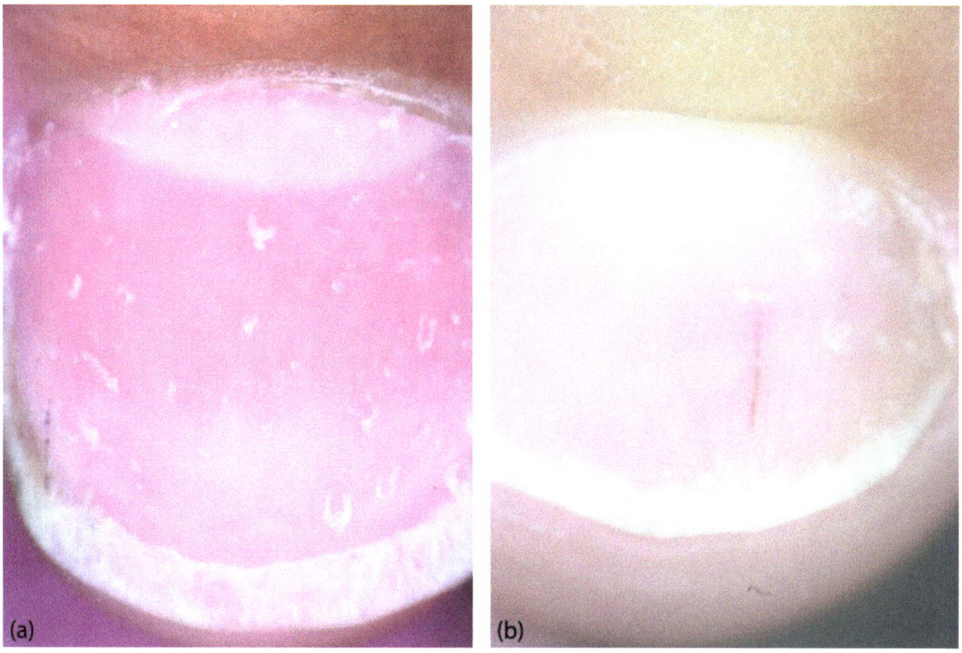

FIGURE 26.1 ×20 Psoriatic pits surrounded and/or covered by scales (a). Note also splinter hemorrhages (b).

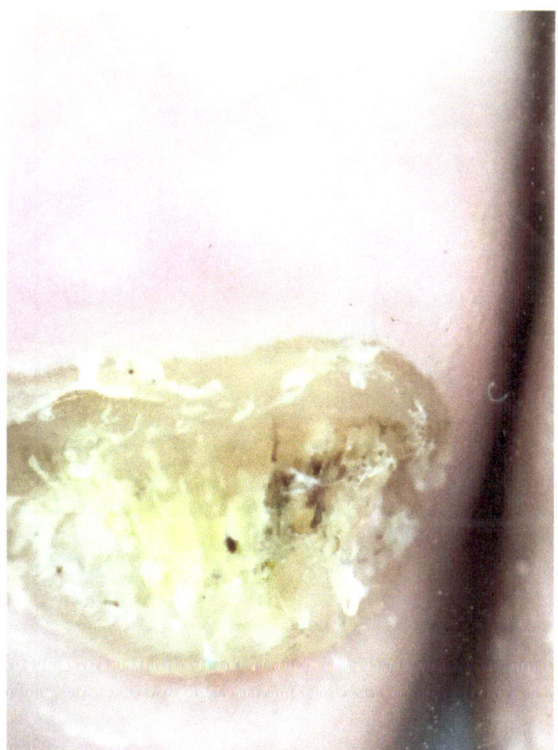

FIGURE 26.2 ×20 Psoriasis. Nail crumbling. Diffuse fragmentation of the nail plate with scaling and hemorrhages.

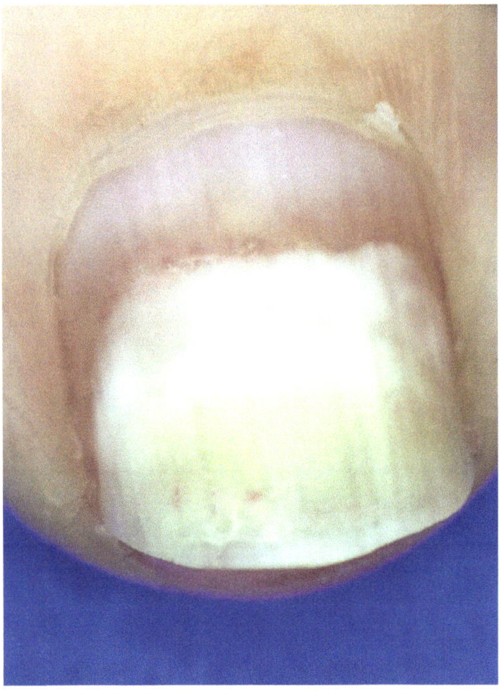

FIGURE 26.3 ×20 Psoriatic onycholysis with erythematous border.

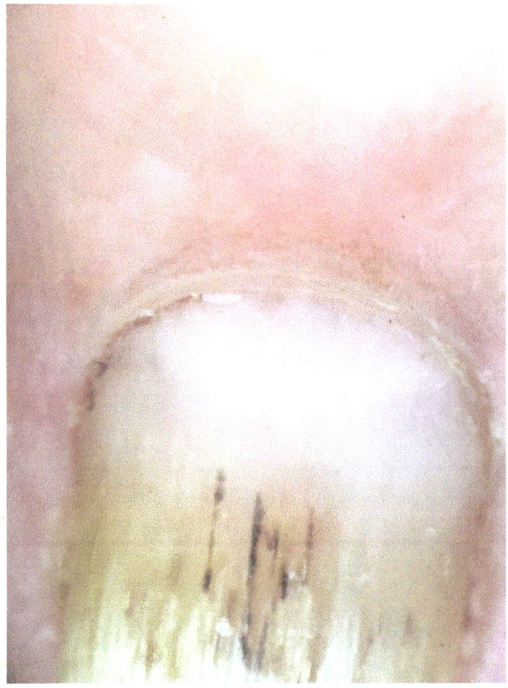

FIGURE 26.4 Psoriasis. ×20 Splinter hemorrhages. Thickness and shape vary along the length of the hemorrhagic lines.

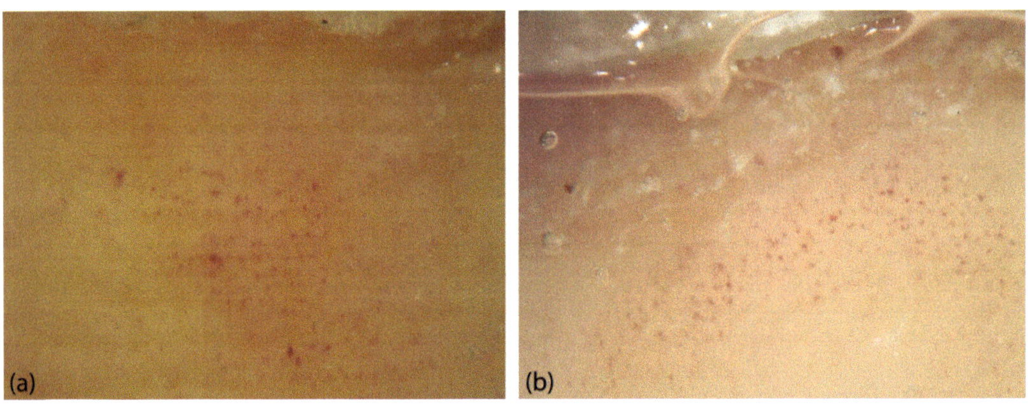

FIGURE 26.5 (a,b) Psoriasis. ×50 Twisted enlarged capillaries at the hyponychium.

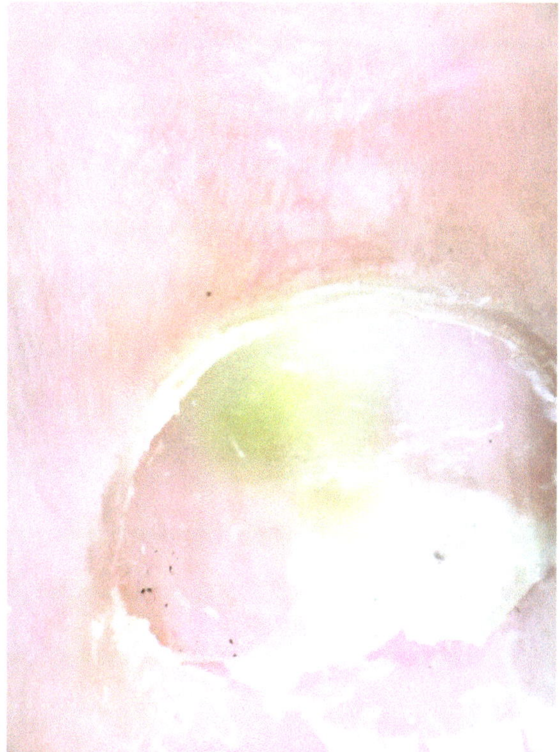

FIGURE 26.6 ×20 Acrodermatitis Continua of Hallopeau. Subungual pustule originating under the proximal nail fold.

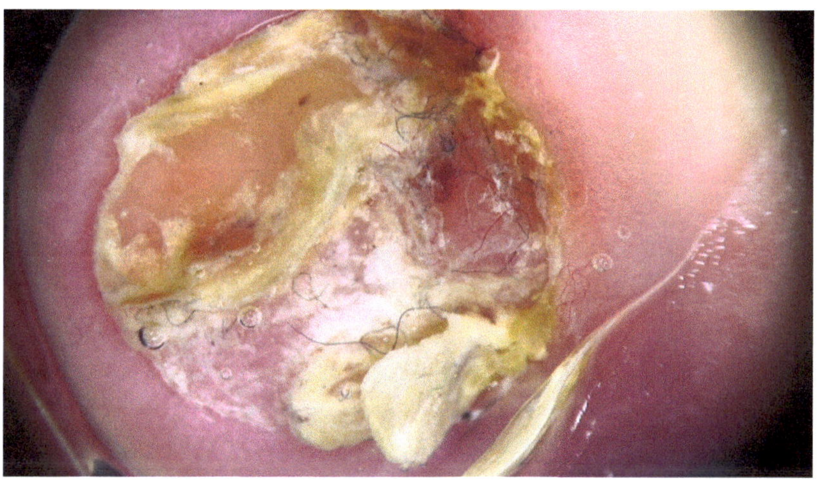

FIGURE 26.7 Parakeratosis pustolosa. ×20 Nail bed scaling and hemorrhagic crusting with embedded textile fibers. Periungual erythema and yellowish scales. Onycholysis with partial destruction of the nail plate.

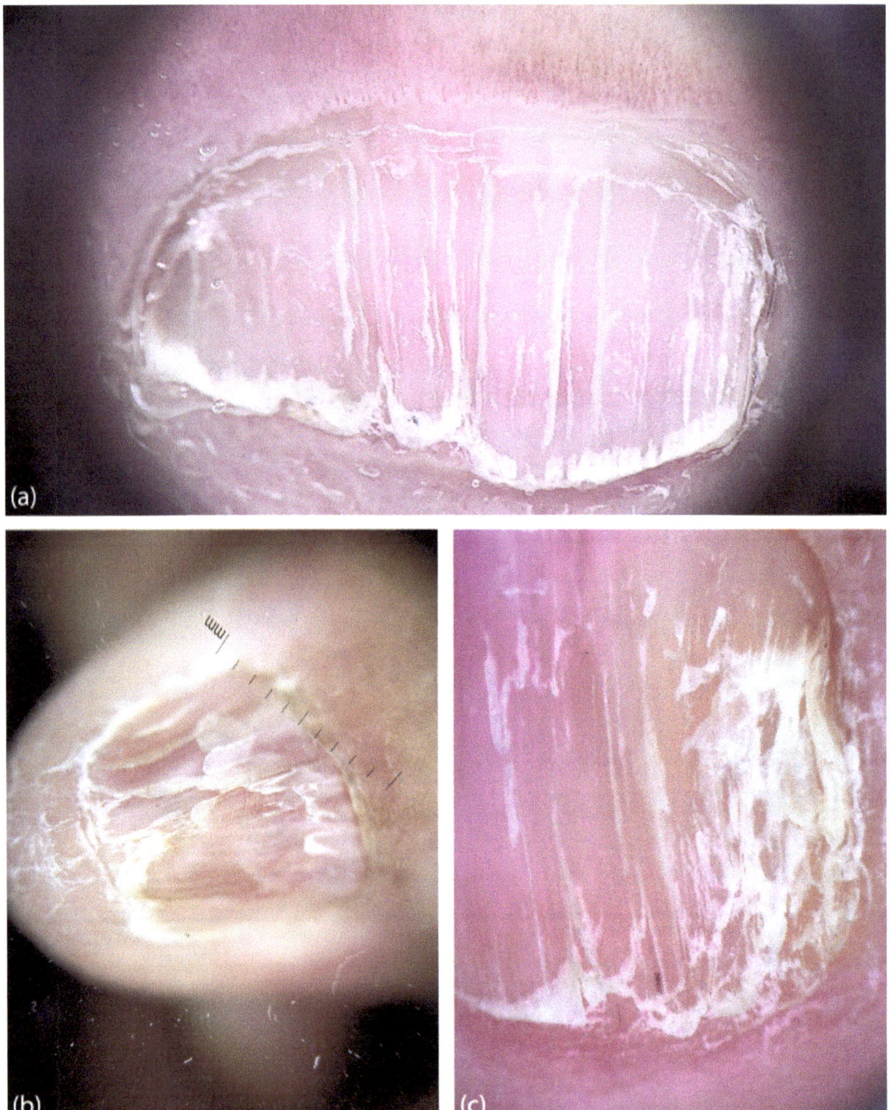

FIGURE 26.8 Lichen planus. ×20 Longitudinal fissures and scaling (a); ×10 also note detachment of the nail plate layers (b); ×20 damage may not affect the nail plate homogeneously (c).

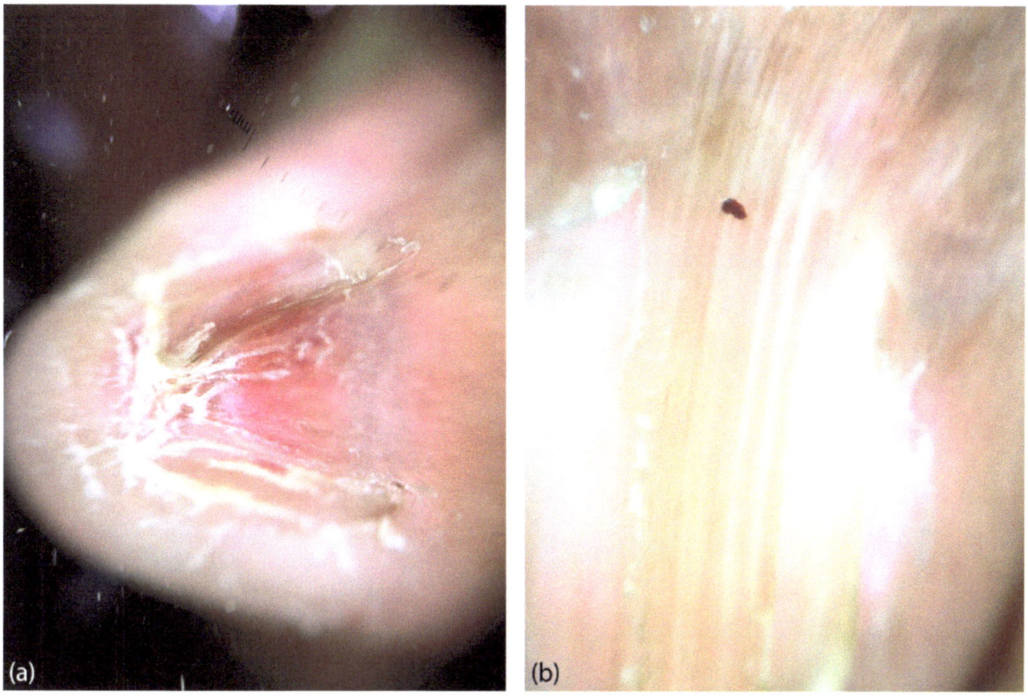

FIGURE 26.9 Lichen planus. ×10 Pterygium has an irregular red-whitish or brownish color; note the nail plate remnants on the sides of the pterygium (a); ×20 the pterygium presents longitudinal linear white lines of fibrosis projecting from the proximal nail fold, also note the cuticle at the sides of the pterygium (b).

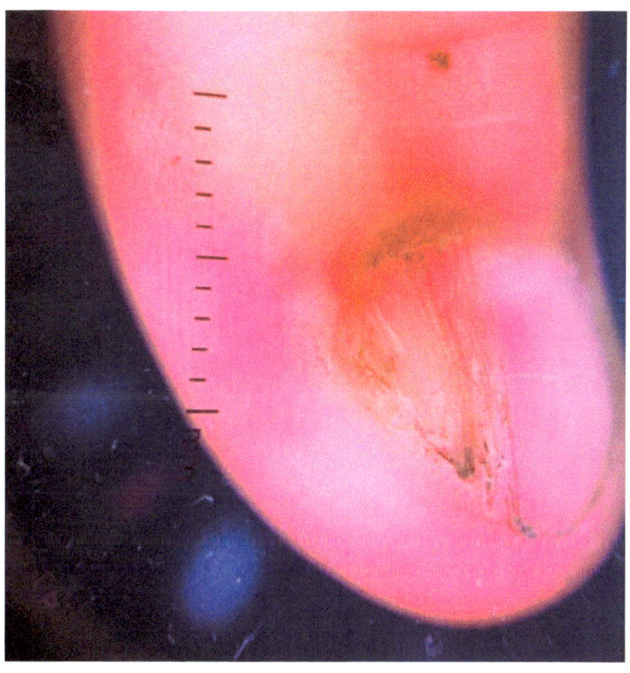

FIGURE 26.10 Lichen striatus. ×10 Longitudinal fissuring limited to one side of the nail plate.

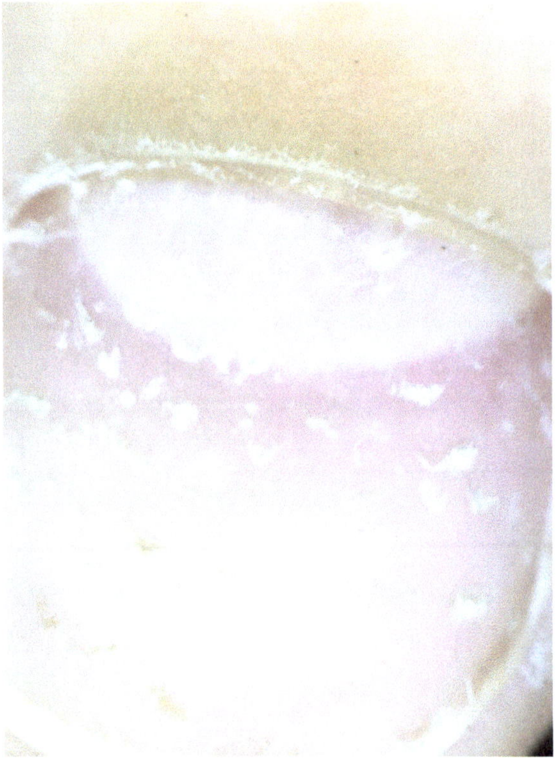

FIGURE 26.11 Alopecia areata. ×20 Pits correspond to superficial spotty white scaling of the nail plate.

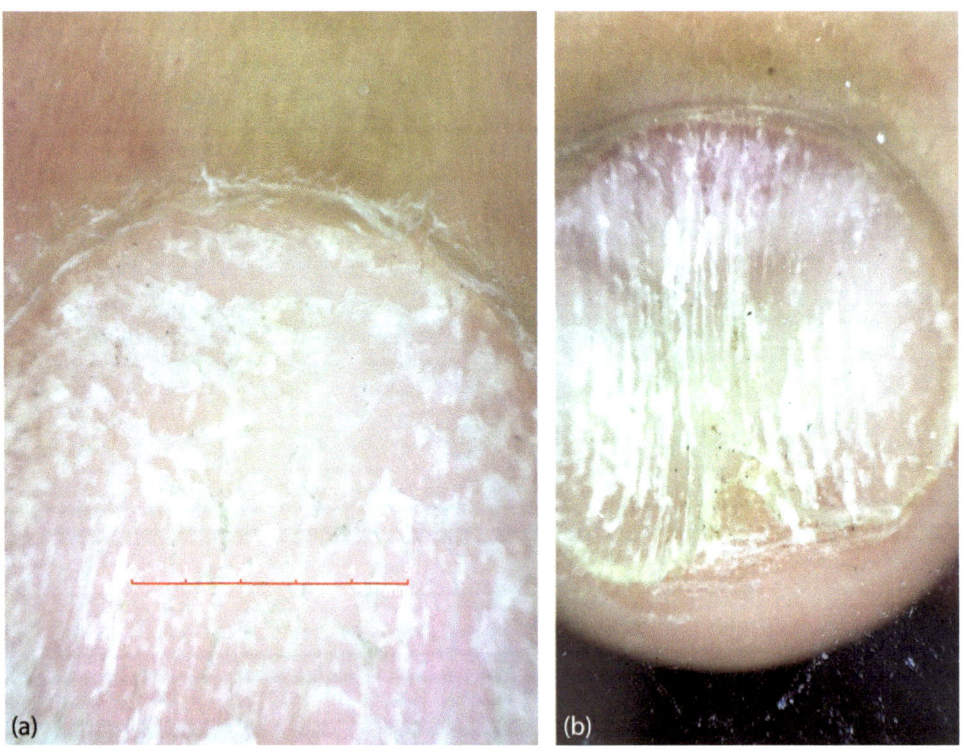

FIGURE 26.12 Trachyonychia in alopecia areata. ×20 Multiple spotty areas filled with scales (a) or multiple thin parallel longitudinal furrows filled with scales (b).

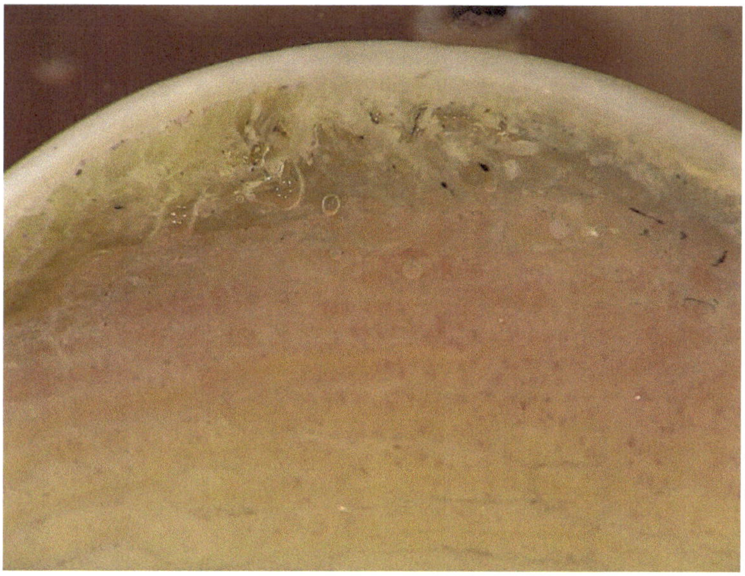

FIGURE 26.13 ×40 Psoriasiform contact dermatitis due to acrylates showing compact hyperkeratosis at the free margin and twisted capillary loops in the hyponychium.

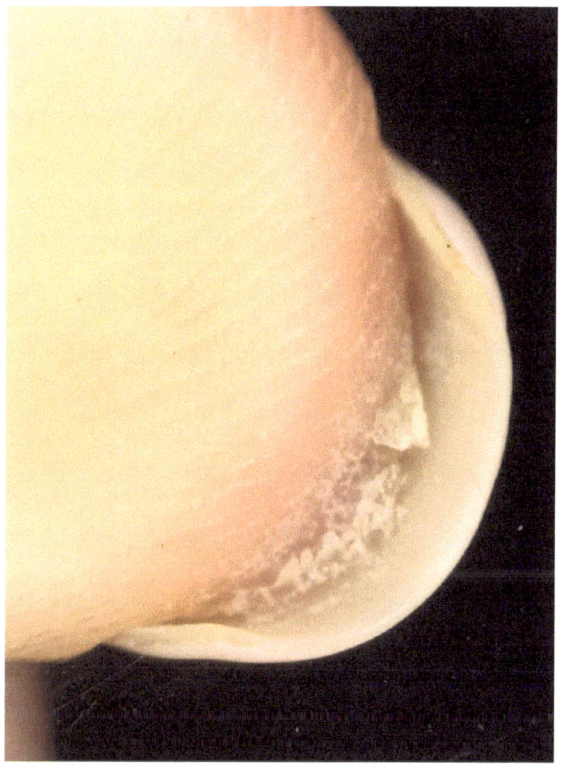

FIGURE 26.14 ×20 Pterygium inversum in a patient using acrylates gel polish.

SUGGESTED READING

Cervantes J, Sanchez,M, Eber AE, Perper M, Tosti A. Pterygium inversum unguis secondary to gel polish. *J Eur Acad Dermatol Venereol.* 2018;32:160–3.

Chen AF, Chimento SM, Hu S, Sanchez M, Zaiac M, Tosti A. Nail damage from gel polish manicure. *J Cosmet Dermatol.* 2012;11:27–29.

Errichetti E, Stinco G. Dermoscopy in facilitating the recognition of acrodermatitis continua of Hallopeau. *J Dermatol.* 2017;44(11):e286–e287.

Errichetti E, Zabotti A, Stinco G, Quartuccio L, Sacco S, De Marchi G, et al. Dermoscopy of nail fold and elbow in the differential diagnosis of early psoriatic arthritis sine psoriasis and early rheumatoid arthritis. *J Dermatol.* 2016;43(10):1217–20.

Farias DC, Tosti A, Chiacchio ND, Hirata SH. Dermoscopy in nail psoriasis. *An Bras Dermatol.* 2010;85(1):101–3.

Gnesotto L, Mioso G, Starace M, Piraccini BM, Naldi L, Sechi A. Nail lichen striatus affecting adjacent nails: a sign of blaschko lines. *Dermatol Pract Concept.* 2023;13(4):e2023208.

Iorizzo M, Dahdah M, Vincenzi C, Tosti A. Videodermoscopy of the hyponychium in nail bed psoriasis. *J Am Acad Dermatol.* 2008;58(4):714–5.

Iorizzo M, Starace M, Pasch MC. Leukonychia: what can white nails tell us? *Am J Clin Dermatol.* 2022;23(2):177–93.

Lencastre A, Lamas A, Sá D, Tosti A. Onychoscopy. *Clin Dermatol.* 2013;31(5):587–93.

Mattos Simoes Mendonca M, LaSenna C, Tosti A. Severe onychodystrophy due to allergic contact dermatitis from acrylic nails. *Skin Appendage Disord.* 2015;1(2):91–4.

Nakamura RC, Costa MC. Dermatoscopic findings in the most frequent onychopathies: descriptive analysis of 500 cases. *Int J Dermatol.* 2012;51(4):483–5.

Sar-Pomian M, Starace MVR, Lencastre A, Piraccini BM, Richert B, Rudnicka L, Trakatelli MG, Iorizzo M. Dermoscopic nail changes in psoriasis, lichen planus, and lichen striatus. *Skin Appendage Disord.* 2024;10(4):273–92.

Yadav TA, Khopkar US. Dermoscopy to detect signs of subclinical nail involvement in chronic plaque psoriasis: a study of 68 patients. *Indian J Dermatol.* 2015;60(3):272–5.

27 Traumatic Nail Disorders

SUBUNGUAL HEMATOMA (FIGURES 27.1–27.3)

Dermoscopy

- Pigmentation is red to black in color, depending on the age of the lesion, with recent lesions often presenting a pink-red color.
- Red color in older lesions may indicate new bleeding from repeated trauma.
- The superficial nail plate is normal or may show onychomadesis.
- Color is homogeneous or may show a combination with purple-black, red-black, brown-black.
- The dark homogeneous pigmentation often masks the lunula and is visible through the cuticles.
- Globules: Located at the periphery, appear as dark-red, small, round, or oval-shaped areas of discoloration, usually arranged in clusters, indicate that trauma is still active.
- Streaks (filamentous distal end): Are linear dark-purple to black lines that extend distally from the pigmentation and result from trauma to the nail bed capillaries.
- Peripheral fading, periungual hemorrhages, and splinter hemorrhages are also common findings.
- Punctate leukonychia: Can be associated.

Although hematomas are benign, they do not rule out the possibility of associated tumors, as spontaneous bleeding can occur in nail unit tumors, including melanomas.

ONYCHOLYSIS (FIGURES 27.4–27.9)

Distal Onycholysis: Look at the Proximal Border

- Sharp and linear proximal border is usually associated with trauma.
- Irregular proximal border with alternation of concavity and convexity (roller-coaster pattern) is usually due to traumatic cleaning under the nail plate.
- Presence of erythematous border surrounding the onycholytic area is seen in psoriasis (see Chapter 26).
- Jagged proximal border with multiple sharp lines projecting to the proximal nail is typical of onychomycosis (see Chapter 29).
- Erosive or exophytic lesions uplifting the nail plate suggest nail tumors (see Chapter 30).
- Green color indicates *Pseudomonas* colonization.
- Red to purple color is characteristic of hemorrhagic onycholysis.
- Debris such as hair fragments, textile fibers, or foreign bodies can be seen within the onycholytic area.
- Presence of twisted capillaries in the hyponychium should be searched in all cases of "idiopathic onycholysis" to rule out nail psoriasis (see Chapter 26).

TRAUMATIC LEUKONYCHIA (FIGURE 27.10)

Transverse leukonychia due to trauma can affect the fingernails, where it is usually due to manicure, or the big toenails, where it is due to the repetitive trauma to the distal edge from the tip of the shoes.

DOI: 10.1201/9780429351433-27

Dermoscopy

- Punctate or transverse opaque white discoloration that does not fade with pressure
- Normal nail surface

SUPERFICIAL FRICTION (WORN DOWN NAILS; FIGURE 27.11)

Superficial friction is consequence of repetitive rubbing.

Dermoscopy

- Thinning of the distal nail plate surface, with convex proximal border and visualization of nail bed capillaries

ONYCHOTILLOMANIA (FIGURES 27.12, 27.13)

Clinical Features

- Onychotillomania usually involves the proximal nail fold with scaling, swelling, and periungual hemorrhages.
- Severe cases also involve the whole nail with partial or complete absence of the nail plate and cuticle, periungual and nail bed scales, periungual and nail bed hemorrhages, and crusts.

Dermoscopy

- The proximal nail fold shows dilated capillaries and cuticular hemorrhages and crusts.
- Scales: Are detected in the nail bed, nail folds, and hyponychium. Keratinization of the nail bed is due to nail plate loss.
- Absence of nail plate: Can be complete or partial.
- Wavy lines: Uneven longitudinal white, reddish-purple, brown, or black lines appearing on different planes.
- Nail bed capillary hemorrhages: The nail plate is absent, and the nail bed and the lunula show reddish-brown or purplish-black pinpoint dots or streaks with an oblique wavy pattern.
- Yellowish crusts: Often seen along with scales and hemorrhages.
- Longitudinal melanonychia: Due to the activation of melanocytes in the distal matrix, can be seen when the nail plate is still preserved.
- Nail bed pigmentation: Longitudinal gray pigmentation of the nail bed, when the plate is absent.

CENTRAL NAIL PLATE DEFORMITIES (FIGURE 27.14)

- Habit tic deformities: The nail plate presents a longitudinal groove with multiple transversal parallel scratches with a scaly surface.
- Heller's deformity: The nail plate shows a central fissure with an inverted Christmas tree pattern.

Nail Changes Due to Nail Care

Manicures can cause nail damage through instruments, nail polish, removers, and artificial nails.

- Transverse ridging or leukonychia
- Onycholysis with roller-coaster border
- Yellowish chromonychia: Can be associated with superficial scaling
- Pterygium inversum: Obliteration of the subungal space, associated with acrylates use (see Chapter 25)
- Keratin degranulation (see Chapter 28)

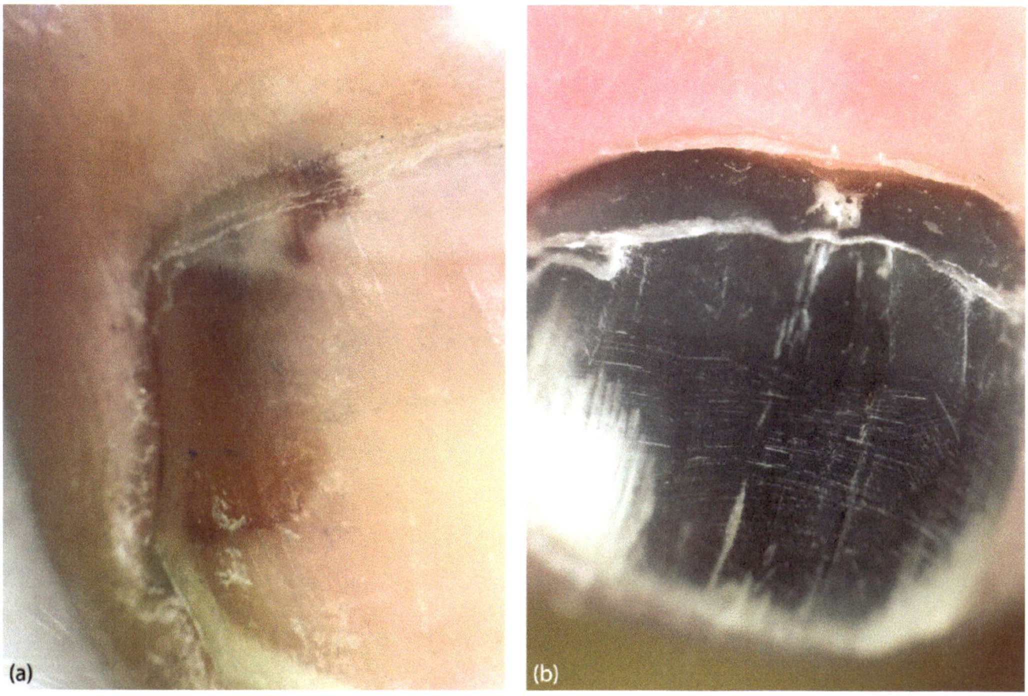

FIGURE 27.1 ×20 Heterogeneous discoloration, ranging from pink to red color, in a recent lesion (a); ×20 homogeneous dark-purple discoloration of the whole nail plate, obscuring the lunula (b).

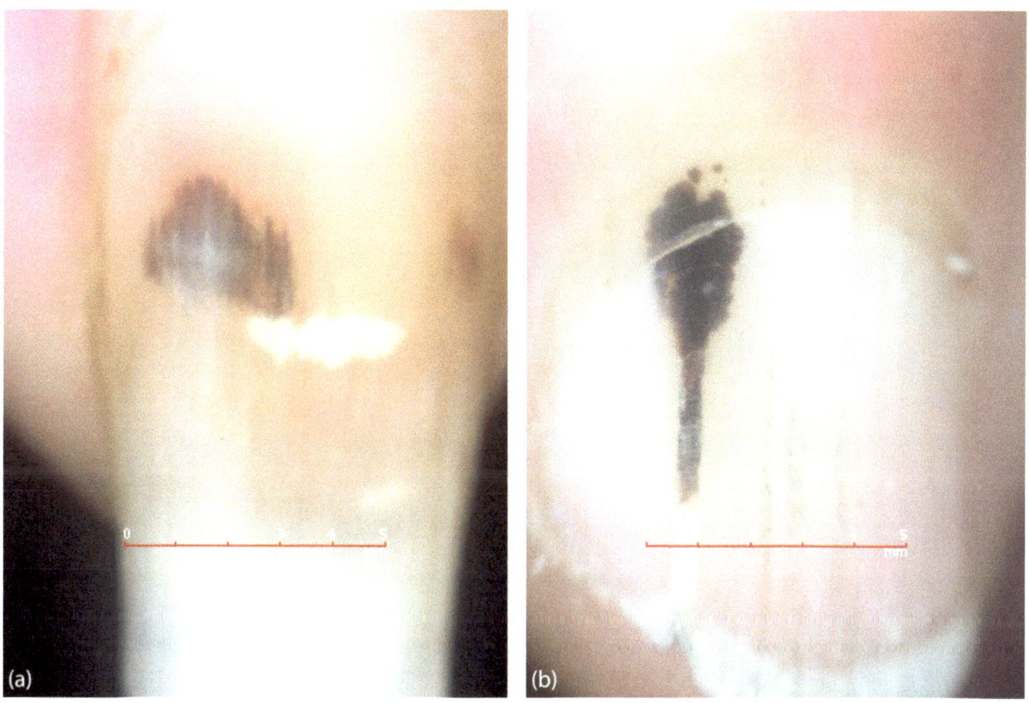

FIGURE 27.2 ×20 Small hematoma with filamentous distal ends associated with leukonychia (a); ×20 small hematoma with satellite globules extending into the proximal nail fold (b).

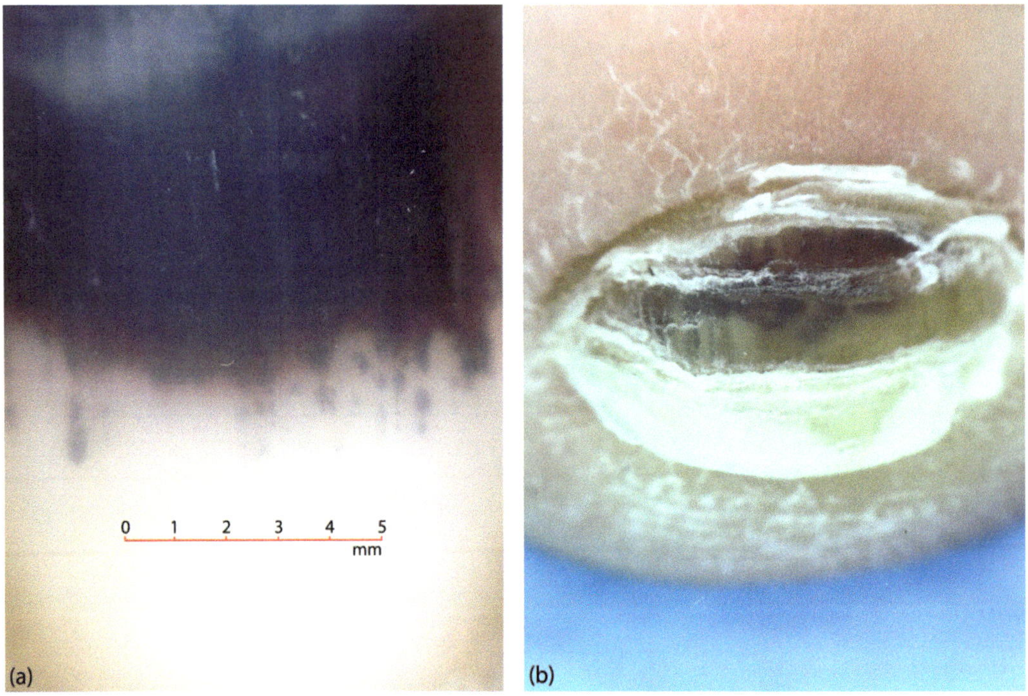

FIGURE 27.3 ×20 Dark purple discoloration with peripheral fading, globules, and streaks in its distal portion. Note the whitish opaque reflection on the nail plate surface (a); ×20 dark purple discoloration with globules associated with onychomadesis (b).

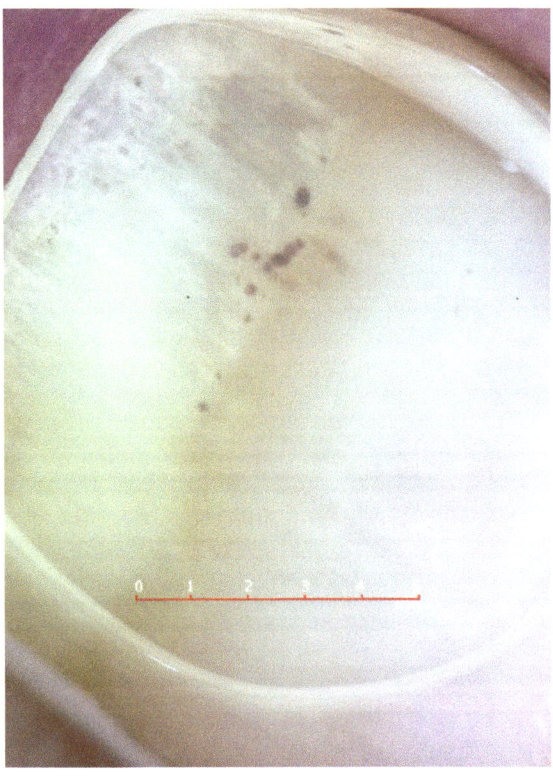

FIGURE 27.4 ×20 Traumatic onycholysis of the toenails. Note sharp proximal borders and round hemorrhagic spots within and around the onycholytic area.

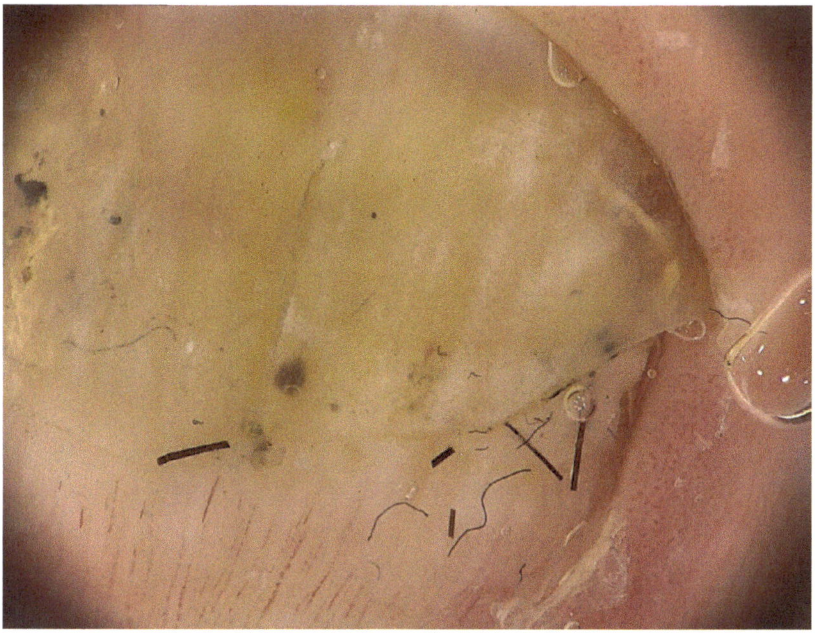

FIGURE 27.5 ×40 Traumatic onycholysis of the fingernails in a hairdresser, dermoscopy shows hair fragments within the onycholytic space.

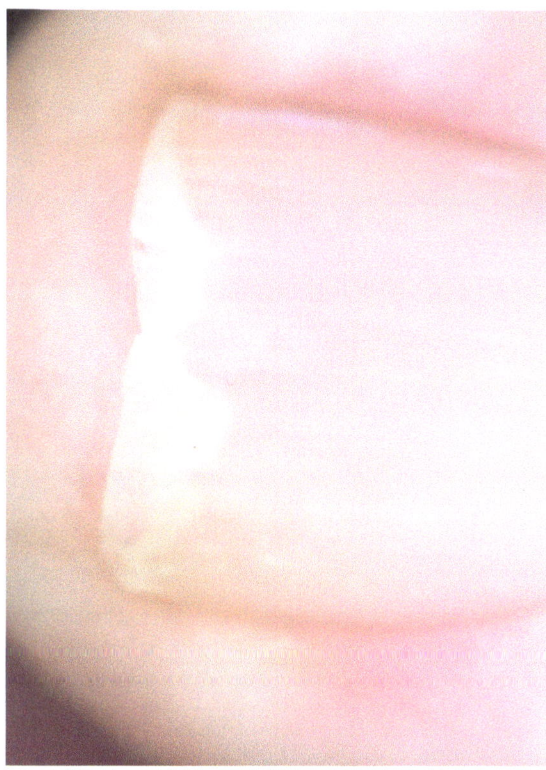

FIGURE 27.6 ×20 Roller-coaster onycholysis. Note that the proximal border is irregular and has multiple convexities.

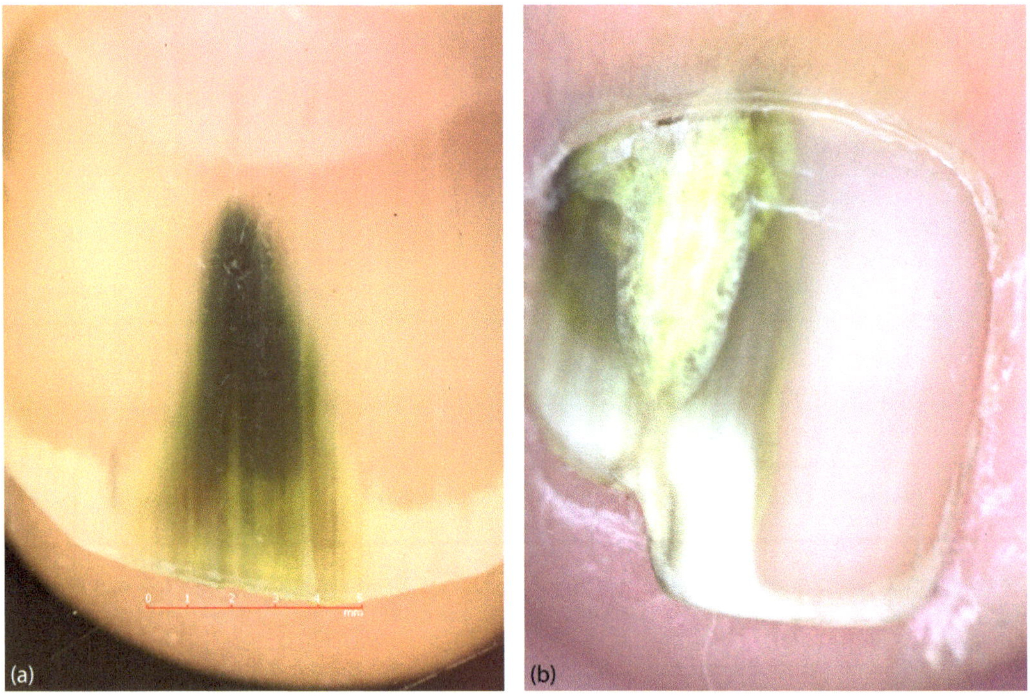

FIGURE 27.7 Pseudomonas colonization. ×20 Green discoloration of distal onycholysis (a); and ×20 proximal onycholysis (b).

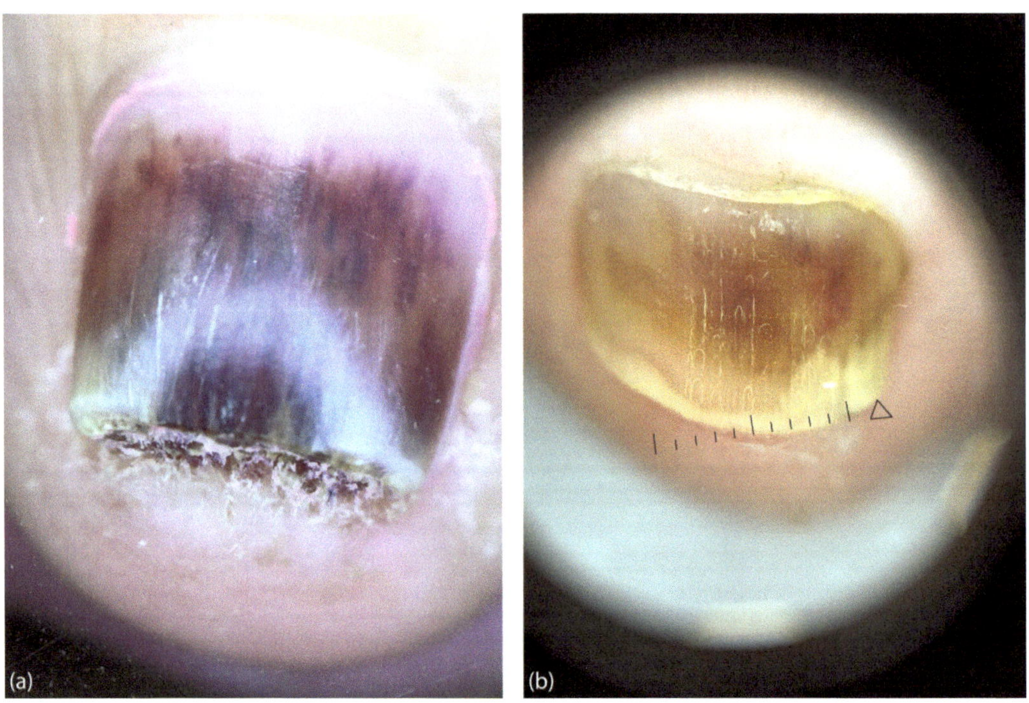

FIGURE 27.8 ×20 Hemorrhagic onycholysis due to anticoagulants (a); ×10 chemotherapy (b).

FIGURE 27.9 Glomus tumor. ×20 Presence of a purple patch under the nail plate close to the onycholysis should raise the suspicion of a subungual tumor.

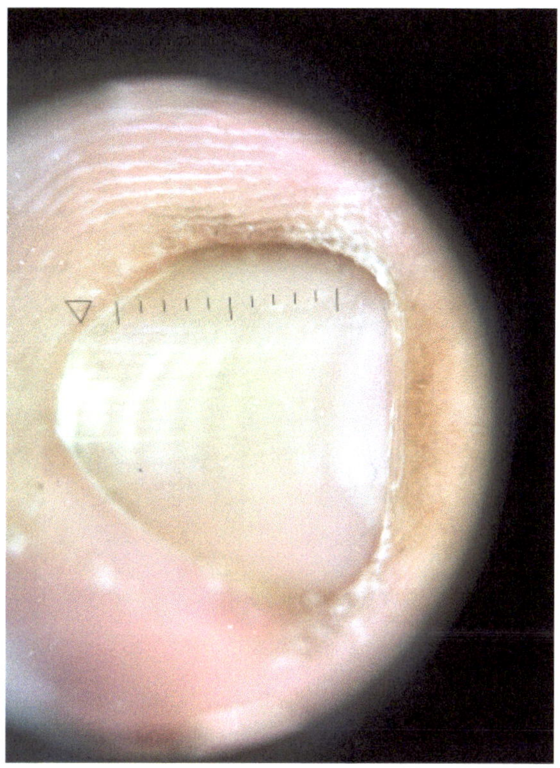

FIGURE 27.10 ×10 Transverse leukonychia.

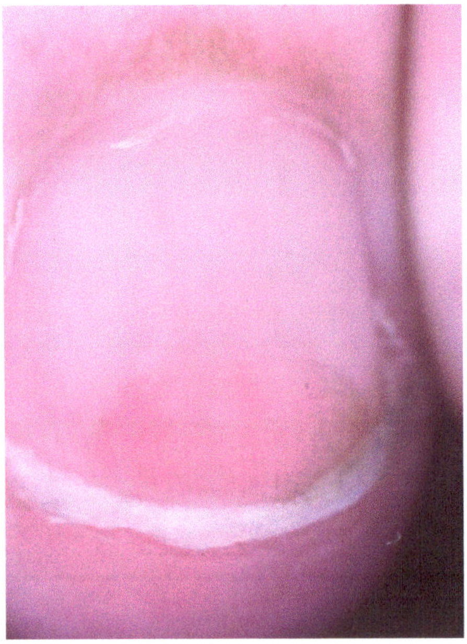

FIGURE 27.11 ×20 Thinning of the distal plate with a pale red background due to visualization of the nail bed capillaries.

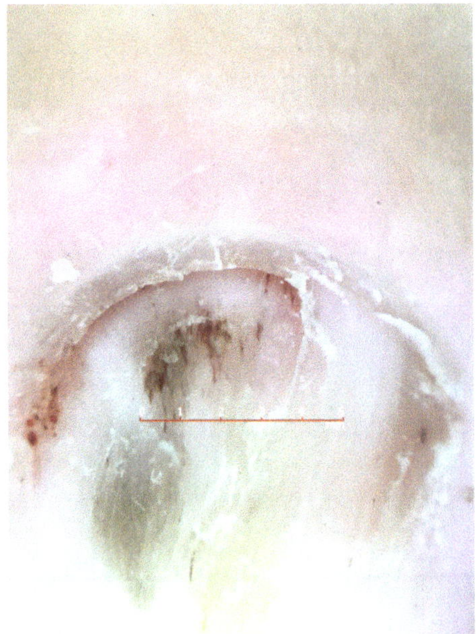

FIGURE 27.12 Onychotillomania. ×20 Periungual hemorrhages, partial destruction of the nail plate, wavy lines, oblique nail bed hemorrhages, and nail bed pigmentation.

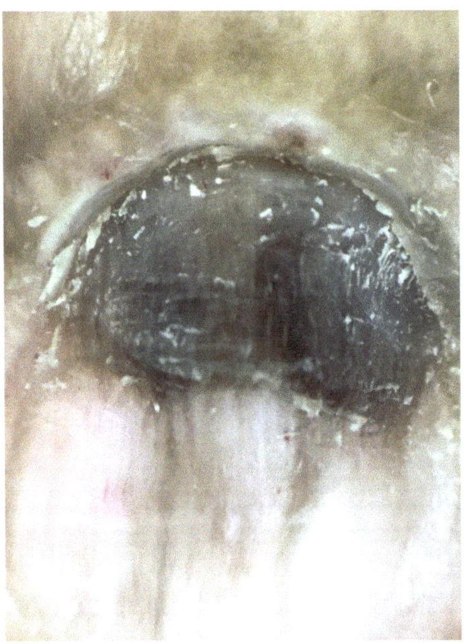

FIGURE 27.13 ×20 Hypopigmented areas with crusting and hemorrhages of the proximal nail fold. Melanonychia of the proximal nail plate. The distal nail plate is absent, and the nail bed shows pigmented wavy lines with a gray hue.

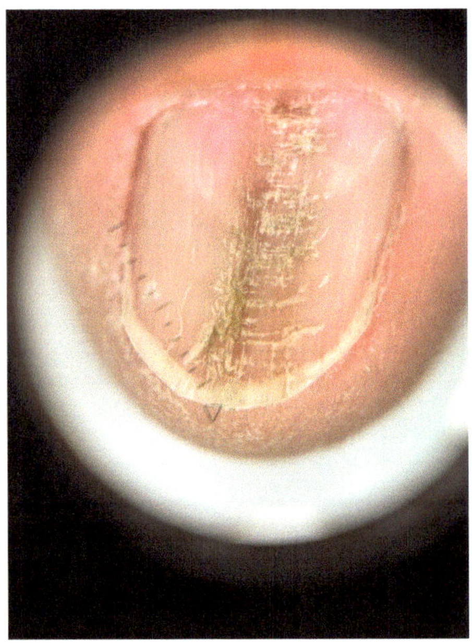

FIGURE 27.14 ×10 Longitudinal groove with multiple transverse parallel white indentations in habit tic deformity. Also note macro-lunula.

SUGGESTED READING

Chen Y, Pradhan S, Lyu L, Xue S. Clinical and dermoscopic characteristics of onychophagia and onychotillomania: a retrospective study of 63 cases. *Clin Exp Dermatol.* 2022;47(5):961–63.

Lencastre A, Lamas A, Sá D, Tosti A. Onychoscopy. *Clin Dermatol.* 2013;31(5):587–93.

Maddy AJ, Tosti A. Dermoscopic features of onychotillomania: a study of 36 cases. *J Am Acad Dermatol.* 201879(4):702–5.

Metin MS, Elmas ÖF. Dermoscopic diagnosis of subungual hematoma: new observations. *Postepy Dermatol Alergol.* 2020;37(4):490–4.

Mun JH, Kim GW, Jwa SW, Song M, Kim HS, Ko HC, Kim BS, Kim MB. Dermoscopy of subungual haemorrhage: its usefulness in differential diagnosis from nail-unit melanoma. *Br J Dermatol.* 2013;168(6):1224–9.

Navarro L. Pattern diagnosis of onycholysis. *JEADV Clin Pract.* 2023;2:213–24.

Piraccini BM, Balestri R, Starace M, Rech G. Nail digital dermoscopy (onychoscopy) in the diagnosis of onychomycosis. *J Eur Acad Dermatol Venereol.* 2013;27(4):509–13.

Wu TP, Morrison BW, Tosti A. Worn down nails after acrylic nail removal. *Dermatol Online J.* 2015;21(1):13030.

28 Brittle Nails

BRITTLE NAILS (FIGURES 28.1–28.4)

- Affects up to 20% of the population during their lifetime, with women being at higher risk.
- Fingernails are more involved than toenails.

There are three clinical presentations, which often combine together:

- Onychorrhexis: Due to longitudinal ridging and fissuring
- Pseudo leukonychia: Due to keratin degranulation
- Onychoschizia lamellina: Due to superficial exfoliation

Dermoscopy

- Onychorrhexis: Presence of parallel longitudinal furrows, filled with scales. Proximal nail plate is less affected. Longitudinal splitting of the distal nail plate can also be present.
- Keratin degranulation: The superficial nail plate shows multiple, longitudinally aligned and interconnected ovaloid depressions resembling the rings of a chain. Each ring is bordered by a collarette of scales that are more prominent in its proximal part.
- Onychoschizia lamellina: The nail plate shows single or multiple horizontal layers of superficial scaling starting from its distal edge.
- Scales are easily stained by exogenous pigments in all variants of brittle nails.

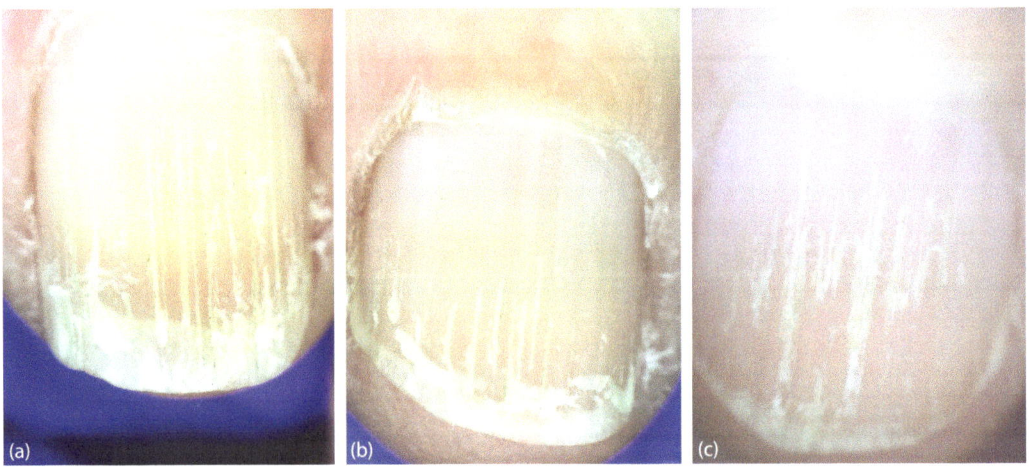

FIGURE 28.1 Onychorrhexis. ×20 Longitudinal ridges filled with white scales, and lamellar splitting of the distal nail (a); the proximal nail plate is not affected (b). Also note ovaloid areas surrounded by white scales due to keratin degranulation (c).

DOI: 10.1201/9780429351433-28

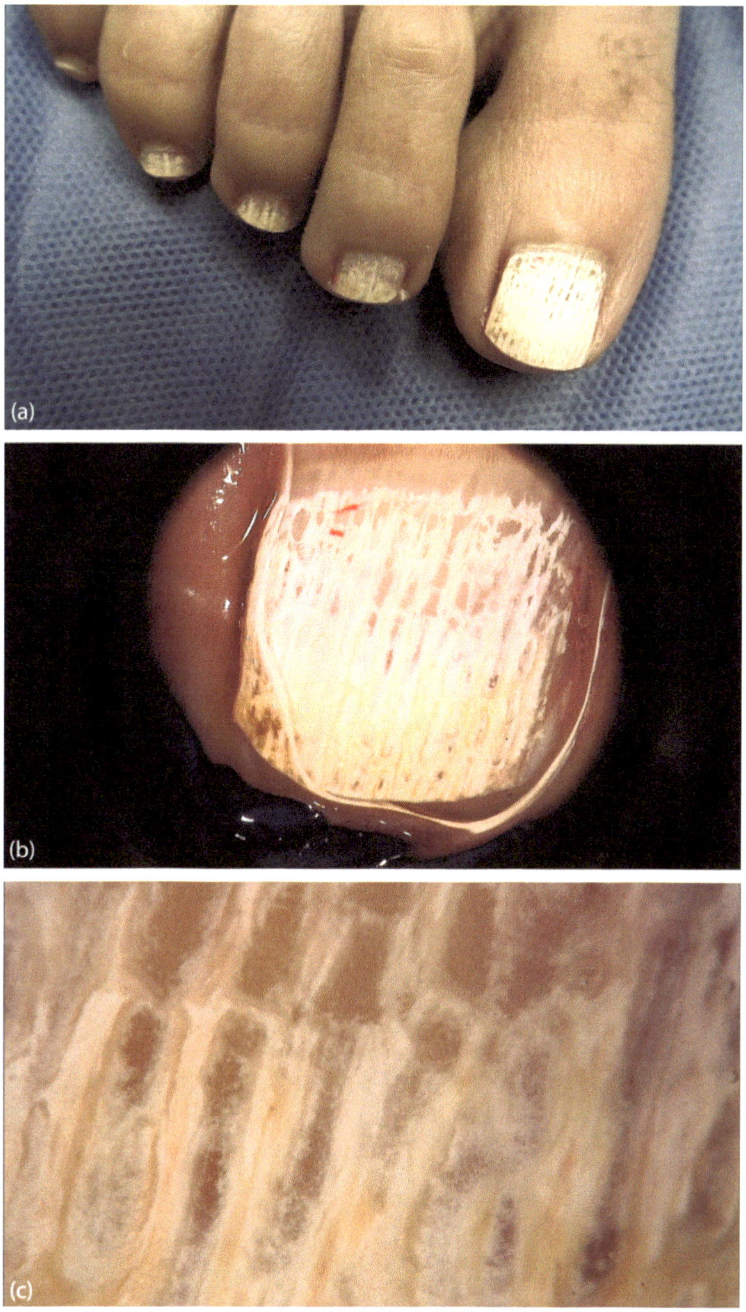

FIGURE 28.2 Pseudo leukonychia from keratin degranulation (a); ×20 multiple longitudinally oriented depressed ovaloid rings surrounded and partially filled by white scales (b); ×50 pattern is better seen at high magnification (c).

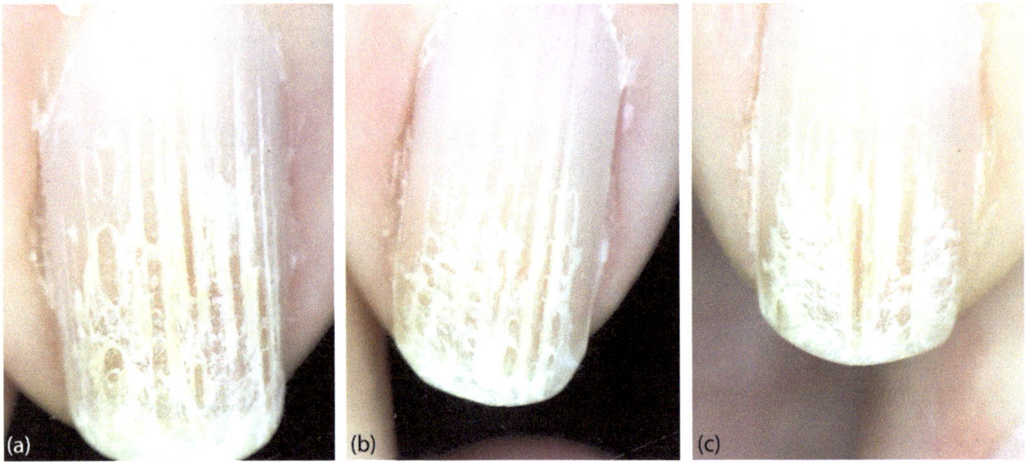

FIGURE 28.3 Keratin degranulation. ×20 Size and depth of the ovaloid depressions varies in different areas of the plate (a,b); ×20 also note transverse parallel raised white scales caused by friction (c).

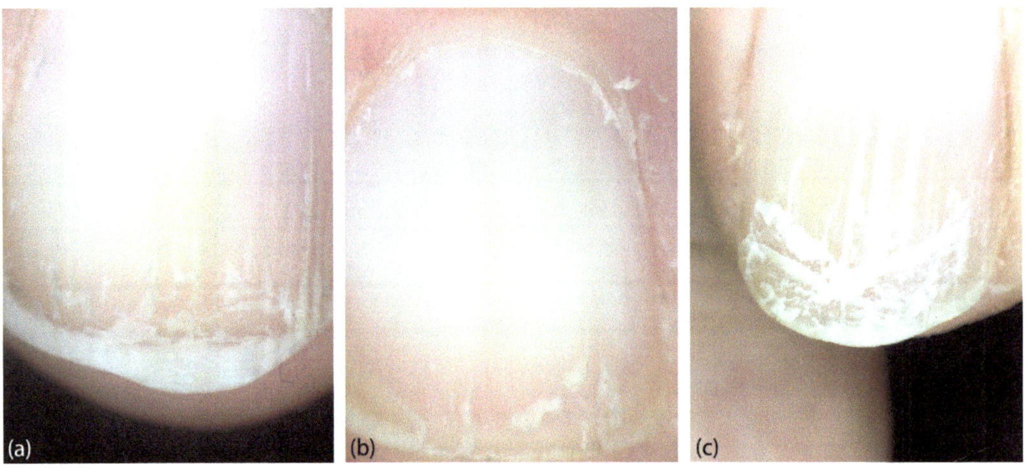

FIGURE 28.4 Onychoschizia lamellina (a,b); ×20 lamellar exfoliation of the superficial nail plate at its distal margin might be associated with onychorrhexis (c).

SUGGESTED READING

Chessa MA, Iorizzo M, Richert B, et al. Pathogenesis, clinical signs and treatment recommendations in brittle nails: a review. *Dermatol Ther.* 2020;10(1):15–27.

Herskovitz I, Nolan BV, Tosti A. Orange chromonychia due to dihydroxyacetone. *Dermatitis.* 2014;25(1):43–4.

29 Onychomycosis

Onychomycoses are fungal nail infections, with *Trichophyton rubrum* being the predominant pathogen, followed by *Trichophyton mentagrophytes* var. *interdigitalis*. The clinical presentation of onychomycosis includes four main patterns, based on the site of fungal invasion.

DISTAL SUBUNGUAL ONYCHOMYCOSIS (DSO) (FIGURES 29.1–29.7)

Dermoscopy

- Onycholysis from onychomycosis differs from traumatic onycholysis because the proximal margin is not sharp but has a jagged appearance, due to the presence of multiple spikes.
- The spikes are sharp, yellow-white thin structures projecting from the onycholytic area into the proximal nail plate.
- White/yellow longitudinal streaks correspond to onycholytic areas filled with fungi. They are parallelly arranged and may involve the entire nail length. Their color may range from white, to yellow, greenish, brown/black.
- The "Aurora Borealis pattern" describes bands of different colors and a veil across the nail plate.
- Dermatophytoma consists of a white or yellow round opaque area in the nail plate, and is often associated with longitudinal streaks or spikes. It corresponds to hyperkeratotic aggregation of fungal filaments and spores.
- Subungual hyperkeratosis: Is friable and presents gaps of different sizes due to the detachment of infected keratin (ruined appearance). The overall picture resembles a cave with stalactites.
- Melanonychia: May present as gray lines due to melanocytic activation or as homogeneous brown/black band of pigmentation due to presence of melanin produced by certain species of fungi. In this case it can involve the whole nail and is often associated with yellowish patches/striae/spikes. Fungal melanonychia is more frequently caused by molds.
- Splinter hemorrhages.
- Fingernail onychomycosis can resemble nail psoriasis both dermoscopically and clinically. The nail plate often shows complete onycholysis with nail plate disruption.

PROXIMAL SUBUNGUAL ONYCHOMYCOSIS (PSO) (FIGURE 29.8)

- Uncommon, often associated with an immunocompromised state, but can rarely occur in the immunocompetent.
- Fungi penetrate the nail matrix via the proximal nail fold and colonize the deep portion of proximal nail plate.

Dermoscopy

- Proximal leukonychia: The proximal nail plate shows a white opaque band emerging from the nail fold. Multiple transverse white bands separated by normal nail can be seen.

WHITE SUPERFICIAL ONYCHOMYCOSIS (WSO) (FIGURES 29.9, 29.10)

- This variant is typically limited to the toenails.
- A deep variant can be observed in children, and in *Candida* sp. and mold infections.

DOI: 10.1201/9780429351433-29

Dermoscopy

- Pseudo leukonychia: The nail surface presents white yellow spots of irregular borders, where the nail plate has lost its shiny texture.
- The yellow white areas of nail plate disruption are associated with fine superficial scales.
- In deep white superficial onychomycosis, dermoscopy shows involvement of deep layers with white patches of nail fragmentation at different levels.

Differential diagnosis includes keratin degranulation due to nail polish, which most commonly affects multiple nails, including fingernails.

ENDONYX

- The primary characteristic is the involvement of the nail plate without affecting the nail bed or matrix.
- The nail plate shows an opaque white discoloration.
- There is an absence of subungual hyperkeratosis and onycholysis

Dermoscopy

- The nail plate shows white cloudy areas with irregular branching at the borders, known as dendritic pattern.
- Diagnosis can be confirmed by dermoscopy of the distal margin showing invasion of the entire nail plate thickness.

CANDIDA ONYCHOMYCOSIS (FIGURE 29.11)

This can be detected in:

- Immunosuppressed patients, including patients with mucocutaneous candidiasis, where it is associated with paronychia and causes total dystrophic onychomycosis.
- Children, where it can cause either white superficial onychomycosis or proximal subungual onychomycosis.

Clinical Presentations

- Total dystrophic onychomycosis may closely resemble trachyonychia in the initial phase of the infection, and then progress to nail crumbling and partial or complete nail plate destruction.

Dermoscopy

- In the trachyonychia-like variety the nail plate shows diffuse superficial scaling with multiple keratin debris oriented longitudinally. The proximal nail is usually more severely affected.
- In severe cases: There is a loss of nail plate and whitish scaling of the nail bed.

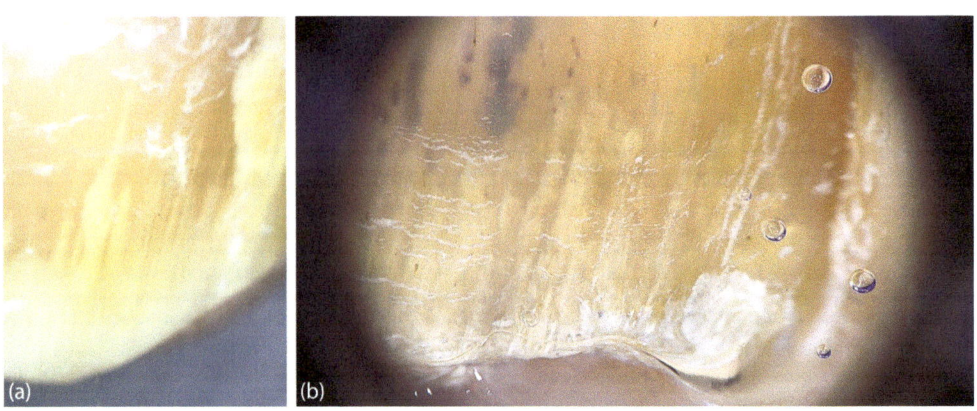

FIGURE 29.1 DSO. ×20 The onycholytic area has a jagged proximal edge with multiple spikes (a); note also splinter hemorrhages (b).

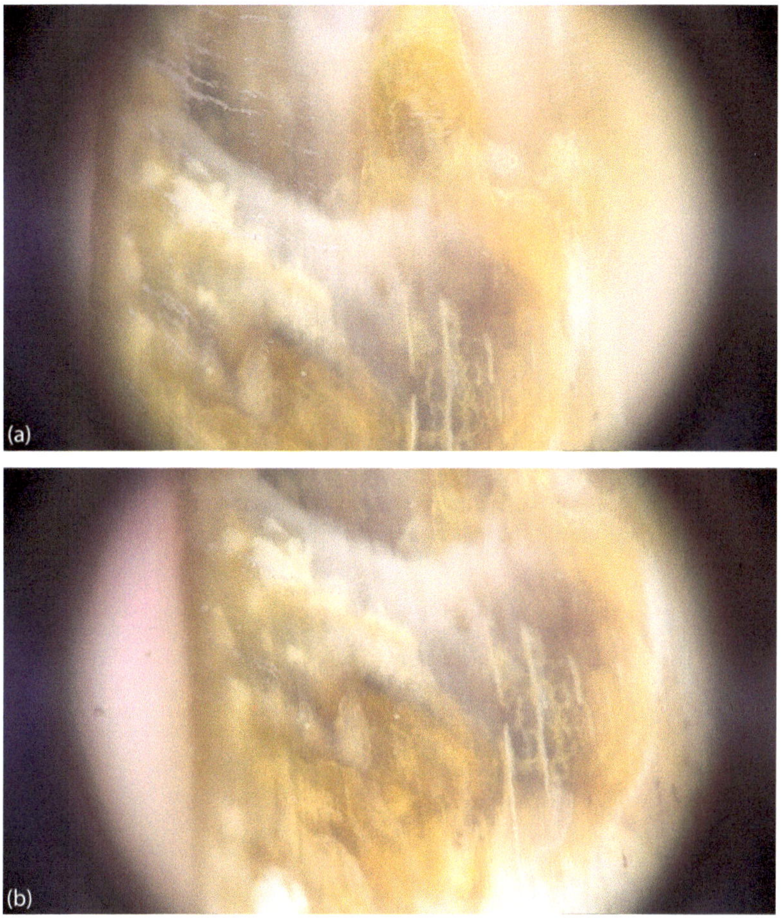

FIGURE 29.2 DSO. ×20 Aurora Borealis pattern (a,b).

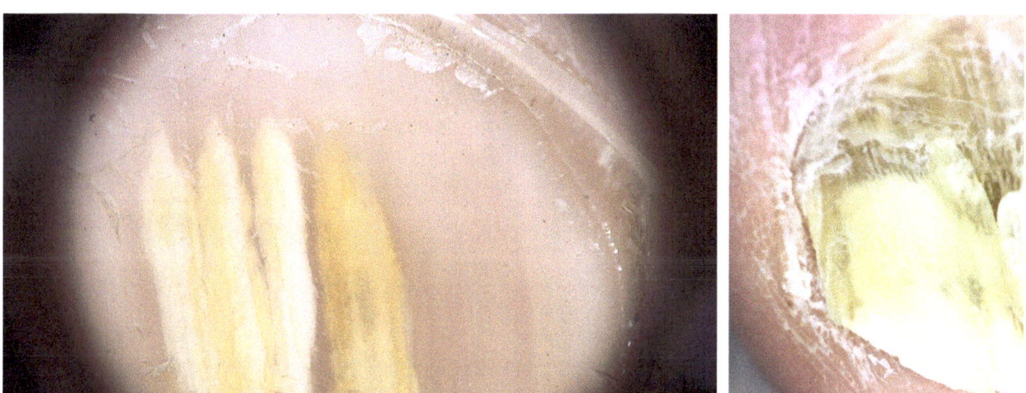

FIGURE 29.3 DSO. ×20 Yellow streaks. These differ from dermathophytoma because the yellow patch is connected with the nail plate distal margin (a,b).

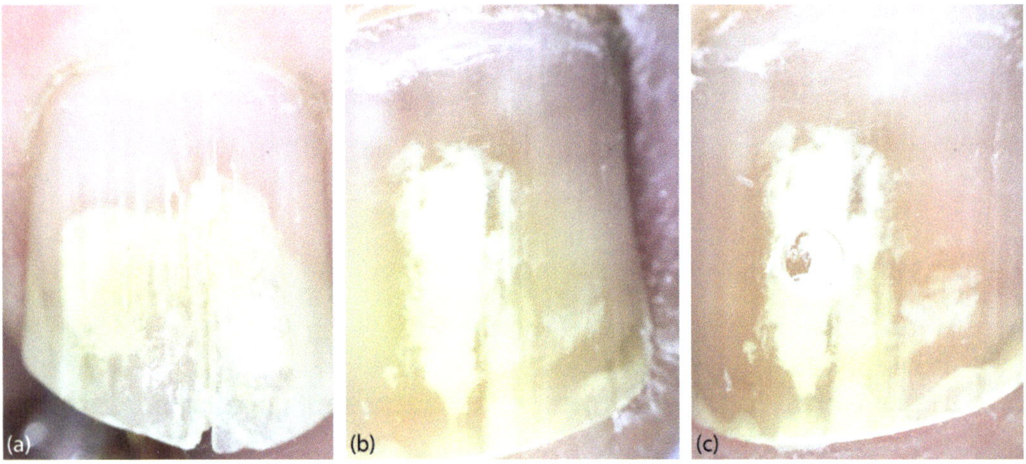

FIGURE 29.4 DSO. ×20 Dermatophytoma: the patch is not connected to the nail plate free margin (a,b); a punch of the nail plate is necessary to confirm diagnosis (c).

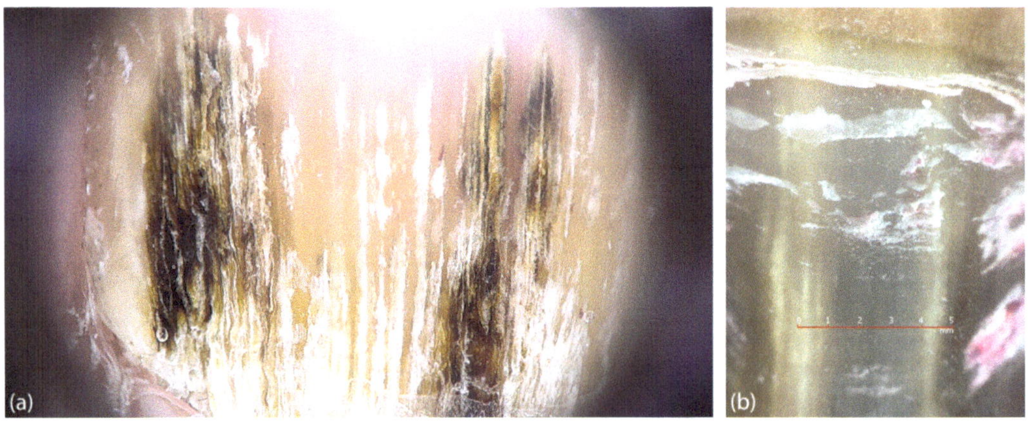

FIGURE 29.5 Pigmented DSO. ×40, ×20 Spikes of yellow discoloration help in making the diagnosis (a,b).

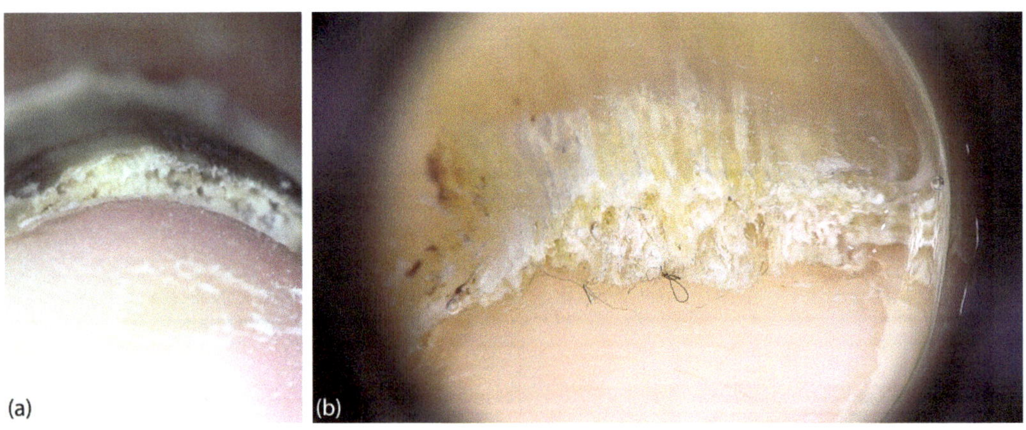

FIGURE 29.6 DSO. ×20 Ruined appearance of the subungual hyperkeratosis (a,b).

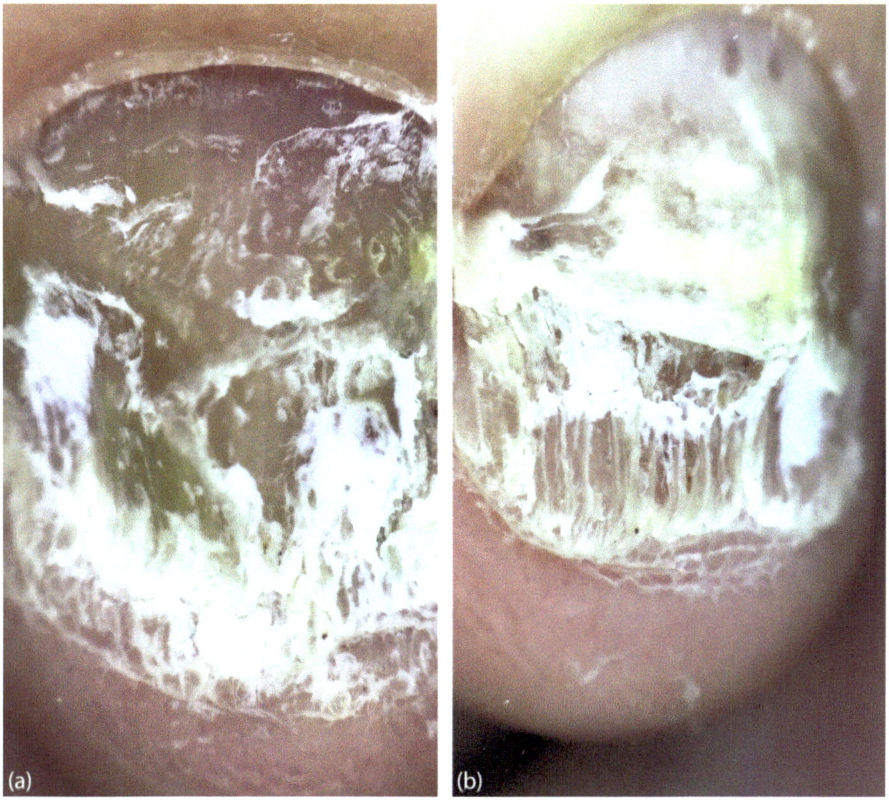

FIGURE 29.7 DSO of the fingernails ×20 (a); the nail plate can be partially or totally disrupted but yellow patches and onycholysis with proximal spikes suggest diagnosis (b).

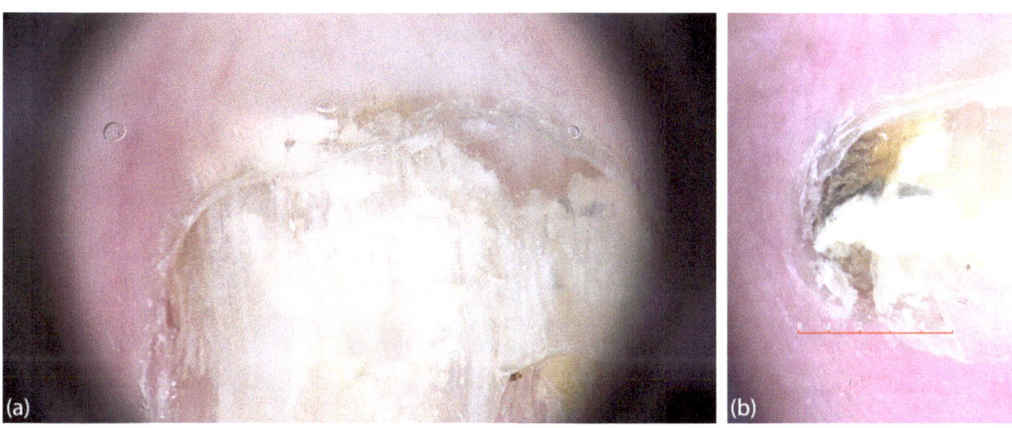

FIGURE 29.8 PSO. ×20 The white patch can be visible through the nail fold (a); ×20 note also frictional melanonychia (b).

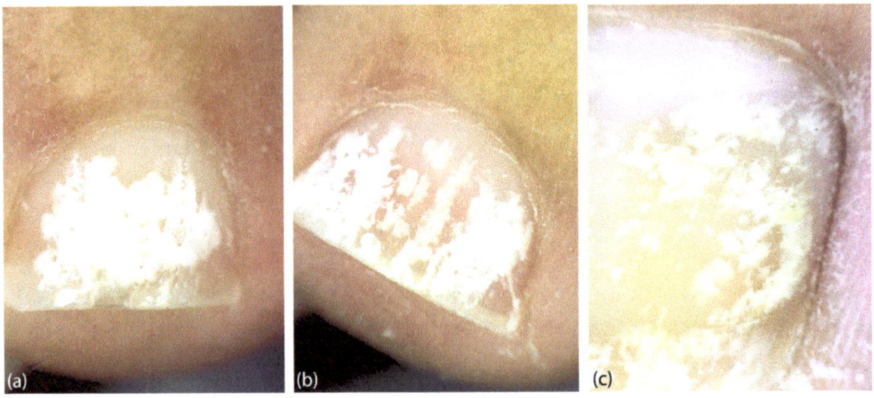

FIGURE 29.9 WSO. ×20 White opaque irregular patches with superficial scaling (a,b); sometimes patches have a yellowish hue (c).

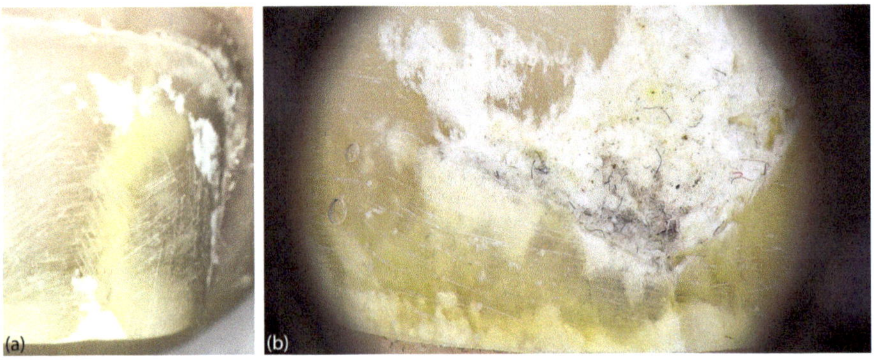

FIGURE 29.10 WSO and DSO. ×20 (a) and ×40 (b). Note superficial scratches as the patient tried to file the nail to get rid of the infection.

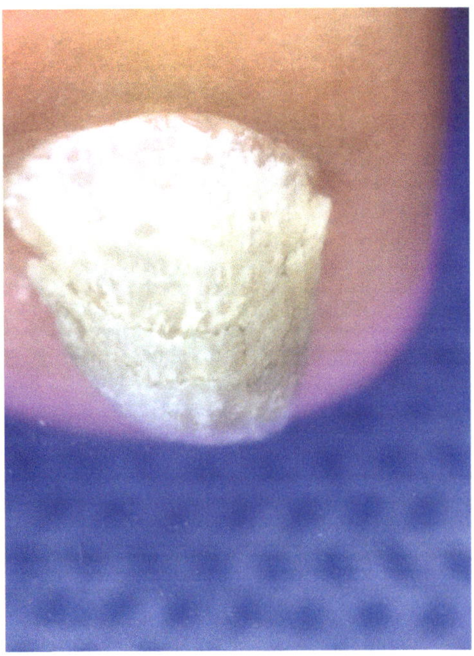

FIGURE 29.11 *Candida* onychomycosis. ×20 White discoloration and fragmentation of the entire nail plate.

SUGGESTED READING

De Crignis G, Valgas N, Rezende P, Leverone A, Nakamura R. Dermatoscopy of onychomycosis. *Int J Dermatol.* 2014;53(2):e97–9.

Finch J, Arenas R, Baran R. Fungal melanonychia. *J Am Acad Dermatol.* 2012;66:830–41.

Gupta AK, Wang T, Cooper EA. Dermatophytomas: clinical overview and treatment. *J Fungi.* 2022;8(7):742.

Jakhar D, Grover C, Kaur I. Dendritic pattern: unique onychoscopic feature in endonyx. *J Am Acad Dermatol.* 2019;81(4):e89–e90.

Piraccini BM, Balestri R, Starace M, Rech G. Nail digital dermoscopy (onychoscopy) in the diagnosis of onychomycosis. *J Eur Acad Dermatol Venereol.* 2013;27(4):509–13.

Starace M, Milan E, Summa G, et al. Onychoscopic characteristics of Trichophyton rubrum and Trichophyton interdigitalis fungal infections: a multicentric study. *Mycoses.* 2024;67(1):e13673.

Verne SH, Chen L, Shah V, Nouri K, Tosti A. Optical coherence tomography features of dermatophytoma. *JAMA Dermatol.* 2018;154(2):225–7.

30 Non-Melanocytic Nail Tumors

- Onychomatricoma
- Onychopapilloma
- Glomus tumor
- Myxoid cyst
- Acquired ungual fibromas/fibrokeratomas
- Viral warts
- Pyogenic granuloma
- Exostosis
- Bowen's disease/Squamous cell carcinoma

ONYCHOMATRICOMA (FIGURES 30.1, 30.2)

Onychomatricoma is a benign fibroepithelial nail matrix tumor that can be diagnosed by dermoscopy.

Dermoscopy

- Longitudinal white/yellow/brown lines aligned along the long axis of the nail plate, corresponding to the channels containing the tumor projections.
- Splinter hemorrhages: Are visualized as linear, interrupted red or brown lines under the nail plate. They are found both in the proximal and distal plate.
- Elongated coiled capillaries of the nail plate: They often form longitudinal loops in the proximal nail.
- Honeycomb (or woodworm)-like cavities at the distal edge: Correspond to the tumor's tunnels.
- Onychomycosis can be associated as fungi can easily penetrate the nail plate channels.

The dermoscopic and clinical features of onychomatricoma are not distinctly different from those of onychocytic matricoma and onychocytic carcinoma, their malignant counterparts. This similarity presents a diagnostic challenge, despite the rarity of the latter two conditions.

ONYCHOPAPILLOMA (FIGURES 30.3, 30.4)

- Onychopapilloma is a benign neoplasm of the distal matrix and the nail bed. It predominantly affects fingernails.
- Multiple onychopapillomas have been associated with BAP1 Tumor Predisposition Syndrome.

Dermoscopy

- Longitudinal erythronychia/leukonychia/melanonychia: The longitudinal band has often a sharp convex proximal border, usually starting from the lunula.
- Splinter hemorrhages are often multiple and visible in the middle and distal nail.
- Subungual keratotic mass has a compact shape and a whitish/brown color, and may contain hemorrhagic vessels. The overlying nail plate is thinned.

A malignant counterpart of onychopapilloma, known as malignant onychopapilloma, has recently been described. The clinical and dermoscopic presentations of malignant onychopapilloma may resemble those of typical onychopapilloma; however, the development of pain in the context of an otherwise typical onychopapilloma may indicate malignancy.

GLOMUS TUMOR (FIGURES 30.5, 30.6)

- Glomus tumors are benign vascular hamartomas originating from the neuromyoarterial cells of the dermal glomus apparatus. The typical subungual localization is due to the abundance of glomus bodies in this area.

DOI: 10.1201/9780429351433-30

- The pain caused by the tumors is always more impressive than the clinical signs, which can be unremarkable.

Dermoscopy

- Irregular red-purple spot.
- Branching or linear vessels inside the erythronychia or the bluish macule suggest the diagnosis.

The final diagnosis of glomus tumor requires imaging techniques.

MYXOID CYST (FIGURES 30.7, 30.8)

- Digital myxoid cysts are common, benign, cystic lesions located on the fingers or toes, containing a clear, gelatinous fluid that originates from the joint and periodically drains spontaneously.
- There are three possible localizations: Over the distal joint (type A), on the proximal nail fold (type B), under the matrix (type C).
- Type A and type B appear as solitary, translucent or skin-colored, dome-shaped papules/nodules, whereas type C is not detectable on visual inspection.
- Both types B and C may cause a longitudinal groove of the nail plate due to extrinsic compression of the nail plate.

Dermoscopy

Nail plate changes:

- Longitudinal grooves
- "Washboard" transverse lines (nail matrix compression is reduced when the cyst drains)

ACQUIRED UNGUAL FIBROMA/ FIBROKERATOMA (FIGURE 30.9)

- Acquired ungual fibrokeratoma is a rare, benign, usually painless, fibrous tissue tumor occurring in the nail unit.
- Patients affected by tuberous sclerosis develop multiple periungual fibromas known as Koenen tumors, starting in adolescence and increasing in number over time. They often recur after excision.

Dermoscopy

- Proximal part can show elongated or punctiform vessels.
- The distal part presents as:
  Keratotic tip characterized by a yellow-brown appearance.
  White, scaly collarette surrounding the central yellow area.
- Nail plate changes: Longitudinal grooving without width variability
- Patients affected by tuberous sclerosis may also present multiple subungual red comets, consisting of hairpin coiled vessels of the middle/distal nail bed.

VIRAL WARTS (FIGURE 30.10)

Warts that develop around the nail are termed periungual, while those developing under the nail are termed subungual.

Dermoscopy

Growth Pattern

- Papillomatous appearance with bleeding spots encircled by whitish keratotic borders (frogspawn)
- Short unsharp projections arising on a rough, irregular surface
- Raised pale multiple papillae with a yellowish color

Vessels

- Dusk-red clods: Typical of the frogspawn pattern
- Dotted vessels
- Hairpin vessels: Are rare

Associated Findings

- Hyperkeratosis of the nail bed: Is typical of hyponychial warts
- Hyperkeratosis of the cuticle: May be observed in warts of the proximal nail fold (PNF)

- Splinter hemorrhages: Are produced by injured nail bed capillaries due to wart's growth under the nail plate
- Onycholysis: Results from the detachment of the nail plate from the nail bed, favored by the subungual growth of the wart

PYOGENIC GRANULOMA (FIGURE 30.11)

Pyogenic granuloma is a common benign vascular tumor frequently affecting the periungual tissues and nail bed.

Dermoscopy

- Homogeneous red or white-red areas
- White collarette: Circular or arc-shaped scaly structure at lesion's borders
- White lines: White streak that resemble a double rail and intersect the lesion
- Ulceration and crusting

In cases of a solitary pyogenic granuloma, particularly when affecting the nail bed, pathology is mandatory to exclude the possibility of malignant tumors such as amelanotic melanoma and Kaposi sarcoma.

EXOSTOSIS (FIGURE 30.12)

Subungual exostosis is a relatively uncommon benign osteocartilaginous tumor. Trauma, chronic irritation, and chronic infection may be implicated in some cases, but the pathogenesis remains unknown.

Dermoscopy

- Hyperkeratosis, onycholysis, ulceration, and vascular ectasia
- White collarette: Circular scaly structure found at lesion's borders

BOWEN'S DISEASE (FIGURE 30.13)

Bowen's disease of the periungual skin and nail bed is a low-grade malignant tumor commonly HPV-related.

Clinical Presentation

1. Wart-like lesion.
2. Erythematous patch or flat plaque of the PNF.
3. Longitudinal erytronychia/melanonychia.
4. In rare cases, the keratotic component is the prominent feature, featuring a cutaneous horn.

Dermoscopy

- Glomerular or dotted vessels with white perivascular halos: Are seen when the scales are removed
- Homogeneous brown-greyish longitudinal band of melanonychia
- Islands of scale and hyperkeratotic, targetoid structures
- Loss of dermatoglyphics

SQUAMOUS CELL CARCINOMA (SCC) (FIGURE 30.14)

- Nail unit invasive SCC is a rare malignant neoplasm that originates beneath or around the nail plate. Despite its slow growth, invasion of adjacent bone is common.
- Clinical presentation is protean and is mainly determined by the tumor localization.

Dermoscopy

Tumor

- Yellowish verrucous mass.
- Unparalleled lateral edges of the nail lesion or fuzzy edges: This feature is particularly useful in distinguishing nail unit SCC from lesions such as onychomatricoma, where the edges are typically parallel.
- Vascular polymorphism: Including dotted, glomerular, and hairpin vessels; it can be a clue to invasive SCC.
- The pigmented band has a homogeneous brown/gray color.

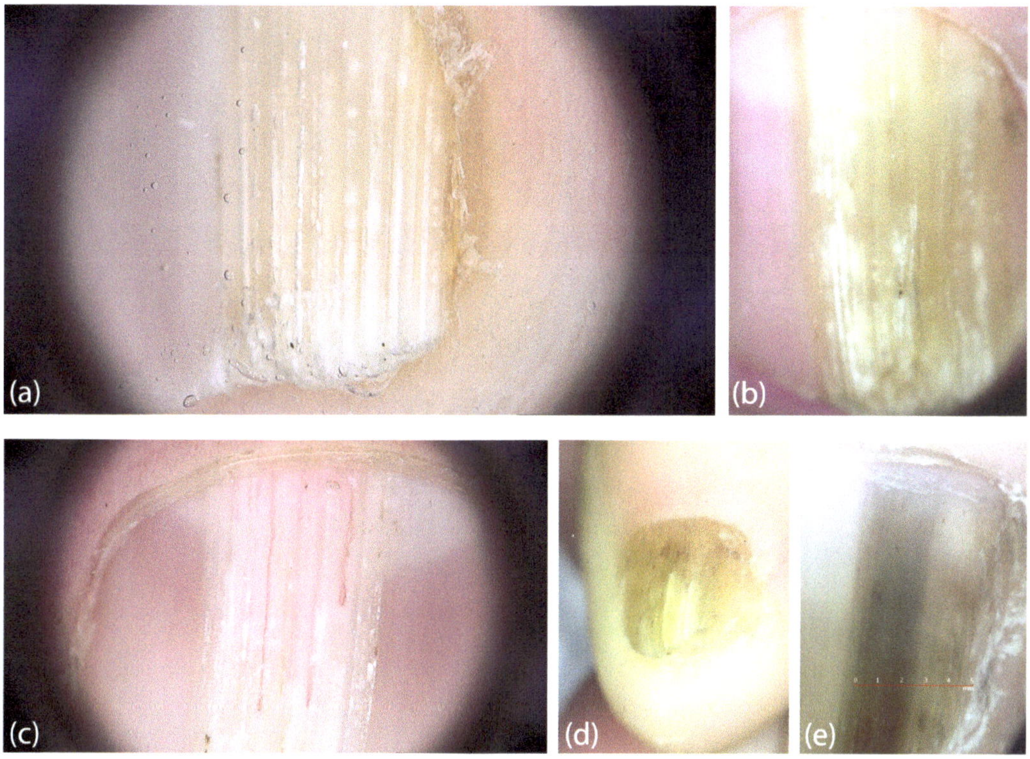

FIGURE 30.1 Onychomatricoma. ×20 Longitudinal white lines within the nail plate (a,b,c,d). Note longitudinal loops in the proximal nail (c) and splinter hemorrhages involving the whole nail length (d). ×20 Gray-brown longitudinal lines and hemorrhages in a patient of color (e).

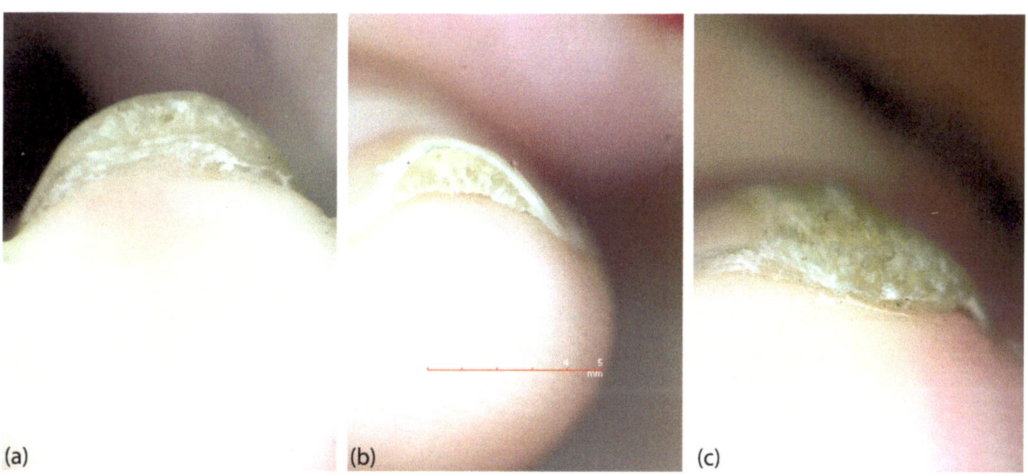

FIGURE 30.2 Onychomatricoma. ×20 Frontal view shows multiple holes with a woodworm-like appearance.

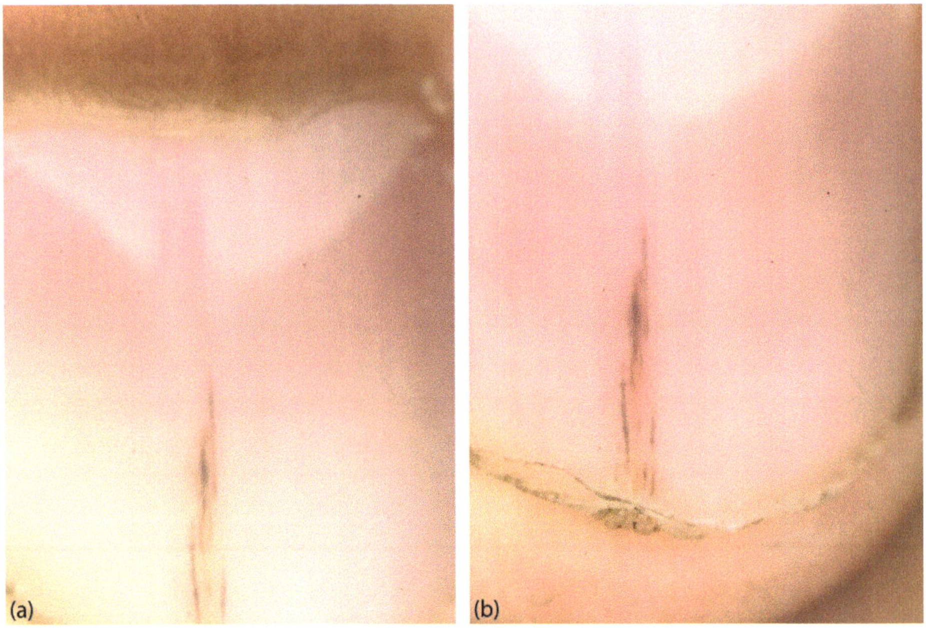

FIGURE 30.3 Onychopapilloma. ×20 Homogeneous, pale red, longitudinal band with multiple splinter hemorrhages (a); ×20 these are prominent in the distal nail, note also the subungual keratotic mass (b).

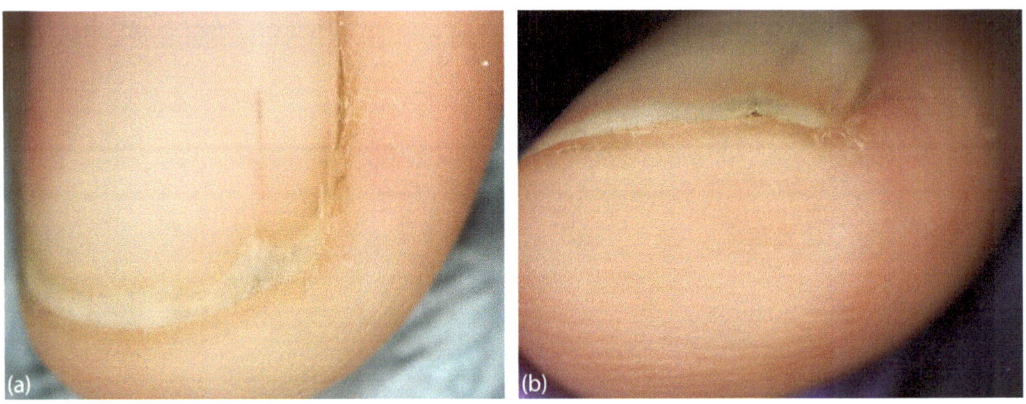

FIGURE 30.4 Onychopapilloma. ×20 Longitudinal leukonychia with splinter hemorrhages and distal onycholysis in correspondence of the keratotic mass (a); ×20 frontal view showing the subungual keratotic mass (b).

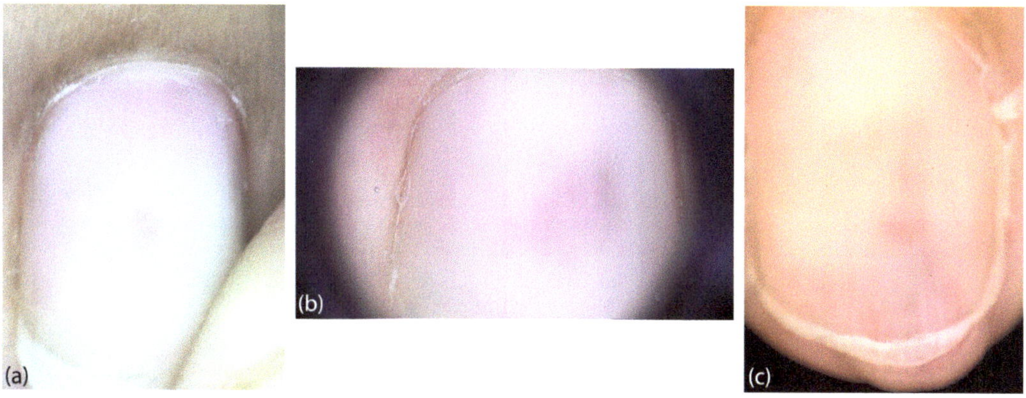

FIGURE 30.5 Glomus tumor. Compression makes the lesion more evident (a). ×20 Red patch in the middle of the nail plate (b); or ×20 in the distal nail plate in case of this subungual nodular lesion (c).

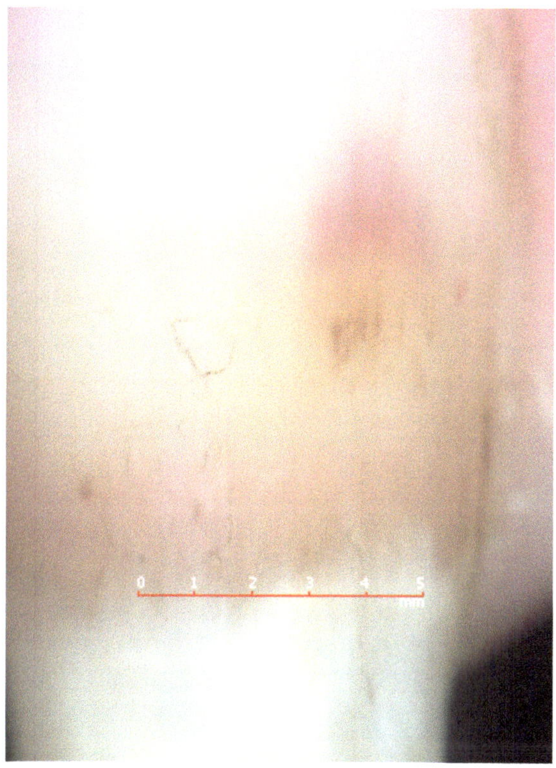

FIGURE 30.6 Glomus tumor. ×20 Presence of linear vessels inside the patch suggests the diagnosis.

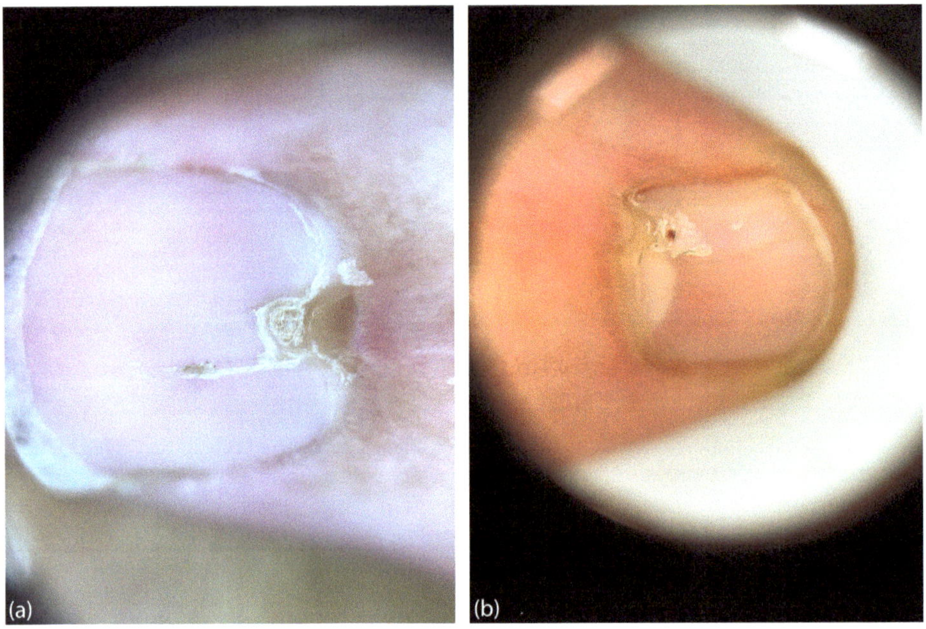

FIGURE 30.7 Myxoid cyst. ×20 (a); ×10 (b) Keratotic plug on the proximal nail fold in correspondence with the cyst opening.

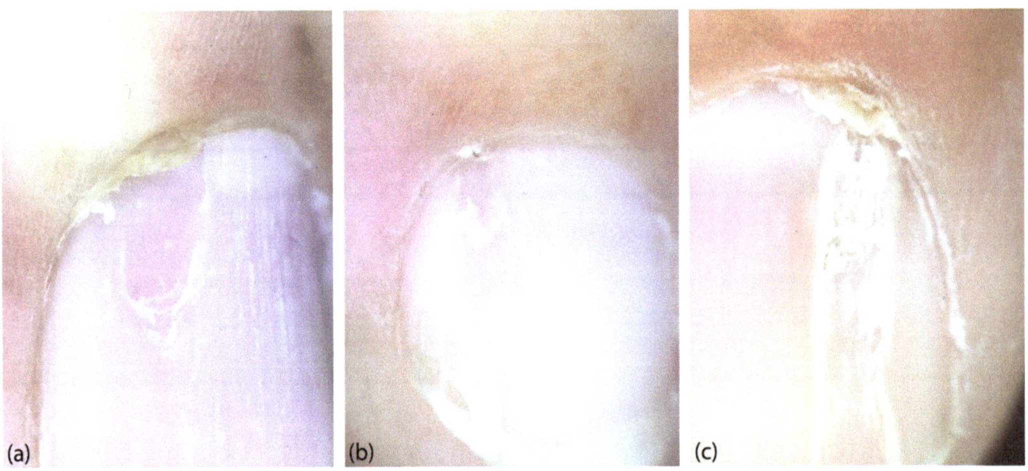

FIGURE 30.8 Myxoid cyst. ×20 Keratotic plug on the proximal nail fold in correspondence with the cyst opening and longitudinal nail plate groove (a); ×20 with washboard transverse lines (b,c).

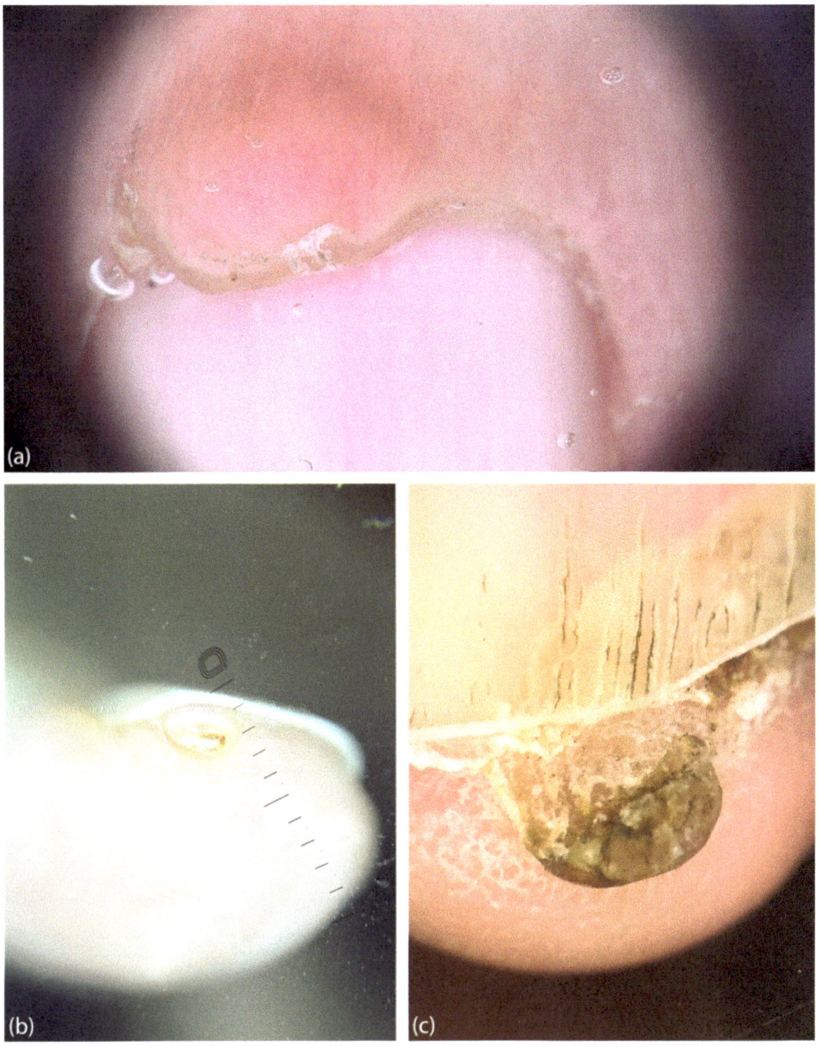

FIGURE 30.9 Ungual fibroma. ×20 Elongated punctiform vessels (a); keratotic tip (b,c). (b) Courtesy of Dr. Paolo Bortoluzzi.

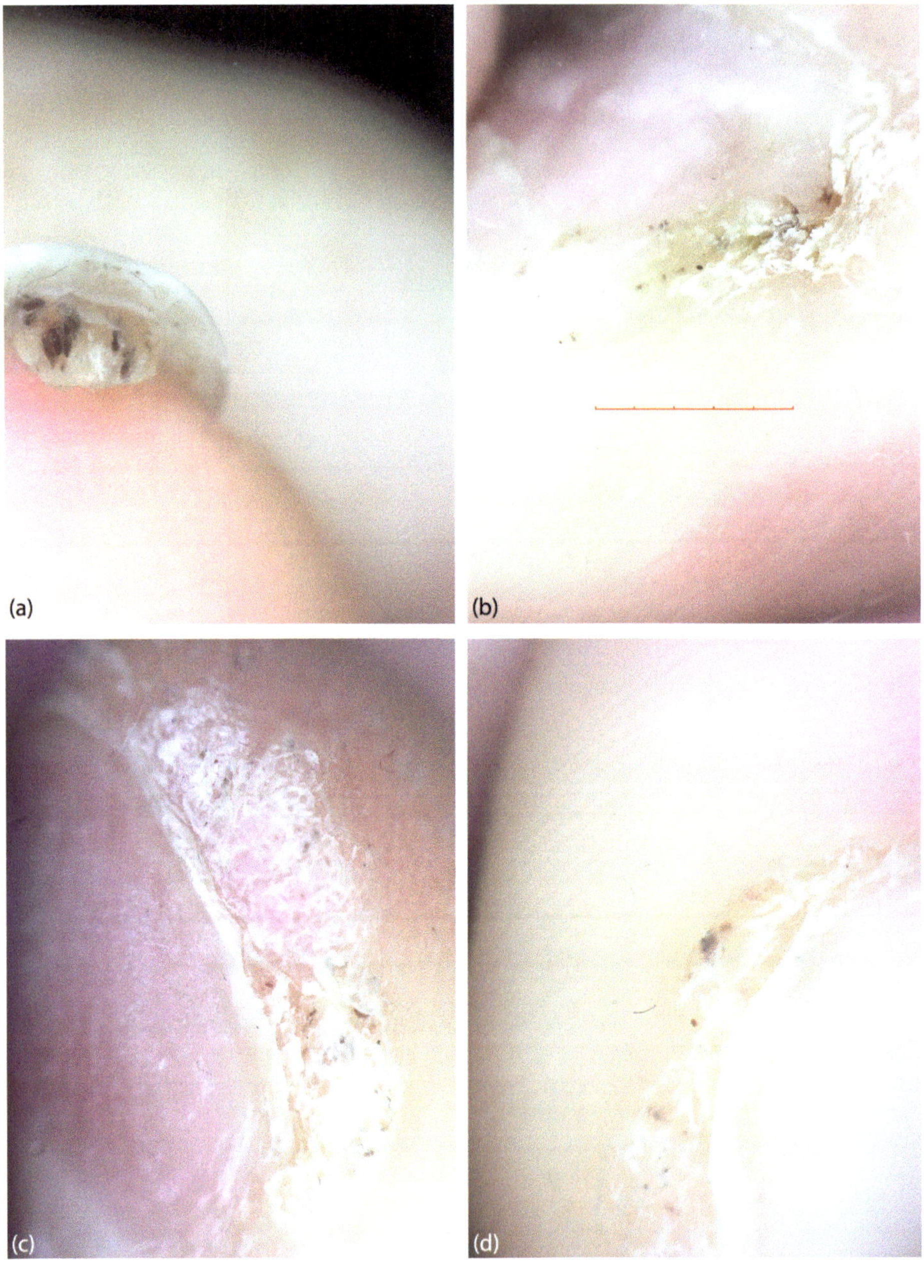

FIGURE 30.10 Warts. ×20 Subungual papillomatous lesion with dusk red clots (a). Hyperkeratotic lesions containing numerous black dotted vessels (b,c). In large longstanding lesions, a biopsy should be done to exclude squamous cell carcinoma even if dermoscopy shows the typical dotted vessels. Hyperkeratotic cuticle with dotted vessels (d).

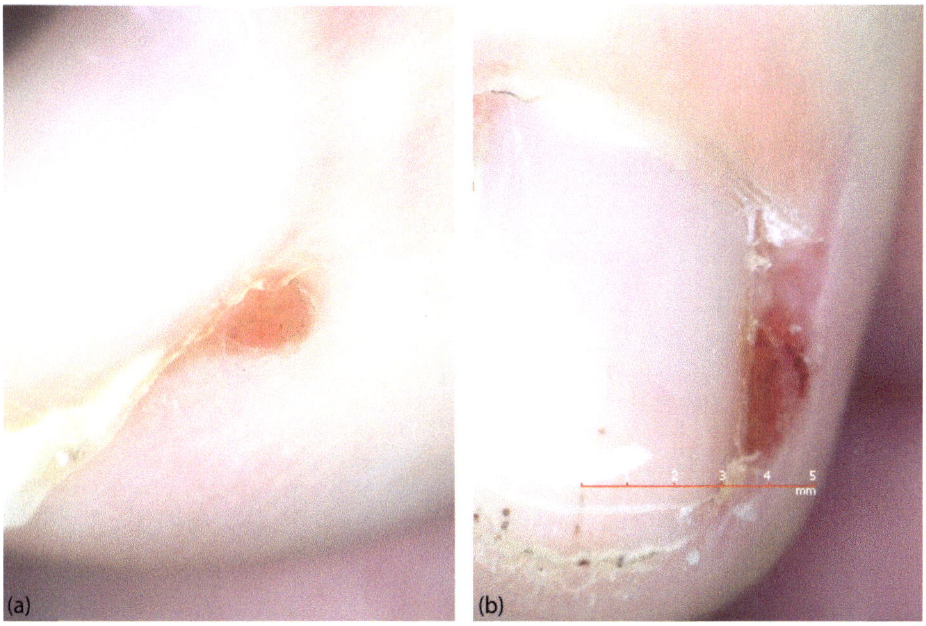

FIGURE 30.11 (a,b) Pyogenic granuloma. ×20 Reddish homogeneous mass with peripheral white collarette.

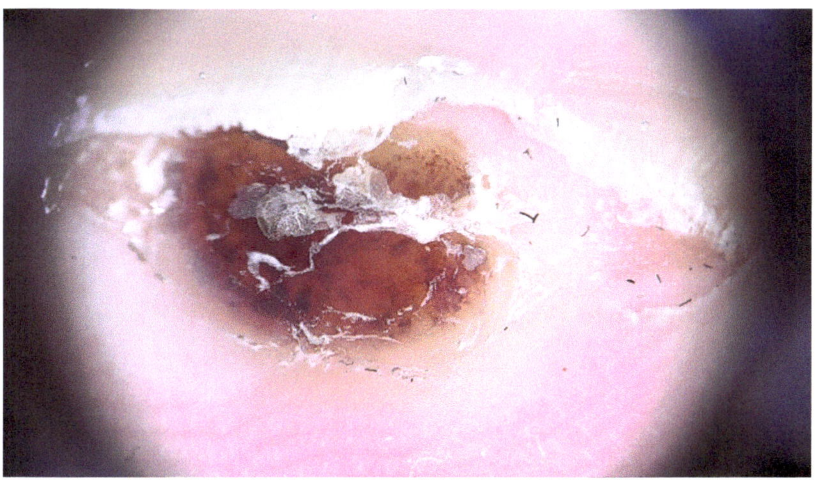

FIGURE 30.12 Exostosis. ×20 Subungual nodule with prominent vessels and peripheral collarette.

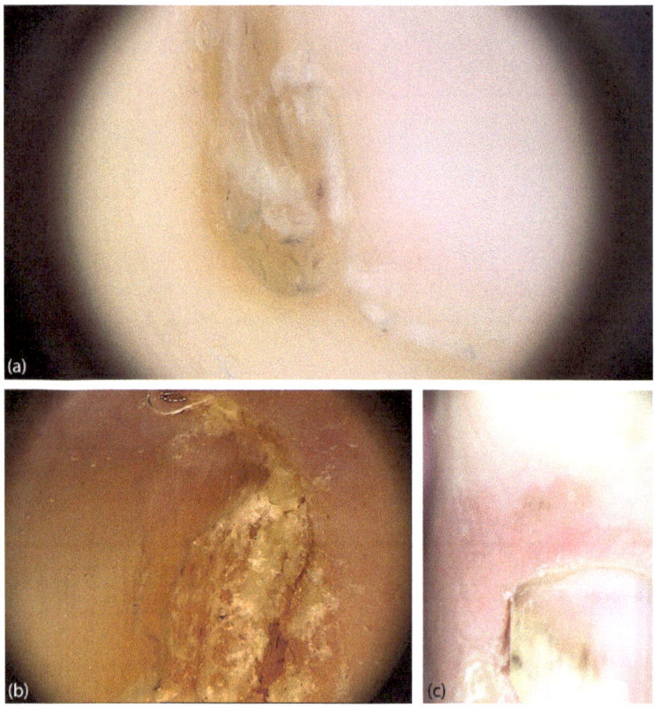

FIGURE 30.13 Bowen's disease. ×20 Wart-like lesions with linear and dotted vessels (a,b); ×20 PNF patch with islands of scale and hyperkeratotic, targetoid structures (c).

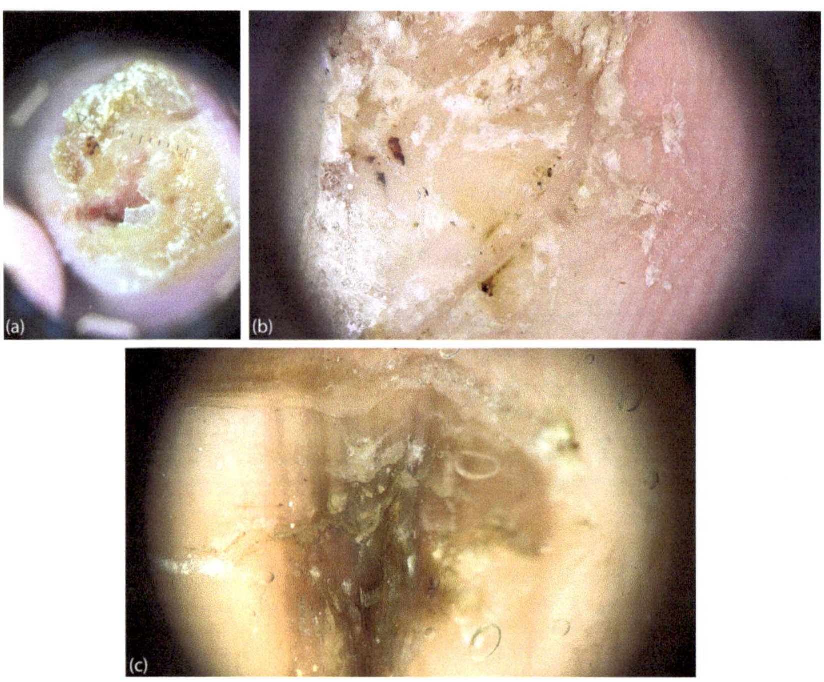

FIGURE 30.14 SCC. ×10 Yellowish verrucous mass (a); ×50 vascular polymorphism (b); ×20 melanonychia can be a prominent feature, particularly in people with skin of color (c).

SUGGESTED READING

Al Rudaisat M, Cheng H. Dermoscopy features of cutaneous warts. *Int J Gen Med.* 2021;14:9903–12.

Bray ER, Tosti A, Morrison BW. Update on squamous cell carcinoma of the nail unit: an human papillomavirus-associated condition. *Skin Appendage Disord.* 2024;10(3):199–206.

Chae JB, Ohn J, Mun JH. Dermoscopic features of digital mucous cysts: a study of 23 cases. *J Dermatol.* 2017;44(11):1309–12.

Curtis KL, Ho B, Jellinek NJ, Rubin AI, Tosti A, Lipner SR. Diagnosis and management of longitudinal erythronychia: a clinical review by an expert panel. *J Am Acad Dermatol.* 2024;91(3):480–9.

Di Chiacchio N, Tavares GT, Tosti A, Di Chiacchio NG, Di Santis E, Alvarenga L, Stuhr P, De Farias D. Onychomatricoma: epidemiological and clinical findings in a large series of 30 cases. *Br J Dermatol.* 2015;173(5):1305–7.

Göktay F, Güldiken G, Altan Ferhatoğlu Z, Güneş P, Atış G, Haneke E. The role of dermoscopy in the diagnosis of subungual glomus tumors. *Int J Dermatol.* 2022;61(7):826 32.

Kallis P, Tosti A. Onychomycosis and onychomatricoma. *Skin Appendage Disord.* 2016;1(4):209–12.

Lebensohn A, Ghafoor A, Bloomquist L, et al. Multiple onychopapillomas and BAP1 tumor predisposition syndrome. *JAMA Dermatol.* 2024;160(8):838–45.

Lencastre A, Lamas A, Sá D, Tosti A. Onychoscopy. *Clin Dermatol.* 2013;31(5):587–93.

Maehara Lde S, Ohe EM, Enokihara MY, Michalany NS, Yamada S, Hirata SH. Diagnosis of glomus tumor by nail bed and matrix dermoscopy. *An Bras Dermatol.* 2010;85(2):236–8.

Ocampo-Garza J, Jacomini Sobral P, Mendes Bretas J, Matana D, Tosti A. Dermoscopic technique for the evaluation of the nail unit. *J Am Acad Dermatol.* 2021;85(2

Piraccini BM, Bellavista S, Misciali C, Tosti A, de Berker D, Richert B. Periungual and subungual pyogenic granuloma. *Br J Dermatol.* 2010;163(5):941–53.

Tosti A, Schneider SL, Ramirez-Quizon MN, Zaiac M, Miteva M. Clinical, dermoscopic, and pathologic features of onychopapilloma: a review of 47 cases. *J Am Acad Dermatol.* 2016;74(3):521–6.

Xie F, Nightingale K, de Berker DA. Dermoscopy of periungual Bowen's disease: a retrospective case series. *Int J Dermatol.* 2024;63(10):1441–43.

31 Melanonychia

Melanocytes, responsible for melanin production, are distributed throughout the nail unit, including the matrix, nail bed, and hyponychium, though their density is notably lower than in other skin regions. The proximal nail matrix predominantly contains dormant melanocytes, while the distal matrix includes both dormant and active, pigment-producing melanocytes. Approximately 50% of melanocytes in the distal matrix produce melanin, which explains why bands of longitudinal melanonychia (LM) mostly originate from this area. LM typically manifests as a longitudinal brown-to-black band of pigmentation along the length of the nail plate.

Melanocytes in the nail bed epithelium are few and do not synthesize melanin, so pigmented lesions in the nail bed are often amelanotic.

Nail pigmentation may result from melanocyte activation or benign or malignant melanocyte hyperplasia, including nevi, lentigo, and melanoma.

MELANONYCHIA (FIGURES 31.1–31.15)

Melanonychia is a brown-to-black band of nail pigmentation: Can be longitudinal, transverse, or diffuse.

Classification

Melanocytic Conditions

- Melanocyte activation: Increased melanin production from the activation of a normal number of melanocytes in the nail matrix
- Melanocyte proliferation/hyperplasia:
  - Nevi: Increased melanin production due to an increased number of melanocytes, organized in nests (benign) in the nail matrix
  - Lentigo: Increased melanin production due to an increased number of single, not-confluent melanocytes (benign) in the nail matrix
  - Melanoma

Non-Melanocytic Conditions

- Subungual hematoma/hemorrhages
- Pigmented onychomycosis
- Pigmented squamous cell carcinoma
- Pigmented onychopapilloma
- Pigmented onychomatricoma

Dermoscopy

Important Clues (Figures 31.2–31.6)

- Purple-red color is suggestive of hematoma (see Chapter 27).
- Background color: Gray, brown, or black.
- Gray color/hue: Is typically associated with melanocytic activation.
- Transverse gray bands are mostly caused by drugs, and often associated with Muehrcke's lines in patients undergoing chemotherapy.
- Red dots due to blood extravasation are suggestive for trauma but do not exclude a bleeding tumor.
- Brown or black bands: Common in both benign and malignant melanonychia; homogeneous brown color is usually associated with benign lesions.
- Band evolution: New or changing single pigmented bands in adults are worrisome, especially those increasing in width, changing in color (becoming darker or more heterogeneous), or associated with abnormalities of the nail plate (splitting, loss, fissuring, grooving).
- In children, these features are normally seen in bands due to nevi, which often also fade or disappear.

DOI: 10.1201/9780429351433-31

- Pigmented dots in the proximal nail fold (PNF) and in the hyponychium are sometimes associated with regressing nevi in children.
- Borders: Blurred borders are more suspicious for malignancy, rather than well-defined borders, which are likely associated with benign conditions.
- Presence of lines of different color (heterogeneous pigmentation), irregular thickness, spacing, and parallelism inside the band of melanonychia is associated with melanoma in adults.
- The same pattern in children is associated with nevi.
- Presence of granules is associated with melanoma in adults but not in children.
- Advanced nail melanoma shows black background, structureless pattern, evident Hutchinson's sign, ulceration, and bleeding.
- Assessment of the nail free edge establishes pigment location/origin.
- Pigmentation location of the free edge: Dorsal nail plate, ventral nail plate, full thickness. Light bands may not have a visible pigmentation of the free edge (see Chapter 25).
- Pseudo-Hutchinson's sign: Pigmentation through the cuticle is more evident with dermoscopy (see Chapter 24).
- A pseudo-Hutchinson's sign of the hyponychium has been reported in benign lesions with linear pigmentation crossing the skin furrows (see Chapter 25).
- The cuticle can be pigmented itself, particularly in case of dark pigmented bands of skin of color. Pigmentation is usually homogeneous.
- Micro-Hutchinson's sign: Pigmentation of the periungual area is not visible to the naked eye. The proximal nail fold shows longitudinal lines projecting from the nail plate.
- Hutchinson's sign: May involve the proximal nail fold or the hyponychium.
- Hutchinson's sign of the proximal nail fold and dorsal digit presents multiple structureless irregularly pigmented areas with scattered globules.
- Hutchison's sign of the hyponychium: The pigmentation follows the parallel ridges pattern as in acral melanoma (see Chapter 25).
- Amelanotic melanoma represents about 25% of nail melanoma. Dermoscopy shows atypical vascularity and focal irregular remnants of pigmentation. Polymorphic vascular structures include milky-red areas, irregular linear vessels, hairpin vessels, and dotted vessels.

MELANONYCHIA DUE TO NON-MELANOCYTIC CONDITIONS

Non-melanocytic causes of melanonychia are very common and can affect individuals across all populations.

Dermoscopy

- Subungual hemorrhage: Red, blue, or black globules and well-circumscribed blotches. The pigmentation typically moves distally as the nail grows (see Chapter 27).
- Fungal Melanonychia: Diffuse brown-black pigmentation, often without the irregular lines seen in melanocytic lesions. It usually spares the matrix and may be associated with yellow longitudinal striae or subungual hyperkeratosis (ruin pattern) (see Chapter 29).
- Bacterial melanonychia: Green-black pigmentation, often starting from the nail folds, typically associated with onycholysis (see Chapter 27).
- Onychopapilloma may present as a longitudinal melanonychia in skin of color, but is associated with a distal keratotic mass underneath the nail plate (see Chapter 30).
- Bowen's disease/squamous cell carcinoma presents an adjacent brown-greyish longitudinal band of melanonychia (see Chapter 30).

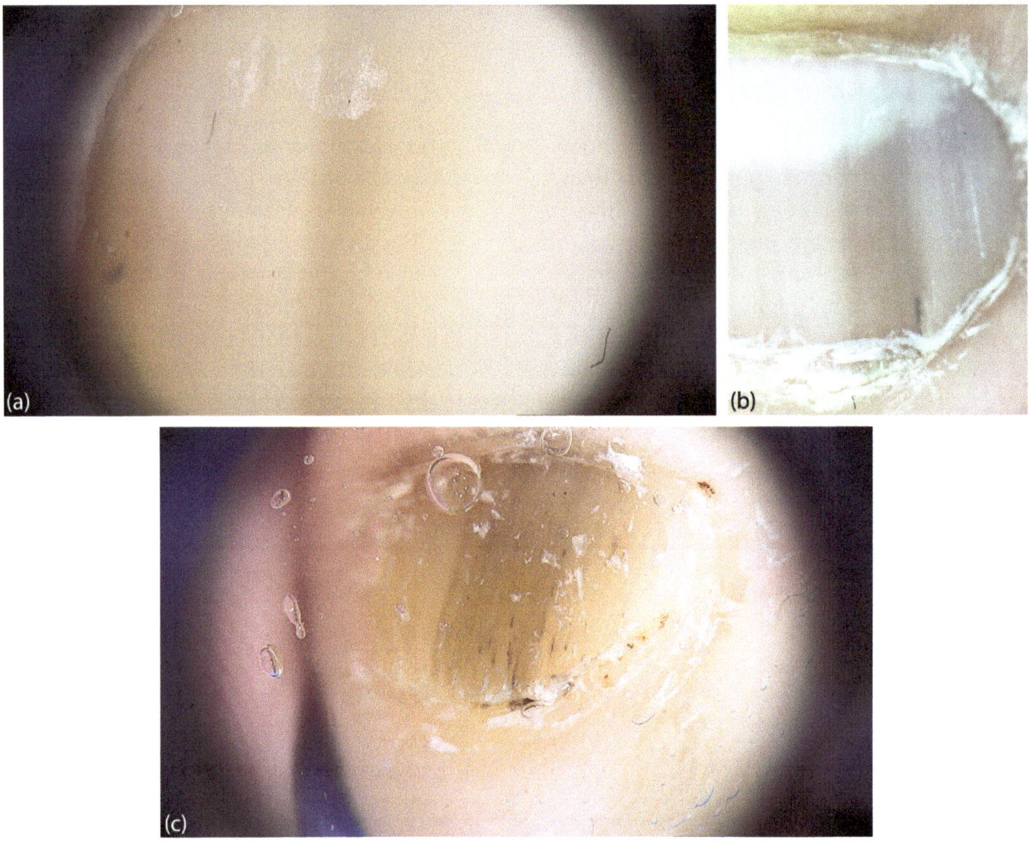

FIGURE 31.1 Melanocyte activation. ×50 The band is gray in color and homogeneous (a); ×20 large band in a patient of color (b); ×20 presence of splinter hemorrhages in this toenail is suggestive for friction melanonychia (c).

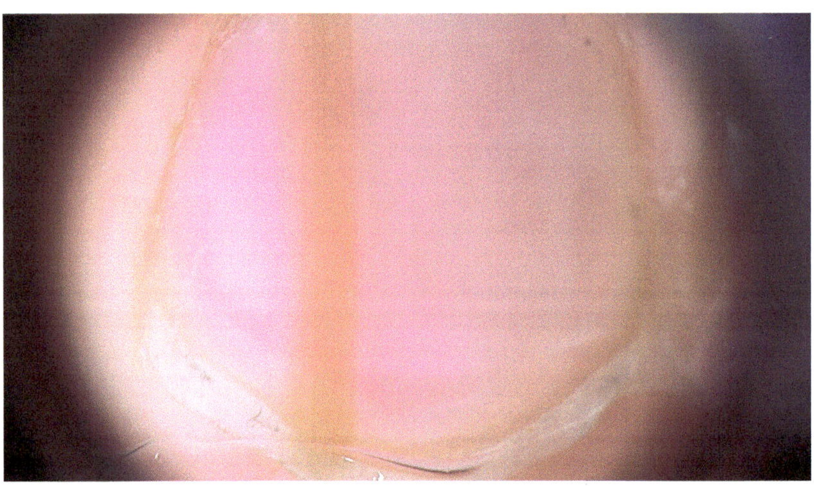

FIGURE 31.2 Nevus in an adult. × 20 Light brown band with regular lines.

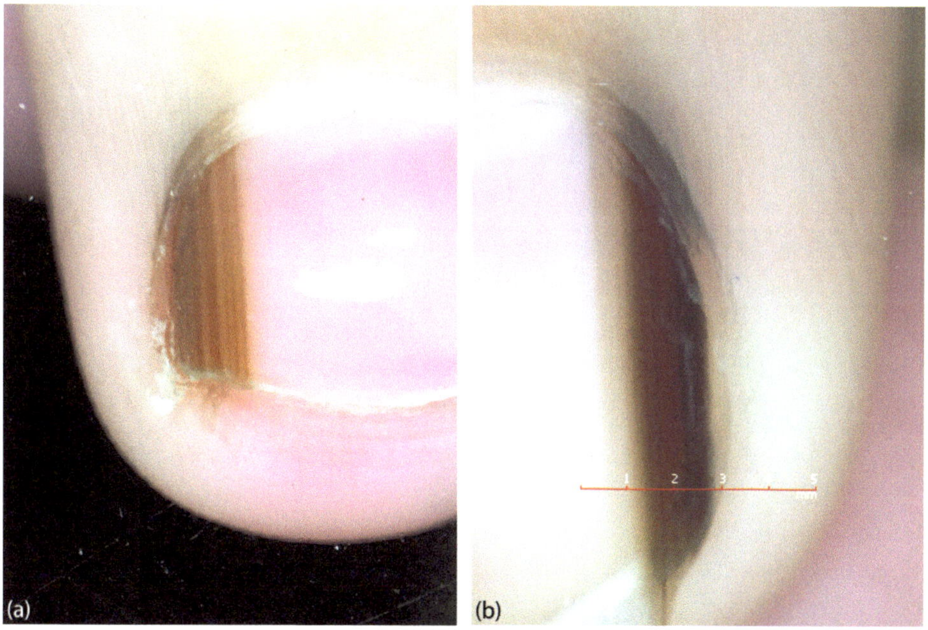

FIGURE 31.3 Nevi in children. ×20 Bands with lines of irregular color and thickness and pseudo-Hutchinson's sign; note patches of true leukonychia in (a).

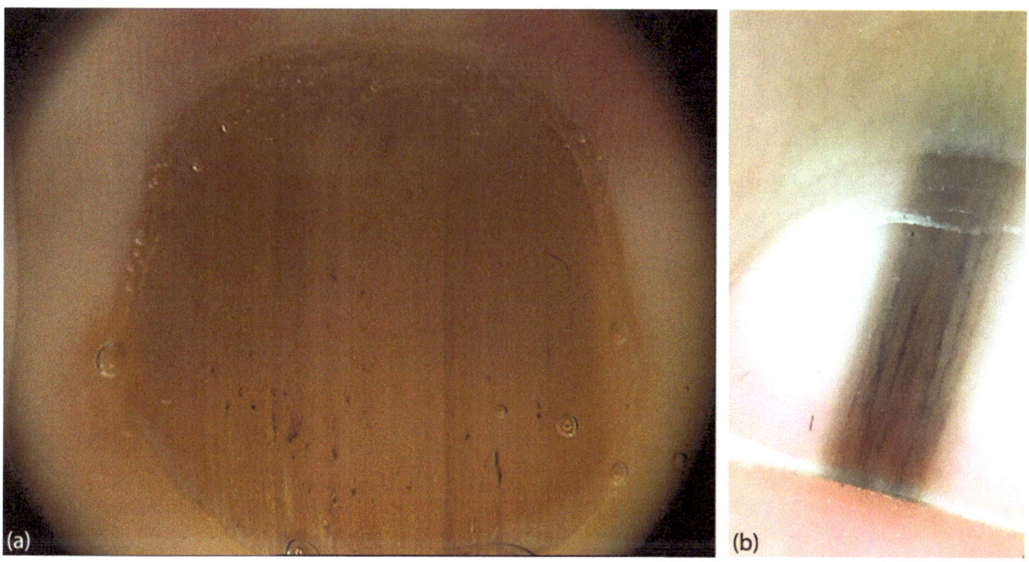

FIGURE 31.4 Nevi in children. ×20 The pigmentation involves the whole plate with irregular lines and presence of granules (a); ×50 brown band with irregular lines and presence of granules (b).

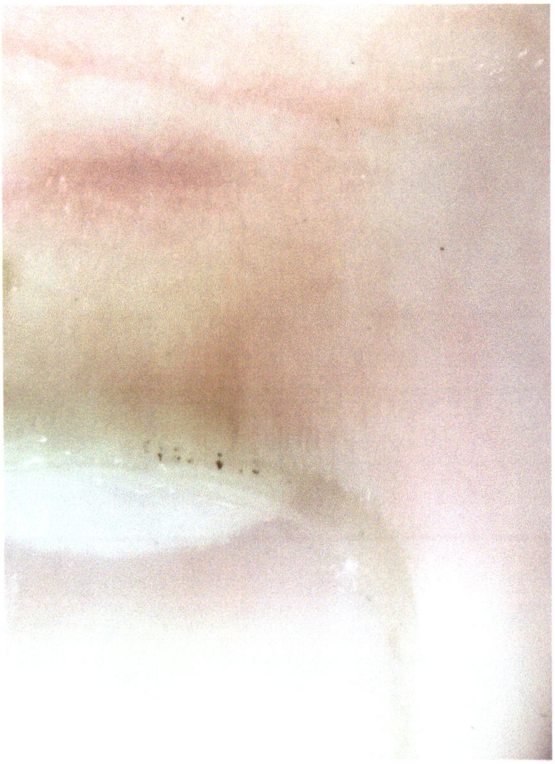

FIGURE 31.5 Nevus in a child. ×50 After fading of the nevus the child developed these pigmented dots in the proximal nail fold.

FIGURE 31.6 Nevus in a child. ×20 (a) and ×50 (b) Light band with granules, the hyponychium shows linear pigmentation crossing the skin furrows.

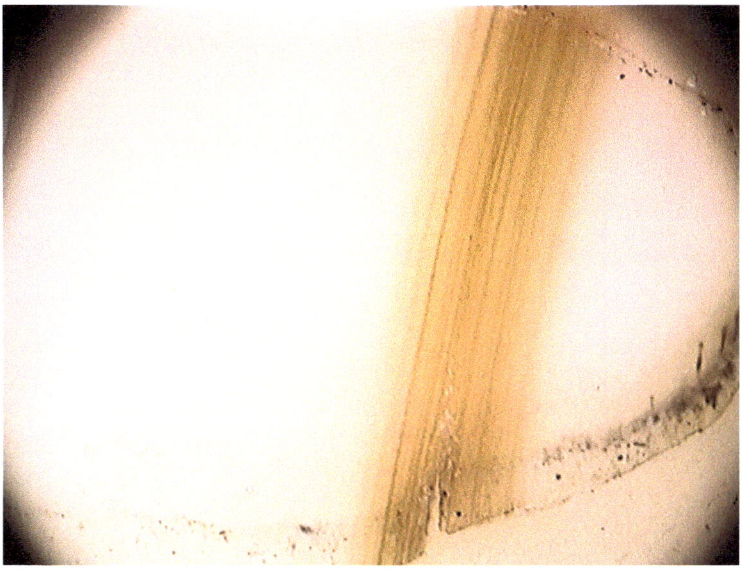

FIGURE 31.7 Nevus in a child. ×20 Nail plate splitting in correspondence of the band.

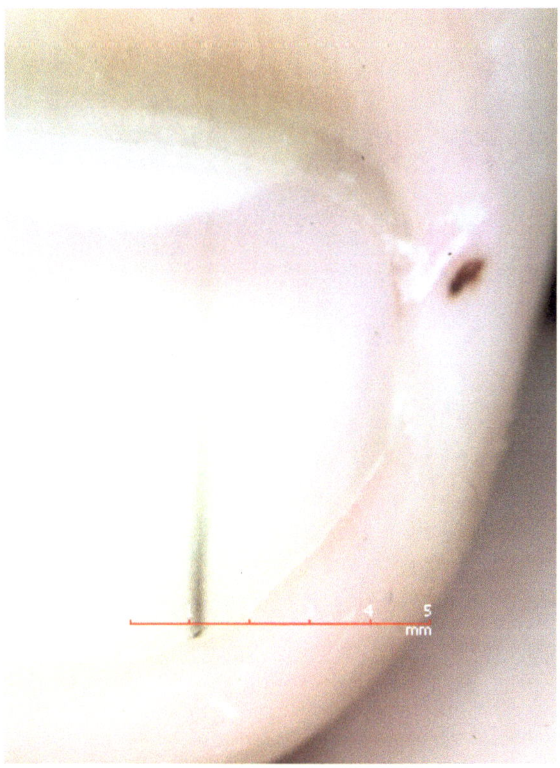

FIGURE 31.8 Nevus in a child. ×20 Pale band with granules and pigmentation of the proximal nail fold.

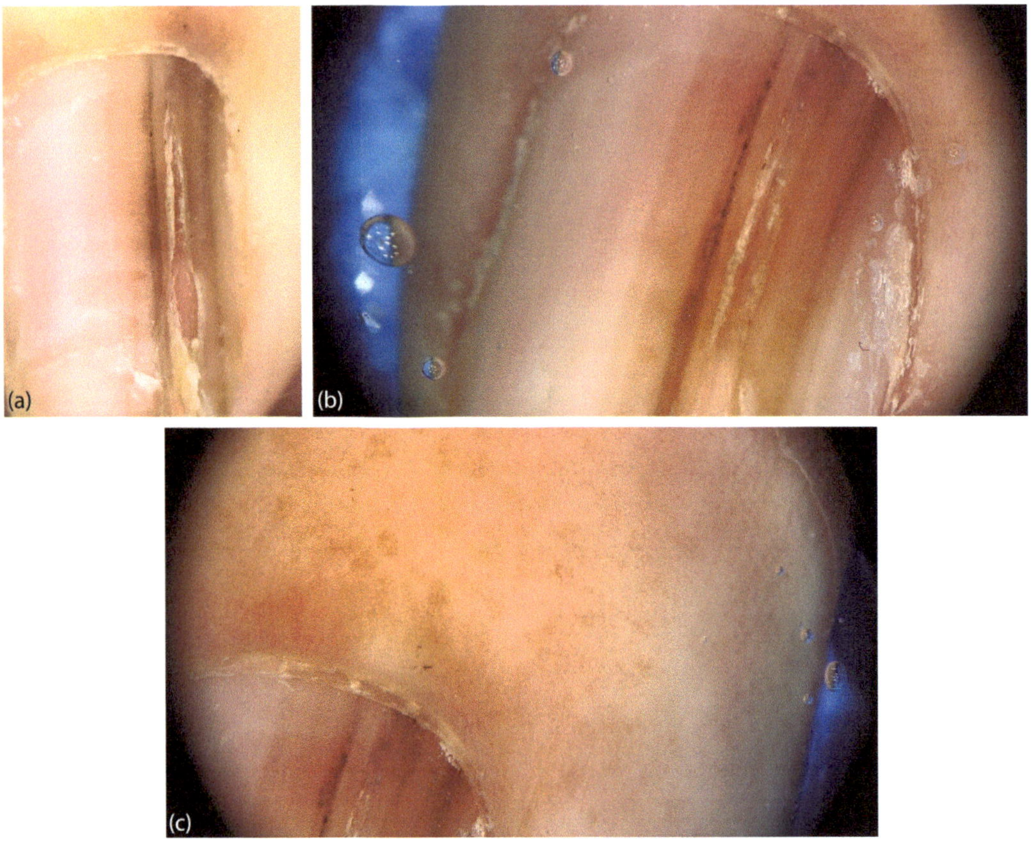

FIGURE 31.9 Nail melanoma. ×20 Dark brown band with lines of irregular color and thickness and nail plate fissuring (a); ×40 presence of granules (b); and ×40 patchy pigmentation of the PNF (Hutchinson's sign) (c).

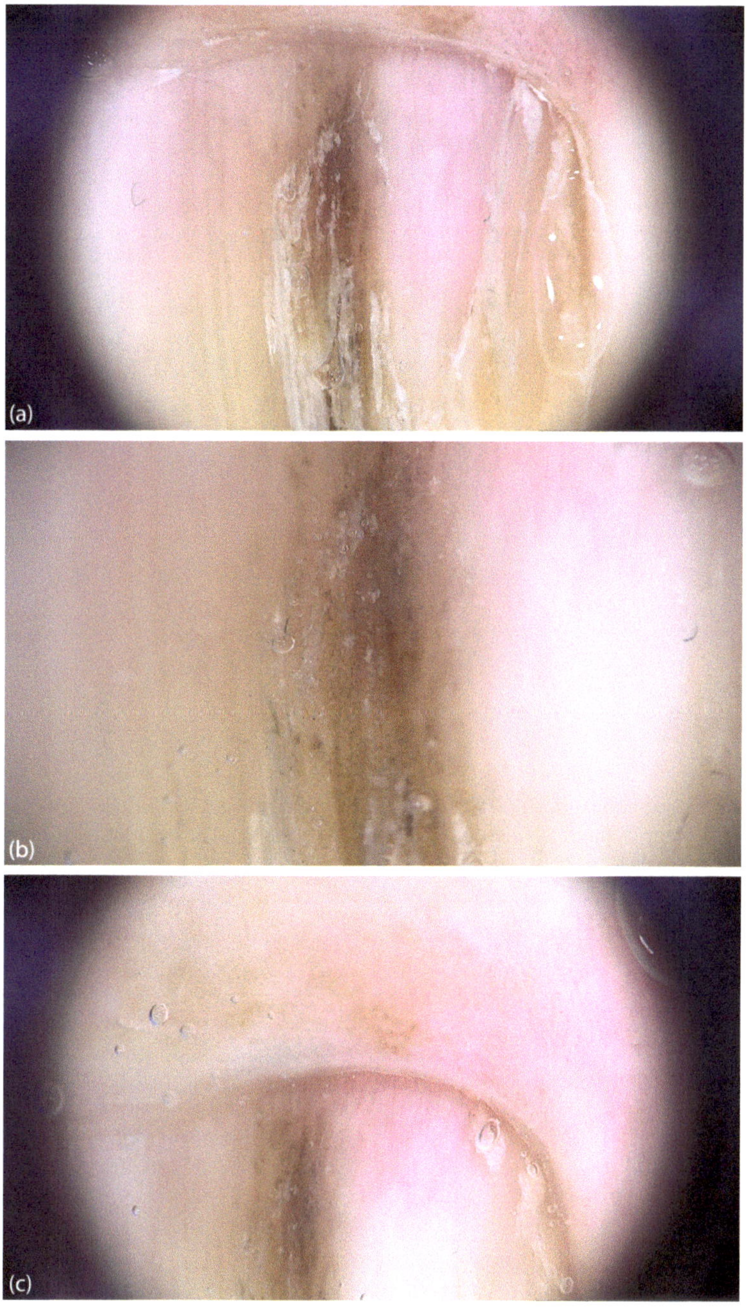

FIGURE 31.10 Nail melanoma. ×20 (a) and ×50 (b) Brown band with multiple granules, nail plate splitting, and exfoliation; the PNF shows multiple structureless irregularly pigmented areas with scattered globules (Hutchinson's sign) (c).

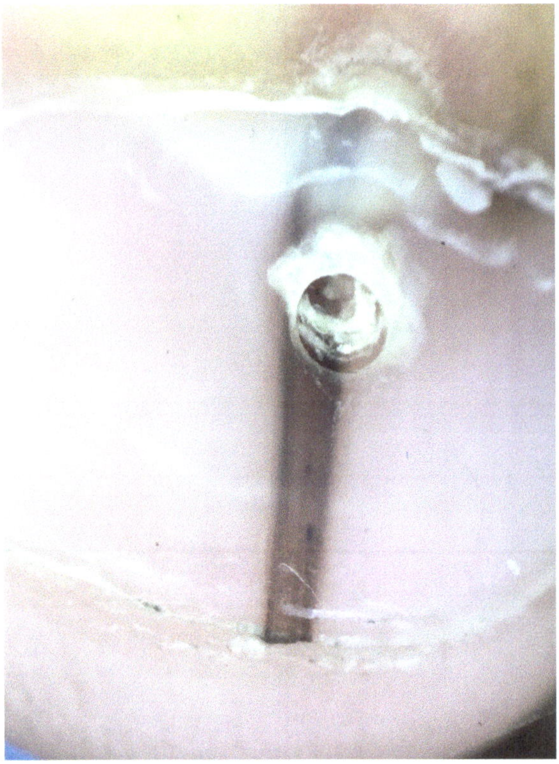

FIGURE 31.11 Nail melanoma in situ. ×20 This patient had a punch biopsy through the nail plate that did not show any pigmentary changes as missed the lesion. The dark band has a triangular shape, irregular borders, and multiple granules.

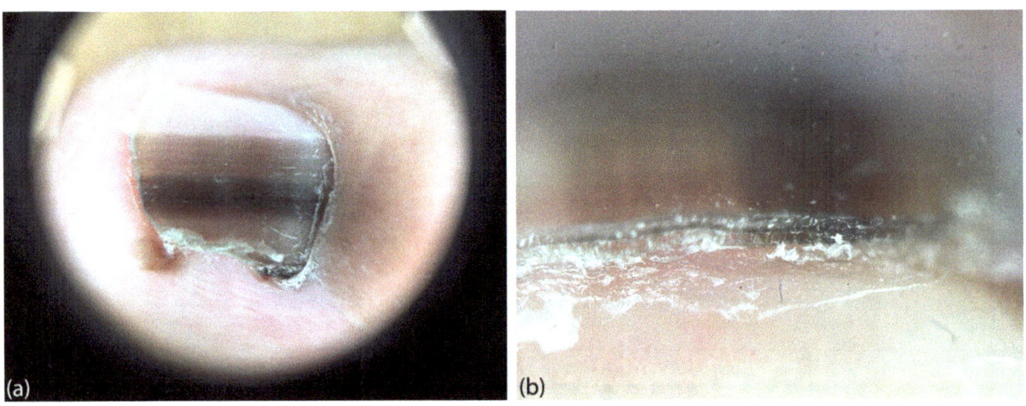

FIGURE 31.12 Nail melanoma. ×10 The band has multiple color and is associated with pigmentation of the proximal nail fold and the hyponychium (Hutchinson's sign) (a); ×20 the pigmentation involves the whole thickness of the nail plate (b).

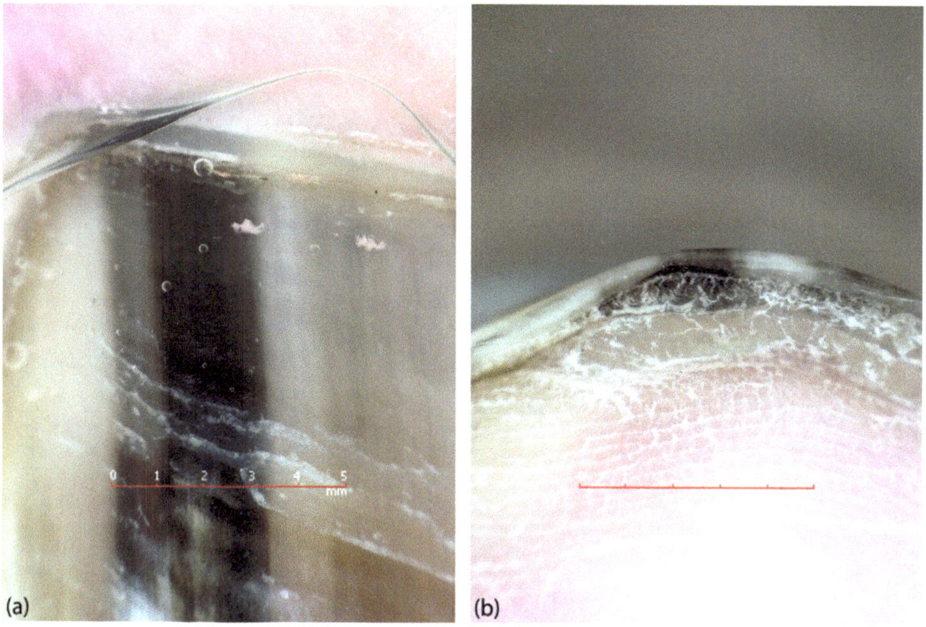

FIGURE 31.13 Nail melanoma. ×20 Dark band with multiple colors and irregular lines (a); distal dermoscopy shows that the pigmentation involves the whole thickness of the nail plate (b).

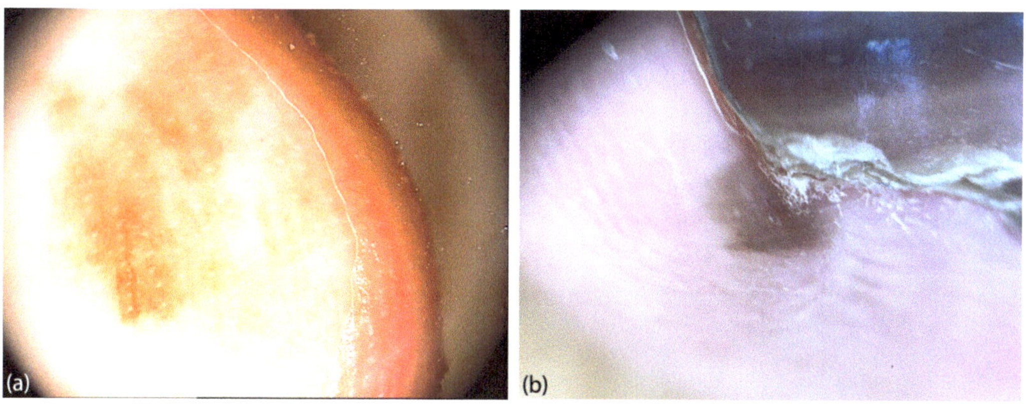

FIGURE 31.14 Nail Melanoma. ×20 Hutchinson sign of the hyponychium, the pigmentation follows the parallel ridges pattern (a-b).

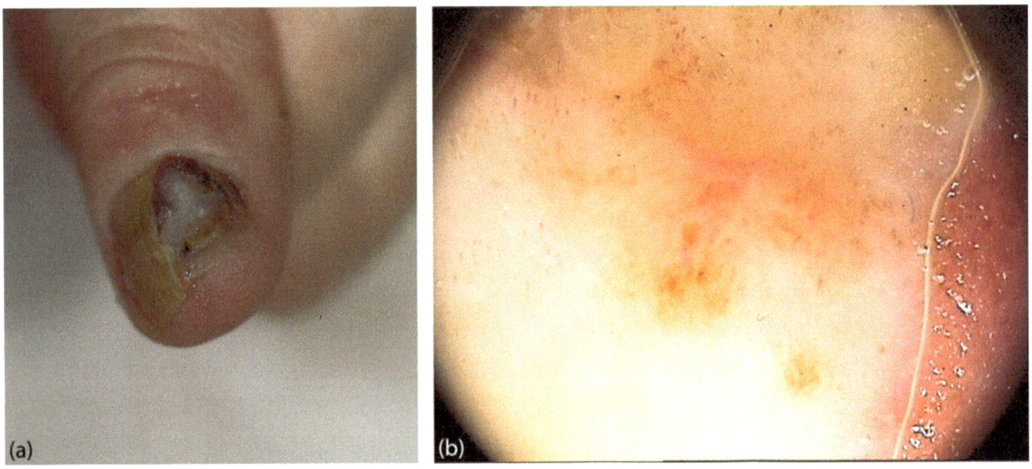

FIGURE 31.15 Amelanotic melanoma (a); ×50 irregular remnants of pigmentation and atypical vascularity (b).

SUGGESTED READING

Algarra-Sahuquillo J, Ramos-Rodríguez D, Santos-E-Silva Caldeira-Marques ML, Mercader-Salvans J, Rodríguez-Rodríguez RN, Hernández-León CN, Guimerá Martin-Neda F. Short brown parallel lines on the proximal nail fold. clinical-dermoscopic-histologic correlation of a melanocytic nevus of the eponychium. *Skin Appendage Disord*. 2023;9(2):147–50.

Di Chiacchio ND, Farias DC, Piraccini BM, Hirata SH, Richert B, Zaiac M, et al. Consensus on melanonychia nail plate dermoscopy. *An Bras Dermatol*. 2013;88(2):309–13.

Di Chiacchio N, Hirata SH, Enokihara MY, Michalany NS, Fabbrocini G, Tosti A. Dermatologists' accuracy in early diagnosis of melanoma of the nail matrix. *Arch Dermatol*. 2010;146(4):382–7.

Di Chiacchio N, Ruben BS, Loureiro WR. Longitudinal melanonychias. *Clin Dermatol*. 2013;31(5):594–601.

Duarte AF, Correia O, Barros AM, Ventura F, Haneke E. Nail melanoma in situ: clinical, dermoscopic, pathologic clues, and steps for minimally invasive treatment. *Dermatol Surg*. 2015;41(1):59–68.

Ko D, Oromendia C, Scher R, Lipner SR. Retrospective single-center study evaluating clinical and dermoscopic features of longitudinal melanonychia, ABCDEF criteria, and risk of malignancy. *J Am Acad Dermatol*. 2019;80(5):1272–83.

Maddy AJ, Tosti A. Spontaneous regression of a nail matrix melanocytic nevus in a child. *Pediatr Dermatol*. 2017;34(5):e254–e256.

Mun JH, Kim GW, Jwa SW, Song M, Kim HS, Ko HC, et al. Dermoscopy of subungual haemorrhage: its usefulness in differential diagnosis from nail-unit melanoma. *Br J Dermatol*. 2013;168(6):1224–9. Erratum in: *Br J Dermatol*. 2013;169(3):727.

Ocampo-Garza J, Bretas JM, Matana D, Sobral PJ, Thompson CT, Zaiac M, Tosti A. Longitudinal melanonychia biopsy: what not to do. *J Drugs Dermatol*. 2018;17(5):587–8.

Oska C, Morrison B, Tosti A. Postinflammatory pigmentation and friction melanonychia. *Int J Dermatol*. 2023;62(9):e474–e476.

Tosti A, Argenziano G. Dermoscopy allows better management of nail pigmentation. *Arch Dermatol*. 2002;138(10):1369–70.

Tosti A, Piraccini BM, de Farias DC. Dealing with melanonychia. *Semin Cutan Med Surg*. 2009;28(1):49–54.

32 Intraoperative Nail Dermoscopy

- Intraoperative dermoscopy involves the removal of the nail plate to allow direct dermoscopic examination of the subungual lesions. It enhances surgical accuracy and guides lesion removal.
- Contact dermoscopy: Can be performed using a translucent sterile adhesive film and immersion fluid.

MELANOCYTIC LESIONS (FIGURES 32.1–32.3)

Melanocyte Activation

- Regular gray pattern: Consists of fine, evenly spaced, parallel gray lines, and its overall appearance is subtle, with a soft gray hue distributed consistently across the lesion. It is associated with melanocytes activation.

Lentigo/Nevi

- Regular brown lines: Uniform in thickness and spacing. These can be a feature either of a lentigo or a melanocytic nevus.
- The presence of globules or blotches is typical of nevi.

Melanoma

- Irregular pattern: Characterized by the presence of longitudinal lines of irregular color and thickness, with or without irregular globules or blotches, and structureless areas.
- This pattern is chaotic and lacks uniformity.

NON-MELANOCYTIC LESIONS (FIGURES 32.4–32.7)

Malignant

Squamous Cell Carcinoma

- Polymorphous vascular patterns with dotted, curved, sagittal, irregular vessels
- Whitish scaly areas
- In keratoacanthoma of the nail, intraoperative dermoscopy can be the only clue for diagnosis of a rapidly growing lesion revealing a volcano shape filled with cheese-like white structures.

Benign

Onychomatricoma

- Crypts ("Sagrada Familia sign"): Consist of small, round, or oval spaces resembling symmetrically arranged cavities, which are detectable on the ventral surface of the reversed nail plate.
- Digitations: Finger-like projections extending from the tumor, seen at the level of the lunula, that match with the cavities of the nail plate (mirror sign)

Glomus Tumor

The lesion can be very well seen and delimitated after nail plate avulsion.

- Irregularly shaped reddish nodule with numerous telangiectatic vessels

Myxoid Cyst

- Opening of the cyst appears as a round to oval structure, with a translucid capsule.

DOI: 10.1201/9780429351433-32

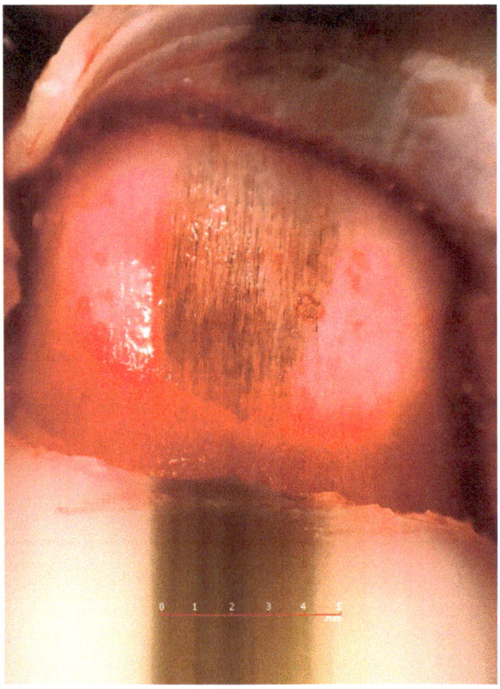

FIGURE 32.1 Nevus. ×20 Regular lines with uniform thickness and spacing. (Courtesy of Dr. Martin Zaiac.)

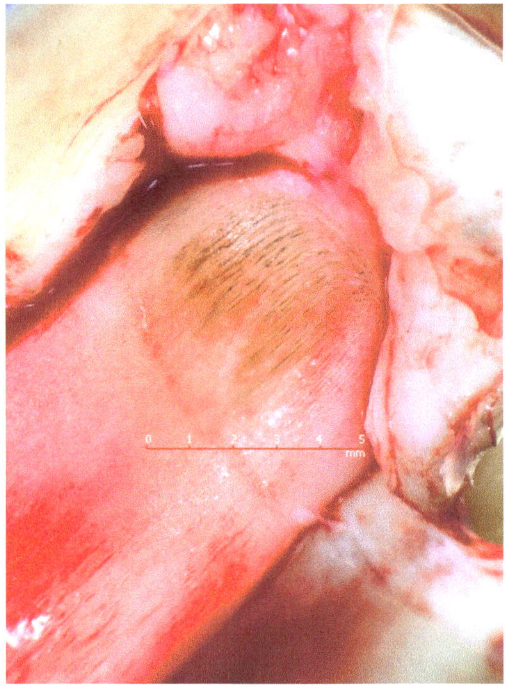

FIGURE 32.2 Lentigo. ×20 Regular brown pattern.

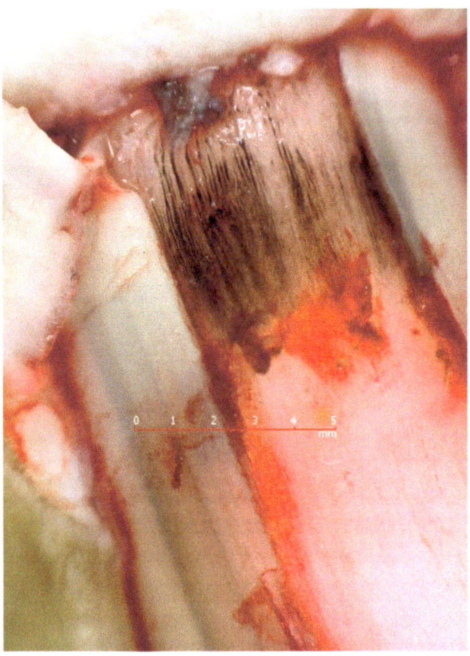

FIGURE 32.3 Melanoma. ×20 Longitudinal lines of irregular thickness, with irregular blotches.

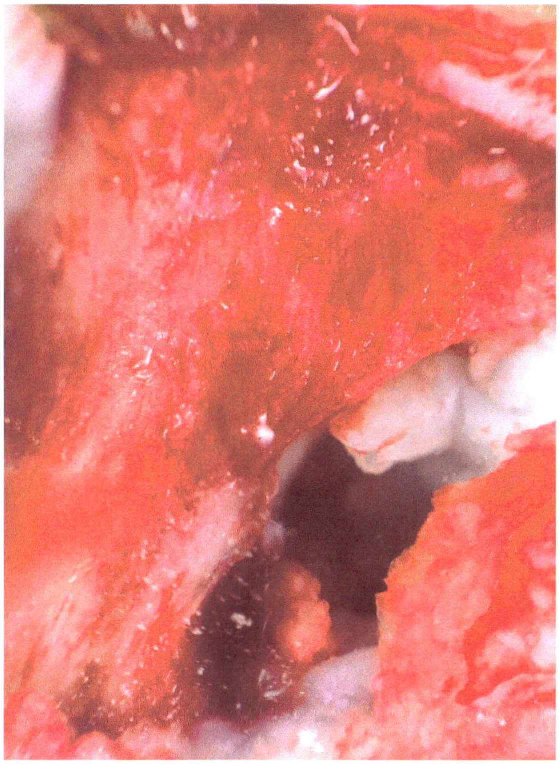

FIGURE 32.4 Keratoacanthoma. ×20 Large cavity filled with cheese-like white structures.

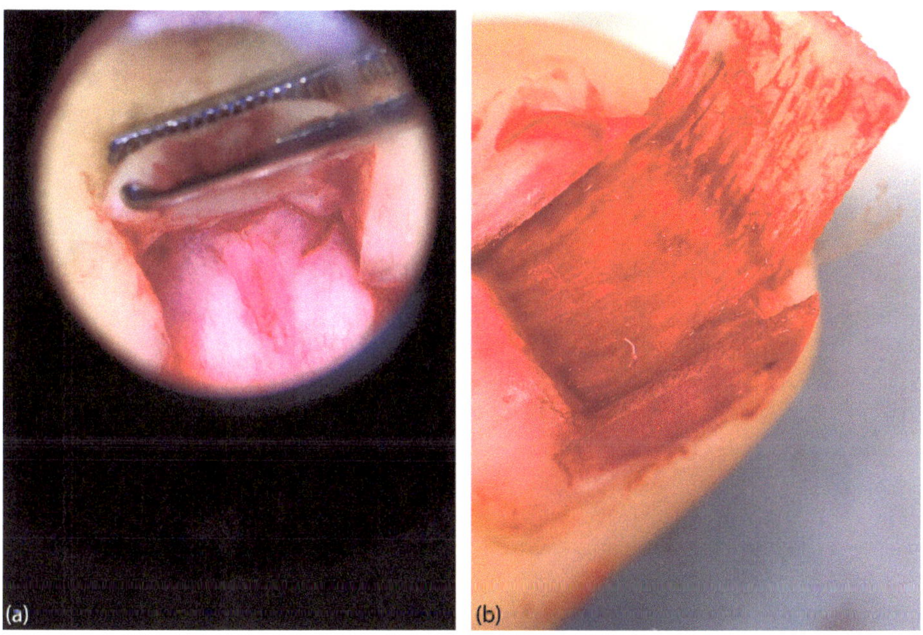

FIGURE 32.5 Onychomatricoma. ×20 Finger-like digitations of the matrix (a); crypts on ventral side of the nail plate (b). (Courtesy of Dr Debora Cadore de Farias.)

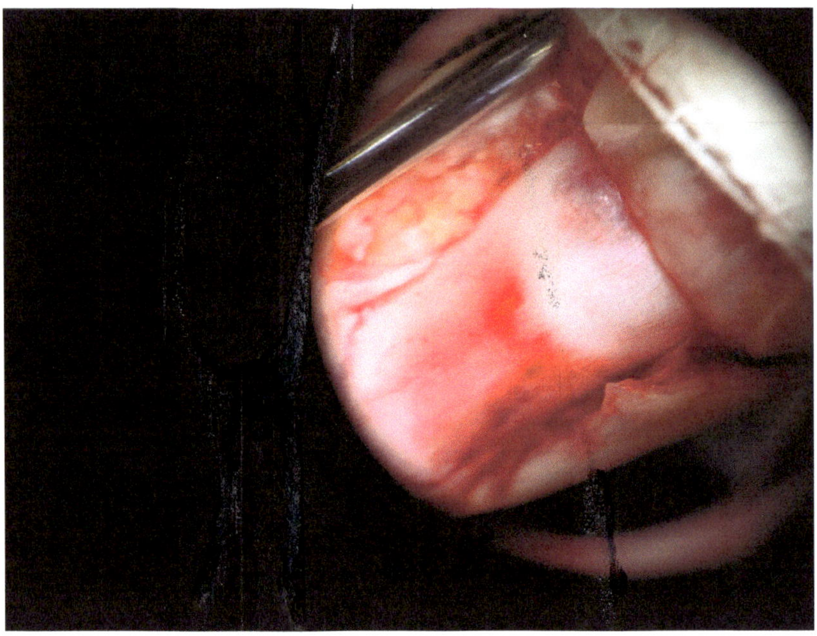

FIGURE 32.6 Glomus tumor. ×20 Erythematous nodule with numerous ramified telangiectatic vessels. (Courtesy of Dr. Debora Cadore de Farias.)

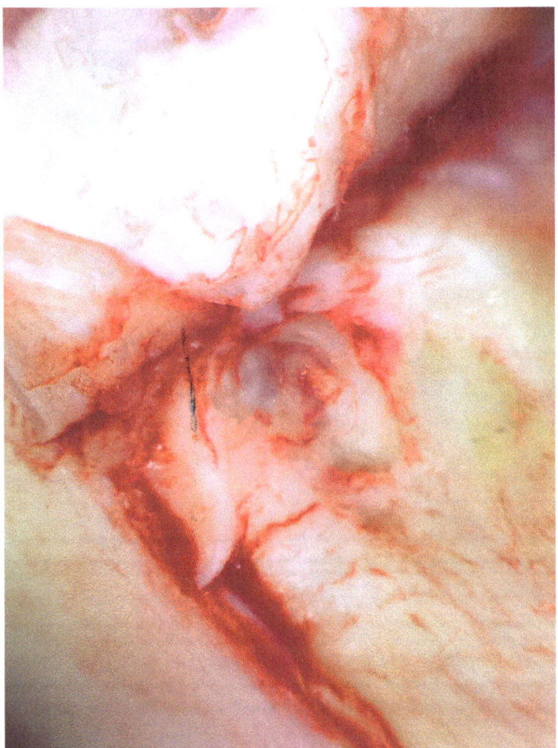

FIGURE 32.7 Myxoid cyst. ×20 Round whitish nodule with a translucid capsule. (Courtesy of Dr. Debora Cadore de Farias.)

SUGGESTED READING

Ginoux E, Perier Muzet M, Poulalhon N, Debarbieux S, Dalle S, Thomas L. Intraoperative dermoscopic features of onychomatricoma: a review of 10 cases. *Clin Exp Dermatol.* 2017;42:395–9.

Hirata SH, Yamada S, Enokihara MY, et al. Patterns of nail matrix and bed of longitudinal melanonychia by intraoperative dermatoscopy. *J Am Acad Dermatol.* 2011;65(2):297–303.

Lee T, Jo G, Mun JH. The usefulness of nail plate and intraoperative dermoscopy in subungual glomus tumor. *Int J Dermatol.* 2018;57:e26–e28.

Rai AK. Role of intraoperative dermoscopy in excision of nail unit glomus tumor. *Indian Dermatol Online J.* 2016;7:448–50.

Simmons BJ, Baker JA, Zaiac M, Cho-Vega JH, Tosti A. Subungual keratoacanthoma in a patient with yellow nail syndrome. *Dermatol Surg.* 2016;42(7):900–2.

33 Connective Tissue Disorders

Nail fold capillaroscopy is an essential diagnostic and prognostic tool for evaluating microvascular alterations in connective tissue disorders. This technique reveals characteristic vascular abnormalities such as dilated capillaries, giant capillaries, and capillary dropouts, which are closely associated with disease activity and severity.

CONNECTIVE TISSUE DISORDERS

- Scleroderma
- Dermatomyositis
- Systemic lupus erythematosus (SLE)

Capillary Patterns

Shape

- Dilated capillaries: Appear wider than normal and are commonly detected in early stages of microangiopathy.
- Giant capillaries: Are wider than typical dilated capillaries, often appearing as large loops.
- Elongated capillaries: Are longer than normal, extending further into the nail fold than typical capillaries; they can be seen in SLE and dermatomyositis.
- Tortuous capillaries: Are twisted or have a wavy appearance, deviating from their normal hairpin or U-shaped structure. These are commonly observed in SLE and dermatomyositis.
- Meandering capillaries: Follow a winding or irregular path, deviating from the typical linear or slightly curved shape. They are typical of SLE.
- Bushy capillaries: Are frayed capillaries, with multiple small branches extending from the main loop, resembling a bush. They are typical of late stages of scleroderma and dermatomyositis.
- Crisscross capillaries: Typically, cross over each other or form a figure-eight pattern; they can be observed in dermatomyositis and SLE.
- Hemorrhages: Are small, pinpoint red or brownish spots near or along the capillaries or within the cuticle.

Density

- Capillary dropouts/avascular areas: Areas where capillaries are significantly reduced in number, creating gaps in the capillary bed. These are seen in scleroderma and dermatomyositis.

Distribution

- Disorganized capillary architecture: Loss of the normal orderly parallel arrangement of capillaries, leading to a chaotic appearance with capillaries oriented in multiple directions.

Scleroderma (Figure 33.1)

- Capillary enlargement, giant capillaries, hemorrhages ramified/bushy capillaries
- Reduced capillary density with avascular areas

Dermatomyositis (Figure 33.2)

- Capillary enlargement
- Bushy capillaries
- Cuticle hemorrhages
- Reduced capillary density with avascular areas

The dermatomyositis pattern is similar to the scleroderma pattern. Diagnosis of dermatomyositis is suggested by finding two or more of the following findings in at least two nail folds: Enlargement of capillary loops, loss of capillaries, disorganization of the normal distribution of capillaries, bushy capillaries, twisted enlarged capillaries, and capillary hemorrhages, often in the cuticle.

DOI: 10.1201/9780429351433-33

Systemic Lupus Erythematosus (Figure 33.3)

- Capillary enlargement with dilated tortuous capillary
- Normal capillary density

In SLE capillary density is normal but capillaries are tortuous, elongated, and dilated.

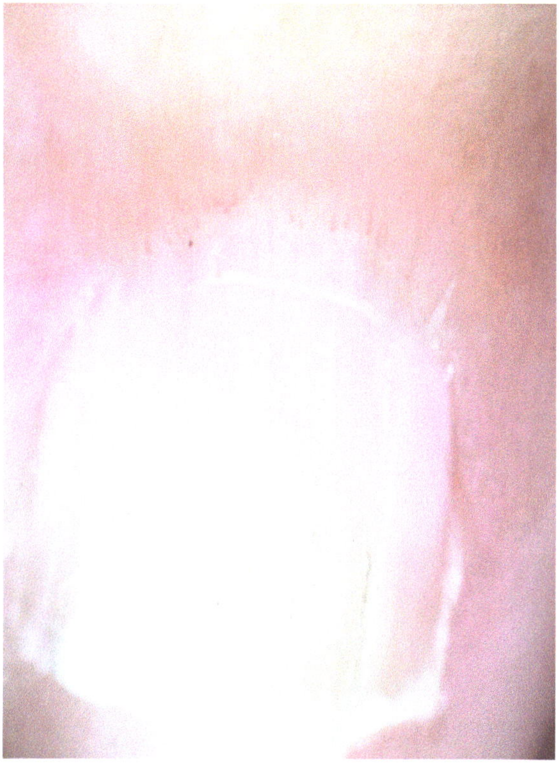

FIGURE 33.1 Scleroderma. ×20 Capillary loss and enlarged capillaries.

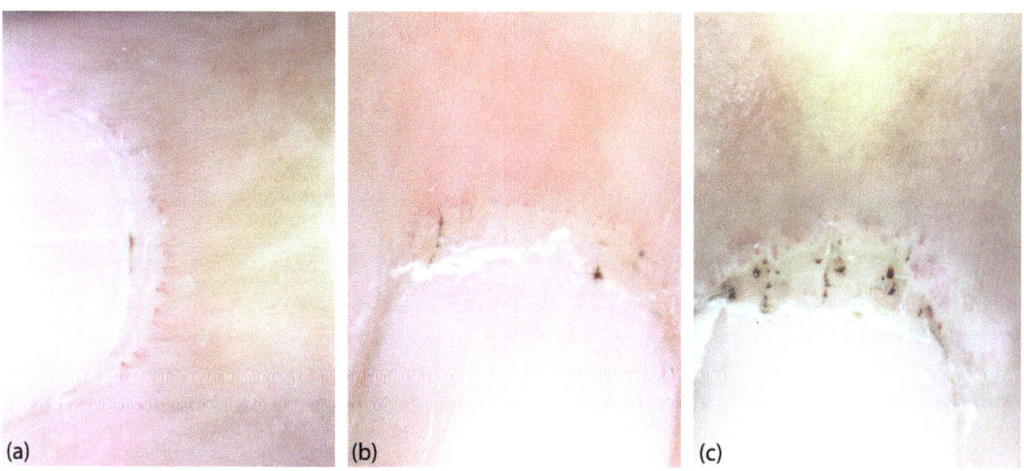

FIGURE 33.2 Dermatomyositis. ×20 Enlarged twisted capillaries (a), capillary loss (b), and cuticle hemorrhages (c).

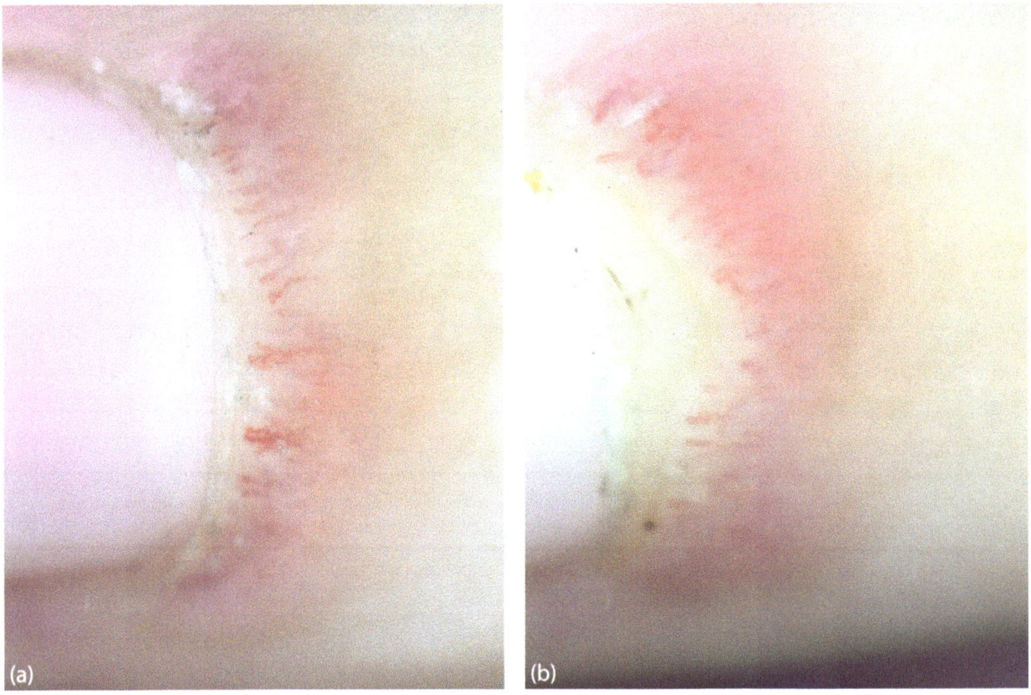

FIGURE 33.3 Systemic lupus erythematosus (a,b). ×20 Enlarged tortuous and meandering capillaries. Normal density.

SUGGESTED READING

Chojer P, Mahajan BB. Nail fold dermoscopy in collagen vascular disorders: a cross-sectional study. *Indian J Dermatol Venereol Leprol.* 2019;85:439.

Hasegawa M. Dermoscopy findings of nail fold capillaries in connective tissue diseases. *J Dermatol.* 2011;38(1):66–70.

Muroi E, Hara T, Yanaba K, Ogawa F, Yoshizaki A, Takenaka M, Shimizu K, Sato S. A portable dermatoscope for easy, rapid examination of periungual nailfold capillary changes in patients with systemic sclerosis. *Rheumatol Int.* 2011;31(12):1601–6.

Ohtsuka T. Dermoscopic detection of nail fold capillary abnormality in patients with systemic sclerosis. *J Dermatol.* 2012;39(4):331–5.

Paudyal A, Yang Y, Zheng M, Zhang X, Wang H, Gong S, Regmi P, Lyu X. Assessment of nail fold capillary changes by hand-held dermoscopy in adult dermatomyositis: a single-centre prospective study. *Australas J Dermatol.* 2023;64(4):514–21.

Index

I

K

L

Q

R

S